ENCYCLOPAEDIA OF
VETERINARY SCIENCE

ENCYCLOPAEDIA OF
VETERINARY SCIENCE

Dr. Anuj Sharma

ANMOL PUBLICATIONS PVT. LTD.
NEW DELHI - 110 002 (INDIA)

ANMOL PUBLICATIONS PVT. LTD.
H.O.: 4374/4B, Ansari Road, Darya Ganj,
New Delhi-110 002 (India)
Ph.: 23278000, 23261597

B.O.: No. 1015, Ist Main Road, BSK IIIrd Stage
IIIrd Phase, IIIrd Block
Bangalore - 560 085 (India)
Visit us at: www.anmolpublications.com

Encyclopaedia of Veterinary Science

First Published, 2006

ISBN 81-261-3038-5

PRINTED IN INDIA

Printed at Mehra Offset Press, Delhi.

Preface

This Encyclopaedia is the perfect guide for those studying Veterinary Science, either at university level or anyone interested in Veterinary Science, such as professional Veterinary scientists and practising personals. It provides a comprehensive coverage of Veterinary Science. The aim of this encyclopaedia is to provide teachers, students and laymen interested in Veterinary Science with clear, concise, and correct definitions and descriptions of the Veterinary Science terms, throughout.

This volume covers all branches of Veterinary Science such as cells, tissues, systems, nutrition, species comparison, principles of disease, disease prevention and diagnosis, zoonotic disease, surgery, decisions in veterinary practice, normal physical parameters, infectious diseases, calculation conversions, activities in cells, organs, processes such as contractility of muscle tissue, coordination through the nervous system, feeding, digestion, excretion, respiration, circulation, reproduction, and secretion.

The Encyclopaedia is to satisfy the immediate technical needs of the user. Concepts are presented in a clear and lucid manner. In terms of its broader objectives, the present book may be viewed as an outline or compendium of Veterinary Science ideas correlated with a large collection of specialized items.

The aim of this volume is to provide a concise repository of number of major concepts in this field. In preparation of this book, the author has freely consulted large number of books and journals so no authenticity is claimed. Author is especially thankful to Anmol Publications Pvt. Ltd., New Delhi for shaping this book in its final form. Suggestions for further improvement of this book are not only welcome but also greatly appreciated.

Author

A

A.I. Artificial insemination, the mechanical introduction of semen into the genital tract of the female.

ABDF Animal Disease Biotechnology Facility.

Abdomen A region of the body between the chest and the pelvis; belly.

Abdominocentesis Placing a needle into the abdominal (belly) cavity to check for the presence of abnormal fluid.

Aber Tail Carried in a semicircle.

Abomasum The fourth or true digestive part of a ruminant's stomach that contains gastric juices and enzymes that begin the breakdown of complex materials.

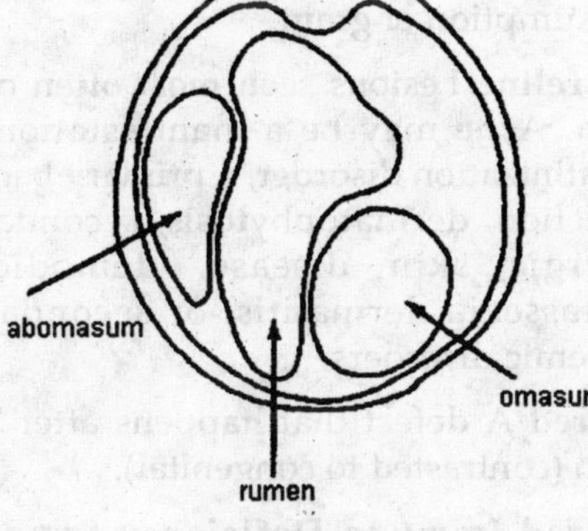

Fig. Abomasum

Abort When a dead embryo or is absorbed or expelled prior to the time when it could survive outside the uterus.

Abortifacients A drug or other agent used to cause abortion. Other agents could be considered as toxins or poisons from plants, trees, etc.

Abortion Expulsion of the fetus (or fetuses) by a pregnant female before the normal end of a pregnancy.

Abrasions Wounds that are not through all the layers of the skin.

Abscess A hole formed by dying tissue that is often filled with puss. A localized collection of pus surrounded by inflamed tissue.

Absence Seizure Also called a Petit Mal Seizure. A seizure of such brief duration that it is difficult to recognize. According to who you talk to, absence seizures are either very rare in dogs or unrecognized.

Acantholysis Seperation of the intracellular bridges in the epidermis. Acantholysis is the characteristic histologic lesion of pemphigus leading to formation of clefts within the epidermis.

Acanthosis Nigricans Thickened, lichenified, seborrheic and greasy lesions which begin as small brown patches in the axilla and progresses to involve the hindlegs, chest and flanks. Most frequently seen in Dachshunds, also in Setters, Lhaso apsos, and others.

Acariasis Infestation with mites.

Accidental host Humans are not part of the life cycle, they accidentally entered into that organisms life cycle and got the disease. Examples: ringworm, rabies.

Accuracy A measure of how good and close a calculated estimate of an animal's genetic value is compared to the unknown true genetic value.

ACE inhibitor Angiotensin-converting-enzyme (ACE) inhibitor: Drug which decreases the function of this particular enzyme. The angiotensin-converting-enzyme changes a compound called angiotensin I to angiotensin II. Angiotensin II is a potent blood vessel constrictor. ACE inhibitors, then, have the effect of dilating blood vessels, since less Angiotensin II is produced.

Acellular vaccine A vaccine containing partial cellular material as opposed to complete cells.

Acetabulum Acetabulum is an anatomical term applied to any cup-like cavity, as that of a bone to receive the protuberant end of another bone.

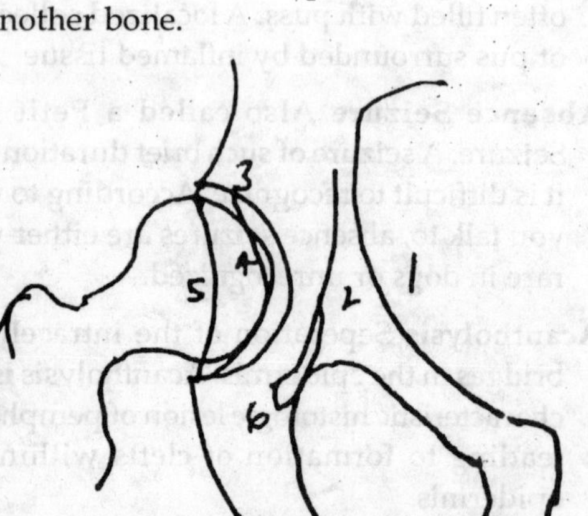

Fig. Acetabulum

Acetonemia (ketosis) A condition characterized by an elevated concentration of ketone bodies in body tissues and fluids. It is more common among high-producing cows in a negative energy balance.

Acetretin A Retinoids which is a synthetic derivatives of vitamin A.

Achondroplasia Improper development of cartilage at the ends of the long bones, resulting in a form of congenital dwarfism. A defect in most breeds and a requisite in others like Dachshunds and Basset Hounds.

Acid A fluid containing a high proportion of hydrogen ions, giving the liquid a sour taste. Measured by pH units, with 1 the most acid, and 14 the least acid. Chemical reactions in the body have to take place at or near neutrality, pH 7.

Acid detergent fiber ADFThe amount of residue (primarily cellulose, lignin and variable amounts of silica) left after boiling a feed sample in an acid detergent solution. The ADF value is used to predict the energy content (TDN, NE) of forages.

Acid Rinse Part of the equipment cleaning process for stainless steel and rubber parts, removes fat, protein and minerals and also reduces bacteria.

Acidosis (grain overload) When the pH of the rumen is abnormally low (<5.5). Signs of disease may include diarrhea, with or without blood. Usually due to over-consumption of grain.

Acne, feline Lesions seen most often on the chin. Acne may be a manifestation of a keratinization disorder, a primary bacterial infection, dermatophytosis, secondary to allergic skin disease, demodicosis, Malassezia dermatitis, or secondary to systemic disorders.

Acquired A defect that happens after being born (contrasted to congenital).

Acquired Immune Deficiency Syndrome (AIDS) A medical condition where the immune system cannot function properly and protect the body from disease. As a result, the body cannot defend itself against infections (like pneumonia). Aids is caused by the Human Immunodifiency Virus (HIV). This virus is spread through direct contact with the blood and body fluids of an infected individual. High-risk activities include unprotected sexual intercourse and intravenous drug use (sharing needles). There is no cure for AIDS; however, research efforts are on going to develop a vaccine.

Acquired Immunity Immunity obtained either from the development of antibodies in response to exposure to an antigen, as from vaccination or an attack of an infectious disease, or from the transmission of antibodies, as from mother to fetus through the placenta or the injection of antiserum. Results in resistance to further infection.

Acral lick dermatitis Acral pruritic nodules - "Lick granuloma". Lesions caused by chronic licking.

Acre Unit of measurement of land area; 4,840 square yards or 43,560 square feet.

Acronym Abbreviation for a phrase. MPL is the acronym for master problem list.

Across Breed Comparison (ABC) An estimate of genetic merit. It indicates the expected difference between the performance of progeny of an individual ram and the average of all rams tested regardless of breed.

ACTH Adrenocorticotropic hormone. A hormone, secreted by the pituitary gland, which stimulates the adrenal gland to work.

Actinic The injurious effects of ultraviolet light.

Action The horse's way of travel, how he moves his legs and degree of animation. The degree of flexion of the joints of the legs during movement; also reflected in head, neck, and tail carriage. High, snappy action is desired in some classes while easy, ground-covering action is the goal in other classes.

Activated charcoal Charcoal which has been treated to increase its adsorptive power (ability to have chemicals adhere to it); used to treat various forms of poisoning.

Activated partial thromboplastin time APPTThe time it takes for plasma to form a fibrin clot after the addition of calcium and a phospholipid reagent. APPT measures the intrinsic coagulation system.

Active immunity The production of antibodies against a specific disease by the immune system. Active immunity can be acquired in two ways, either by contracting the disease or through vaccination. Active immunity is usually permanent, meaning an individual is protected from the disease for the duration of their lives.

Acuminate Abruptly narrowing to sharp point.

Acupoint Specific locations at which treatment by acupuncture is delivered.

Acupressure Therapy which involves pressing points on the body with the fingers to alter the internal flow of chi in order to strengthen it, to calm it, or to remove a blockage of the flow. The acupressure points are aligned along the body meridians.

Acupuncture The Chinese practice of inserting needles into specific points (acupoints) along the "meridians" of the body. It is used to relieve pain, to induce surgical anesthesia, and for preventative and therapeutic purposes. The insertion of the needles stimulates the acupuncture points and alters the flow of chi.

Acute Disease An illness that manifests rapidly.

Acute Having a sudden and generally severe onset. See also Chronic.

Acute renal failure ARFAn acute suppression of renal function. The most common causes of ARF are renal ischemia and nephrotoxicity.

Acute tubular necrosis ATNAcute death of the epithelial cells lining the renal tubules due to ischemia or toxins.

Ad libitum (ad lib.) At pleasure. Commonly used to express feed available on free-choice basis.

Adaptive immunity Known as immune components of the immune system that are acquired after birth; the response of antigen-specific lymphocytes to antigen, including the development of immunological memory. Also referred to as learned or acquired immunity.

Addison's disease The pituitary gland produces a hormone that triggers the adrenal gland to produce corticosteroids. If there is a problem with the adrenal gland, or a pituitary tumor, the process breaks down and not enough corticosteroids are produced. Characterized by weakness, weight loss, anorexia, and fatigue.

Additive Genes Effects Members of a gene pair that have the ability to be expressed equally are additive genes. The gene pair is expressed as the sum of the individual effects of the genes in the pair.

Adenocarcinoma A form of cancer that occurs in the prostate gland.

Adenoids Adenoids is the pathological enlargement of the lymphoid tissue.

Adenovirus A family of DNA viruses that is used as a vehicle for the delivery of genes in many forms of gene-therapy.

ADF Acid Detergent Fiber; an indicator of relative digestibility of forages.

ADG See average daily gain.

Adhesion The sticking together of internal organs during the healing process following inflammation, causing restriction of movement and pain.

Adhesion molecule A molecule that mediates the binding of one cell to other cells or to extracellular matrix proteins. Integrins, selectins, members of the immunoglobulin superclass family, and CD44 and related proteins are all adhesion molecules important in the operation of the immune system (see CAM's and ICAM).

Adin Acid Detergent insoluble nitrogen. Undigestible dietary protein or nitrogen.

Adipose tissue Adipose tissue is a form of connective tissue in which the constituent cells are modified to enable them to contain droplets of oil. (Fat).

Adjusted 100-Day Weight This weight is the 50-day adjusted weight plus the postweaning 50-day weight gain (postweaning ADG x 50).

Adjusted 50-Day Weight This weight is calculated from an actual weight taken between 35 and 65 days of age. All lamb weights are then adjusted to the equivalent of a 50-day old ram lamb raised as a single from a mature ewe (4-5 years of age).

Adjuvant 1.A substance added to a drug product formulation that affects the action of the active ingredient in a predictable way In immunology, a vehicle used to enhance antigenicity; e.g. a suspension of minerals (alum, aluminum hydroxide or phosphate) on which antigen is adsorbed; or water-in-oil emulsion in which antigen solution is emulsified in mineral oil sometimes with the inclusion of killed mycobacteria to further enhance antigenicity.

Adnexa Structures bound to the skin such as sebaceous and apocrine glands.

Adrenal glands The adrenal glands are a pair of glands on the kidneys which secrete adrenalin and other hormones.

Adrenaline A hormone produced by the adrenal glands that elevates heart and respiration rates; also called 'epinephrine.'

Adrenergic Communication between the nerves and muscles that uses epinephrine as the 'messenger.' Adrenergic stimulation is what is involved in the 'flight or fight' response, which means the body is alerted to a danger of some sort and prepares to basically run or fight. Adrenergic stimulation results in an increased heart rate, sweating, and increased blood pressure.

Adsorbent A solid substance which attracts other molecules to its surface.

Adult stem cell Refers to stem cells derived from adults, but also to stem cells derived from fetuses.

Adulticide Medication formulated to kill adult forms of a parasite.

Adverse events Undesirable experiences occurring after immunization that may or may not be related to the vaccine.

Adverse reaction to food An abnormal clinical response attributed to an ingested food or food product.

AED (Anti epileptic drug) Also called anticonvulsant or antiseizure drugs. Examples would be phenobarbital and potassium bromide.

Aerobic Needing oxygen to live. See also Anaerobic bacteria.

Aerobic bacteria Bacteria that require oxygen to survive and grow.

Aerobic Requiring oxygen For example, many microorganisms require oxygen for the oxidation of food materials.

Afe Au Lait Usually used to describe Poodles, this color is the typical color of the French coffee of the same name, which is about equal parts of coffee and milk. It may be described as rich, well-saturated light brown. Color definitions may vary by breed. Always check the breed standard for the definitive color description.

Affenpinscher A breed of small dogs of European origin, having wiry, shaggy hair and a tufted muzzle.

Afghan Hound A large, slender hunting dog having long, thick hair, a pointed muzzle, and drooping ears.

Aflatoxin Toxin produced by the fungi Aspergillus flavus and Aspergillus parasiticus.

Afterbirth The placenta and allied membranes with which the fetus is connected with the mother. It is expelled from the uterus following parturition.

Agalactia Failure to secrete milk following parturition.

Age (of the horse) Computed from January 1 of the year in which the horse is foaled.

Age and Month of Calving Factors Factors used to eliminate the environmental effects of different ages and months of the year at calving. These factors standardize lactation records for genetic evaluations.

Age at Last Calving Age determined by subtracting the cow's birth date from her most recent calving date.

Age specific data base The minimum amount of information that is planned to be collected on all patients of a certain age; for example pediatric or geriatric databases.

Aged A horse which is ten years old or more

Agglutination An abnormal clumping of red blood cells. Often seen in patients with immune-mediated anemia.

Agonist A drug which when attached to a receptor causes an effect.

Agriculture The utilization of biological process on farms to produce food and other products useful and necessary to man. Both a "way of life" and a "means of life" for people involved in this industry.

AI (Artificial Insemination) The technique that involves breeding of females without the males being physically present.

AI Daughter Female offspring of an artificially inseminated dam.

Aid An aid is an action by a part of the rider's or handler's body to a part of the horse's body to cause the horse to react in a particular way. An aid is almost never used alone but always used in conjunction with other aids. A rider's natural aids are his or her mind, seat, weight, upper body, legs, hands, and voice. The combined use of all of the rider's aids simultaneously produce a smooth, balanced response from a horse. A handler's natural aids are the mind, hands, and overall body language. Examples of Artificial Aids (which are extensions, reinforcements, or substitutions for the natural aids) are whips, spurs, and nosebands.

Aids Signals from the rider to the horse with with his hands, seat, weight, legs and voice, to tell the horse what to do. . Natural aids are the mind, voice, hands, legs, and weight. Examples of artificial aids (which are extensions, reinforcements, or substitutions of the natural aids) are whips, spurs, nosebands, draw reins and martingales.

Alanine Aminotransferase ALT (SALT)Also known as serum alanine aminotransferase (SALT). An enzyme found in hepatocytes (liver cells) released with cellular injury including cellular hypoxia.

Albino An animal that is completely white because it lacks the ability to make pigment. Its eyes are pale blue or pink.

Albumin A protein in the blood responsible for the maintenance of osmotic (water) pressure in the blood; also binds (attaches) to large molecules in the blood and serves to transport them; produced by the liver; also called 'serum albumin.'

Aldosterone A hormone secreted by the adrenal gland that stimulates sodium (and therefore water) retention and potassium excretion; important in blood pressure maintenance.

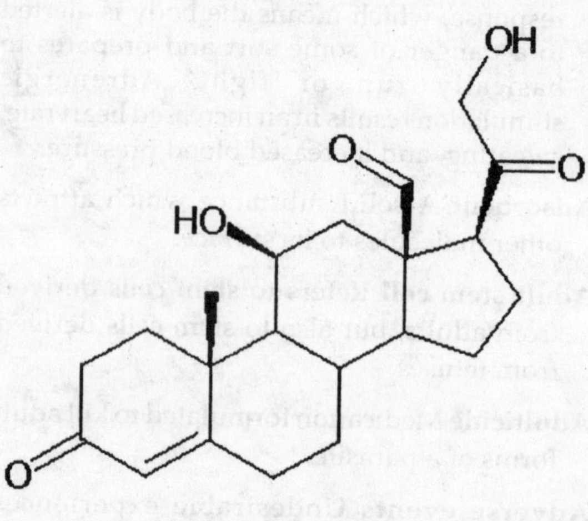

Fig. Aldosterone

Alektorophobia Fear of chickens.

Alfalfa (medicago sativa) A leguminous plant used primarily for hay, usually high in protein and calcium.

Alimentary Another term for the gut or intestinal tract. The alimentary tract runs from the mouth, through the esophagus to the stomach, duodenum, small intestine, large intestine, rectum, and anus.

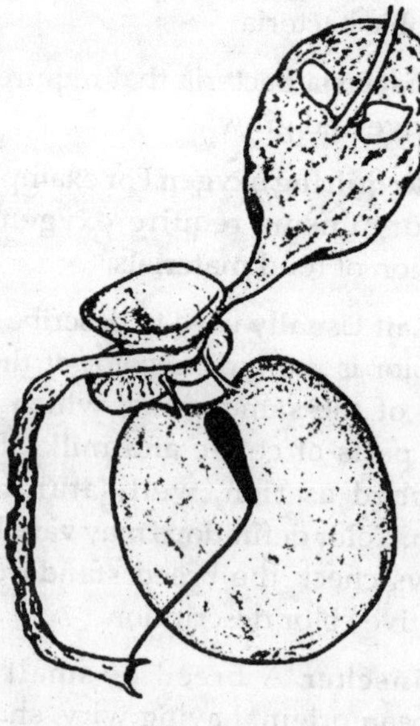

Fig. Alimentary Canal

Alkaline A substance with very few hydrogen ions, and a pH over 7. Lye is strongly alkaline.

Alkaline phosphatase AP SAPAlso known as serum alkaline phosphatase (SAP). An enzyme found in many tissues but most often elevated in serum in response to cholestasis, bone remodeling or glucocorticoid excess.

All in, all out management system A management system where the entire population is removed from a single area, the area is thoroughly cleaned and disinfected, and then the pigs are moved back in.

Allbreed (AB) An "allbreed ring" at a show is a ring in which cats of all breeds are judged and ranked against each other. An "allbreed judge" is a judge who is licensed to judge allbreed rings. Compare with specialty.

Alleles Any one of a series of two or more different genes that may occupy the same locus on a specific chromosome. As autosomal chromosomes are paired each autosomal gene is represented twice in normal somatic cells. If the same a. occupies this a. If the a.'s are different, the individual or cell is heterozygous for both a.'s.

Allergen A substance that causes an allergic reaction, e.g., pollen.

Allergic contact dermatitis ACDDermatitis caused by caustic or irritating substances. No prior sensitization is required.

Allergy Immunological hypersensitivity to certain foreign antigens.anemia reduction of red blood cells or hemoglobin. The red cells contain the protein 'hemoglobin' which binds oxygen in the red blood cell. This allows the transport of oxygen from the lungs to the tissues. Symptoms include weakness, reluctance to exercise, pale mucus membranes, and tachycardia (abnormally rapid heart rate).

Alley A walking area for cattle within a barn such as a loafing alley, feeding alley or cross alley (walkway) from a barn to the milking parlor.

Alley Scraper A "V" shaped mechanical blade that is dragged over an alley by chain or cable to pull manure to collection channel at the end of the alley (or possibly the center of the barn). The blade then collapses and is drawn back to the opposite end of the alley.

Allo Other; differing from the normal or usual.

Alloantigen An antigen that occurs in some but not other members of the same species. Isoantigen is sometimes used in this sense.

Allodynia Pain from a stimulus that would normally be non-painful.

Allopathy The traditional approach to treatment that most veterinarians practice; treating the disease by supressing its symptoms or attempting to destroy the microbes associated with the condition; the opposite of homeopathy. Sometimes called the Western approach.

Aloe A tropical herb. The translucent gel from the inner leaves is used externally to relieve burns, skin irritations, and infections. Aloe gel taken internally provides relief from stomach disorders. It is thought to act by inhibiting bradykinin, and thus assist with pain. Aloe gel is used in beauty aids and moisturizers because the polysaccharides it contains help to smooth, soften, and protect the skin. The yellow juice called latex found just beneath the leaf surface acts as a powerful laxative.

Alopecia A loss of hair or baldness.

Alopecia Baldness Loss or deficiency of hair, natural or abnormal.

Alpha virus genus One of the genera of the family togaviridae that was formerly classified as part of the group A arboviruses and includes viruses that cause eastern equine, western equine and Venezuelan encephalitis.

Alpha reductase An enzyme that catalyzes the conversion of testosterone to dihydrotestosterone.

Alter To spay or neuter a cat. An "alter" is an altered cat.

Alula A small winglike group of feathers at the bend of the wing, supported by the anteriormost digit.

Alum precipitate An adjuvant (see adjuvants).

Aluminum hydroxide An adjuvant which is a common component of killed vaccines, included to increase the ability of the vaccine to stimulate an immune response.

Alveolus Microscopic sac-like structures within the lung. The airways terminate in these sac-like structures. When blood in the lung contacts the alveoli, the blood takes up oxygen and empties waste gases that will be removed during breathing.

Amateur Rider over eighteen who does not get paid for riding. An individual who rides or exhibits a horse in competition, who does not derive profit from such activities and does not do so as a profession.

Amateur Owner Class open to horses whose owner or member of owner's immediate family is the rider.

Ambient In the environment. Commonly used: "ambient temperature" = temperature in the current environment.

American Animal Hospital Association AAHA An international association of over 17,000 veterinary care providers who treat companion animals. The association was established in 1933. Over 2,800 veterinary hospitals voluntarily participate in the AAHA hospital evaluation program.

Amino acids Nitrogen-containing compounds that are the building blocks from which protein are made.

Aminobisphosphonate A type of bisphosphonate drug, which is (ironically) a potent inhibitor of osteoclast-mediated bone resorption and also a potent inhibitor of angiogenesis (new blood vessel formation) – a process that is necessary for new bone formation.

Aminoglycoside A class of antibiotics which act by interfering with bacterial protein synthesis within the bacteria which results in the death of the bacteria. Antibiotics in this class include gentamicin (Gentocin), kanamycin, neomycin, streptomycin, tobramycin, and amikacin. Many of these antibiotics are not well-absorbed from the animal's digestive system, so are often administered as injections, or used topically.

Amiodarone A class III antiarrhythmic drug.

Amitosis Amitosis is the anatomical term given to cell reproduction by direct division. The nucleus becomes constricted in the middle, forming an hour-glass shape and then divides into two. This is followed by a division of the whole protoplasmic mass of the cell; two daughter cells are thus formed, each containing a nucleus. Direct division occurs in leucocytes and bone-cells, and in the epithelial cells lining the urinary bladder.

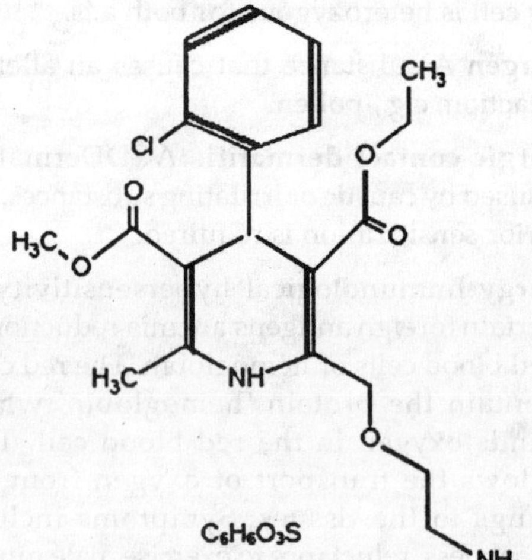

Fig. Amitosis

Amitraz Mitaban, A treatment for demodectic mange. Mechanism of action is unknown, probably a monamine oxidase inhibitor.

Amlodipine A long-acting calcium channel blocker that is the drug of choice for management of hypertension in cats.

Ammonia A colorless pungent gas, NH_3, composed of nitrogen and hydrogen; its compounds are used as fertilizers.

Ammonium An ion (NH^{4+}) derived from ammonia (NH_3).

Amnion The inner most layer of the membrane surrounding the embryo in the uterus. The sac formed by this membrane contains amniotic fluid.

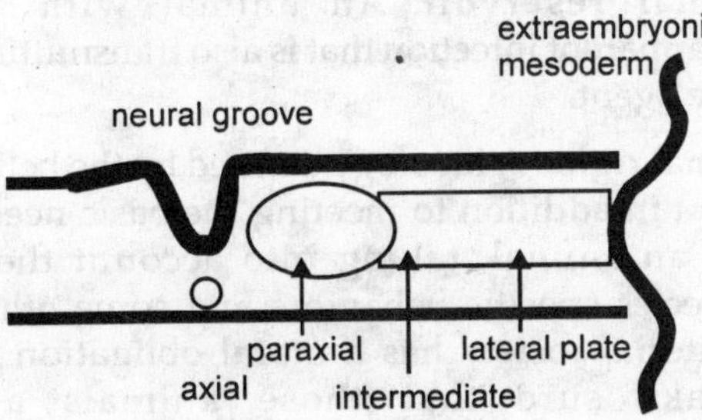

Fig. Amnion

Amniotic vesicle Another name for the embryonic vesicle.

Amphotericin B Systemic antifungal drug.

Amylase An enzyme produced by the pancreas that contributes to digestion of food. Lack of amylase results in a large amount of greasy stool being passed.

Amylopectin A branched chain of glucose molecules. An animal's EPD is ½ of it's EBV and is equal to ½ (Sire EPD + Dam EPD).

Anabolic steroid A type of steroid (not a corticosteroid like prednisone, cortisone, or dexamethasone) which promotes the building of tissues, like muscle.

Anaerobic bacteria Bacteria which only live in an environment in which there is no or little oxygen, e.g., Clostridium tetani which causes tetanus.

Anaerobic treatment lagoon A structure to treat animal waste by predominantly anaerobic biological action using anaerobic or facultative organisms, in the absence of air, for the purpose of reducing organic matter in wastes.

Anagen The phase of the hair cycle during with the hair is synthesized.

Analgesia Refers to the absence of pain in the presence of stimuli that would be expected to be painful. In clinical practice we use the term analgesia to mean a reduction in pain.

Analgesic A drug administered to reduce the perception of pain.

Anamnestic response The memory of immune cells which allows for more rapid and intense production of antibody the second time a host animal sees an antigen. Also called a secondary immune response.

Anaphase Anaphase is the 3rd stage of mitosis cell reproduction. The centromeres split into 2 halves which repel each other.

Anaphylaxis Anaphylaxis is a rare, life-threatening, immediate allergic reaction to something ingested or injected. If untreated, it results in shock, respiratory and cardiac failure, and death. May also be referred to as anaphylactic shock or anaphylactoid reaction. Symptoms of anaphylaxis include breathing difficulty, loss of consciousness and a drop in blood pressure. This condition can be fatal and requires immediate medical attention.

Anatomy The physical structure of the body. Understanding the words used to express positioning on a dog's body helps a great deal in understanding veterinary lingo. For the directions below, the dog is standing in the center of a room with his head facing the north wall.

Anconeus The Anconeus is a muscle in the human arm. It assists the Triceps in extending the elbow-joint.

Ancylostomiasis Hookworm dermatitis.The etiological agents are migrating 3rd stage larvae of Ancylostoma canium or Uncinaria stenocephala.

Androgen A hormone which produces male sexual characteristics, e.g., testosterone.

Anemia The lack of red blood cells in the body. Anemia can be the result of loss, destruction, and/or decreased production of red blood cells.

Anesthesia Loss of sensation induced by a drug. This can be loss of sensation in a body part which is called local anesthesia or loss of consciousness with general anesthesia.

Anestrous period The time when the female does not cycle or exhibit estrus (heat); the non-breeding season.

Angiogenesis The formation of new blood vessels.

Angiography The x-ray of vessels after injecting a contrasting fluid.

Angiotensin-converting-enzyme inhibitor (ACE inhibitor) Drug which decreases the function of this particular enzyme. The angiotensin-converting-enzyme changes a compound called angiotensin I to angiotensin II. Angiotensin II is a potent blood vessel constrictor. ACE inhibitors, then, have the effect of dilating blood vessels, since less Angiotensin II is produced.

Angulated With an angle.

Animal health trust A registered charity which provides specialist veterinary clinical and laboratory services concerning cats, dogs and horses and including infectious disease surveillance in horses. Other services include research related to disease problems including post mortem examinations, laboratory tests, and outbreak investigatiopns. Results of their work are published.

Animal Improvement Programs Laboratory (AIPL) A Department of Agriculture research service computing laboratory that calculates genetic evaluations of cows and sires using data collected through the DHI system.

Animal Legal Defense Fund A group of private attorneys who have joined together who all have the common goal of promoting the welfare and right of animals.

Animal model An animal sufficiently like humans in it anatomy, physiology, or response to an injury that is used in medical research in order to obtain information that can be extrapolated to human medicine.

Animal reservoir An animal with an inapparent infection that is also transmitting the agent.

Animal rights A ideology defined by the belief that in addition to meeting the basic needs of an animal, taking into account their species specific behaviors and some other criteria, society has a moral obligation to make sure that those animals are appropriately cared for and handled.

Animal Unit A unit of measurement of livestock, the equivalent of one mature cow weighing 1,000 pounds. The measure is used in making comparisons of feed consumption and grazing.

Animal unit month (AUM) Amount of forage used by an animal unit (one cow and her calf) for one month.

Animal Welfare Information Center A federally funded group that was originally set up with the Health Research Information Act and part of that was to mandate the Animal Welfare Information Center place to go and look for alternatives to the use of animals in research.

Animal well being A state in which the animal is existing with in a range of acceptable environmental and psychological specifications.

Animals rights A belief in the total elimination of use of animals in our society, period. Human life is equated to animal life.

Anisocoria Pupils that are unequal in size. The problem may be caused by diseases of the eye or the nerves to the eyes.

Anisocytosis Varied sizes of red blood cells. May be an indicator of regenerative anemia.

Anisodactyl Three toes in front and one behind, as in perching birds.

Ankle The ankle is the joint connecting the foot with the leg.

Anopheles The genus of mosquito that transmits malaria.

Anorexia A loss of appetite or desire to eat.

Antagonist A drug which when attached to a receptor blocks the receptor from being stimulated by an agonist drug.

Ante-mortem Before death.

Ante mortem inspection A check on live animals which are about to be slaughtered, to make sure the animals are treated humanely and are not suffering from any disease which would make the meat unfit for human consumption. It is carried out at the slaughterhouse by a veterinary surgeon working for the Meat Hygiene Service.

Antenna An antenna is a sensory organ found on the head of insects.

Anteriad Toward the front.

Anterior Positioned in front of another body part, or towards the head of the animal. Opposite of posterior.

Anterior chamber Space between the cornea and iris and filled with aqueous.

Anterior uveitis Inflammation of the iris and ciliary body.

Anthelmetics Medications given to remove or kill worms. Also called wormers.

Anthropomorphism Projecting human needs or wants on to an animal.

Anti idiotype Antibodies to the variable regions of the antibody-binding site. Anti-idiotypes contain the internal image of the tumor antigen and are capable of inducing antibody responses to the original antigen.

Anti neoplastic Inhibiting or preventing growth and spread of tumors.

Anti angiogenic The property of preventing the formation of blood vessels.

Antibiotic A metabolic product of one microorganism or a chemical that in low concentrations is detrimental to activities of specific other microorganisms. Examples include penicillin, tetracycline, and streptomycin. Not effective against viruses. A drug that kills microorganisms that cause mastitis or other infectious disease.

Antibiotic Residues The presence of traces of antibiotics or their derivatives in milk or meat.

Antibiotic Test Kit Test kit for use on the farm to detect residues of antibiotics in milk before the milk is picked up for delivery to the plant.

Antibodies An infection-fighting protein molecule in blood or secretory fluids that tags, neutralizes, and helps destroy pathogenic microorganisms (e.g., bacteria, viruses) or toxins. Antibodies, known generally as immunoglobulins, are made and secreted by B-lymphocytes in response to stimulation by antigens. Each specific antibody binds only to the specific antigen that stimulated its production.

Antibody isotypes Also known as immunoglobulin isotypes. (See immunoglobulin) Different immunoglobulin isotypes are called IgM, IgD, IgA, and IgE.

Antibody mediated immunity Immunity that results from the activity of antibodies in blood and lymphoid tissue (also called humoral immunity).

Antibody titer A measurement of the amount of antibodies in the blood. The test to measure antibodies is usually performed by making a number of dilutions of the blood and then measuring at what dilution there is sufficient antibody to react in the test. For example, a titer of 1:8 (one to eight) means the blood can be diluted to one part blood and seven parts saline and still produce a positive reaction in the test. The higher the titer (1:16 is higher than 1:8), the more antibody is present.

Anticholinergic Stopping the communications between certain nerves and muscles of the body including those of the gastrointestinal tract and heart. These nerves are called 'parasympathetic' nerves and do such things as constrict the pupils of the eye, stimulate contractions of the muscles in the intestine, and slow the heart rate. Anticholinergic drugs would have the effect, then, of dilating the pupil, slowing contractions of the intestines, and increasing the heart rate.

Anticholinesterase A drug that blocks the enzyme acetylcholinesterase; this results in stimulation of the parasympathetic nervous system.

Anticoagulants Drugs that reduce the ability of the blood to clot. Also called blood thinners.

Anticonvulsant A drug used to prevent or decrease the severity of convulsions.

Antidiuretic hormone ADH A hormone produced by the hypothalmus and stored in the pituitary gland. ADH regulates the ability of the collecting ducts of the kidneys to reabsorb water. In the absence of ADH the animal voids large amount of urine.

Antiemetics Drugs administered to reduce vomiting.

Antifungal Drugs administered to kill or inhibit the growth of fungi (plural of fungus).

Antigen Any substance, which can generate the formation of a specific antibody (a protein created by the immune system to protect the body). For vaccines, the term antigen refers to a vaccine component that induces protection for one single disease (e.g., the measles antigen induces protection against measles).

Antigen presenting cell Antigen-processing cells ingest antigen and chop it into small fragments that are then packaged within the major histocompatibility complex molecules and shuttled to the surface of the cell membrane for presentation. Professional antigen presenting cells are dendritic cells, macrophages, and B cells.

Antigen processing Before the immune system can respond to an antigen it must be able to recognize the antigen. It is able to do so through antigen processing. Macrophages are the major antigen processing cells others include B-lymphocytes.

Antimicrobial A compound which, at low concentrations, exerts an action against microorganisms and exhibits selective toxicity towards them. The term antimicrobial includes any substance of natural, synthetic or semi-synthetic origin which is used to kill, or inhibit the growth of, microorganisms (bacteria, fungi, protozoa and viruses). Antimicrobials include antibiotics, disinfectants, preservatives and other substances (e.g. copper, zinc).

Antimicrobial agent Any substance of natural, synthetic or semi-synthetic origin which at low concentrations kills or inhibits the growth of micro-organisms but causes little or no host damage.

Antimicrobial class Antimicrobials with a related molecular structure, often with a similar mode of action. Variations in the properties of antimicrobials within a class often arise as a result of the presence of different side chains of the molecule, which confer different patterns of pharmacokinetic and pharmacodynamic behavior on the molecule.

Antimicrobial growth promoter Antimicrobial agents used for the purpose of increasing daily weight gain or feed efficiency.

Antimicrobial resistance Antimicrobial resistance is the result of microbes changing in ways that reduce or eliminate the effectiveness of drugs, chemicals, or other agents to cure or prevent infections.

Antimicrobial resistance genes Genes in microorganisms, which confer resistance to antimicrobials. These are often located on mobile genetic elements thereby enabling transmission from resistant to susceptible strains.

Antiprotozoal An agent that kills protozoa, which are one-celled organisms such as Giardia.

Antipruritic Relieves itching.

Antipyretics Drugs that suppress a fever in an attempt to bring the temperature to normal.

Antiseptic A chemical that inhibits the growth of microorganisms without killing them.

Antispasmodic An agent that relieves or decreases spasms in muscle. The muscle could include 'smooth muscle' which is the type of muscle in intestines that causes them to contract and move food through the digestive system.

Antitoxin A substance that acts against specific toxins. it produced by the body and carried in the bloodstream.

Antitussive Cough suppressant.

Anuria The condition of complete failure in the function of the kidneys such that no urine is produced.

Anus The muscular tissue at the end of the rectum that keeps stool in the rectum until the animal defecates.

Aorta The aorta is the largest artery in the human body. It carries blood from the heart to the arms, legs and head.

AP AM/PM Abbreviations commonly used to describe alternate morning/evening monthly types of testing plans. Milk weights and samples are collected at the morning milking for 1 month and at the evening milking the following month.

Apheresed Apheresis- Infusion of a patient's own blood from which certain cellular or fluid elements have been removed. [G.aphaeresis, withdrawal]

Aplastic anemia A serious condition in which red blood cells, white blood cells, and platelets are not produced in sufficient quantity.

Apoptosis Single deletion of scattered cells by fragmentation into membrane bound particles that are phagocytosed by other cells; believed to be due to programmed cell death. [G. a falling or dropping off, fr. Apo, off + ptosis, a falling].

Appointments The type of tack for the horse and attire for the rider or handler that is

Apteria Plural of apterium.

Apterium Unfeathered area between feather tracts.

Aquaculture The (usually commercial) captive raising of fish, corals, and other aquatic life for aquariums, food, and scientific purposes.

Aquatic Pertains to living in or near water.

Aqueous The clear liquid produced by the cells of the ciliary body which fills the anterior chamber (between the cornea and iris) and the posterior chamber (between the iris and lens).

Aqueous humor The fluid found within the eyeball which provides nourishment to the interior eye structures and keeps the eyeball inflated.

Areolar tissue Areolar tissue is a generalised form of connective tissue in which the constituent cells are separated by a semi-fluid matrix in which both white connective tissue and yellow elastic fibres are found.

Arm A group of participants in a clinical trial, all of who receive the same treatment, intervention or placebo. The other arm(s) receive(s) a different treatment.

Arm The arm is a limb extending from the shoulder of an animal.

Aromatherapy The essential oils of plants are used to promote relaxation and help relieve the symptoms of certain ailments. Essential oils are extremely concentrated fragrant extracts which are cold-pressed or steam-distilled from blossoms, leaves, or roots. These oils are applied through massage, mixed with water and used as compresses on the skin, added to a bath, or diffused into the air and inhaled. The essential oils should not be ingested.

Arrested development The parasites "hibernate" in the host as a fourth stage larva, and then in spring, they come out.

Arrhythmia Any variation from the normal rhythm of the heart beat.

Artery Blood vessels that carry blood from the heart to the organs and tissues. Arteries contain more oxygen and nutrients than veins and are under higher pressure.

Arthralgia Joint pain.

Arthritis Inflammation of a joint. Caused by abnormal stress on a normal joint, or by normal stress on an abnormal joint. Polyarthritis is immune mediated, and is arthritis in multiple joints. Autoimmune disease Failure of the immune system to differentiate the body's own cells from foreign substances, triggering an inflammatory response against self. This can be in the form of a very specific immune attack, such as the destruction of pancreatic islet cells resulting in diabetes mellitus, or a broad immunologic injury such as lupus.

Articular Pertaining to a joint.

Artificial insemination Placement of fresh or frozen male semen into the female mechanically without normal sexual contact.

Artificial Rearing Raising a kid on milk or milk replacer.

Artificial vagina AVA rubber cone attached to a collection tube that is used to collect semen.

ARU Animal Resources Unit.

As fed basis An expression of feed nutrient content with moisture included. Nutrient content on an "as fed" basis is always lower than on a "dry matter" basis.

Ascarid Roundworm.

Ascaris Large white intestinal parasite; in the horse the common ascaris is Paracaris equorum.

Ascites The accumulation of fluid in the peritoneal cavity. Some define ascites as fluid of any type including blood, bile and other exudates. Others define ascites as including only pure transudates.

Ascorbic acid A substance found in many fruits and vegetables, especially citrus fruits (oranges and lemons) and tomatoes. It is water soluble, and vitamin C excesses are excreted through the kidney. It is synthesized within the bodies of most animal species, except primates, guinea-pigs, fruit bats, and some fish. These species which do not synthesize vitamin C require it in their diet. Vitamin C helps to potentiate the antioxidant effect of vitamin E, but in excessive doses, it can cause flatulence and diarrhea.

Aseptic Preventing or free from contamination by microorganisms.

Aseptic packaging Method of filling packages without allowing the entry of microorganisms. Commonly used for sterile milk products to provide improved keeping quality.

Ash The inorganic mineral elements of animals and plants, determined by burning off the organic matter and weighing the residue (ash).

Aspirate Withdraw fluid or cells through the use of suction - usually the suction produced by pulling back on the plunger of a syringe attached to a needle which is inserted into the area to be sampled. Also the breathing in of a fluid or foreign substances.

Aspiration Inhaling food or other materials into the airways.

AssessmentYour interpretation of patient data. For example what is the significance of nucleated RBCs.

Association The degree to which the occurrence of two variables or events is linked. Association describes a situation where the likelihood of one event occurring depends on the presence of another event or variable. However, an association between two variables does not necessarily imply a cause and effect relationship. The term association and relationship are often used interchangeably.

Astragalus An herbal remedy from the root of the plant Astragalus membranaceus. Astragalus enhances many bodily functions. Western herbalists believe it to stimulate the immune system and generally strengthen the body by speeding metabolism, promoting tissue regeneration, and increasing energy. It is used to help treat chronic colds, AIDS, cancer, and chronic fatigue. In traditional Chinese medicine, astragalus is regarded as sweet and slightly warm; it is used to treat general weakness, loss of appetite, spontaneous perspiration, diarrhea, and blood abnormalities or deficiencies from excessive bleeding. The Chinese species is the source of the medicine called huang qi.

Astride When a rider sits on a horse with one leg on either side of the horse.

Astrocytes A type of glial cell that has many functions, on of which is to create a scar around the injury site.

Asymptomatic A term used to decide a condition in which no symptoms are present.

Asymptomatic infection The presence of an infection without symptoms. Also known as inapparent or subclinical infection.

Asystole Cardiac arrest.

Ataxia Uncoordination that is caused by temporary or permanent neurological impairment. A side-effect of some AEDs that can diminish with time.

Athymic Lacking a thymus. The thymus is the site of production of T lymphocytes, a vital part of the adaptive immune system.

Atlas In anatomy, the 1st cervical vertebrae is called the atlas because it supports the globe of the head.

Atoll A coral island consisting of a reef surrounding a lagoon.

Atopy Allergic inhalant dermatitis or atopic dermatitis. Allergens are true antigens which are usually inhaled or penetrate the skin as complete allergens or haptens. Allergens may also be ingested or injected.

ATP Adenosine triphosphate; a compound used for energy by cells.

Atresia Regressing or shrinking in size.

Atria The heart has 4 chambers; the two chambers that make up the top of the heart are the atria.

Atrial fibrillationA heart condition in which the atria (chambers of the heart that receive the blood) contract rapidly, irregularly, and independently of the ventricles (the chambers of the heart that pump the blood). This greatly decreases the efficiency of the heart and its ability to move blood.

Atrial flutterA heart condition in which the atria (chambers of the heart that receive the blood) contract rapidly, irregularly, and independently of the ventricles (the chambers of the heart that pump the blood). This greatly decreases the efficiency of the heart and its ability to move blood.

AtriumThe two chambers of the heart that receive blood. The right atrium receives blood from the body. The left atrium receives oxygenated blood from the lungs.

Atrophy A defect or failure of nutrition or physiologic function manifested as a wasting away or reduction in the size of cell, tissue, organ, or body part.

Atropine A parasympatholytic drug which competitivly blocks acetylcholine at muscarinic receptors and increases sinus node automaticity and atrial-ventricular conduction resulting in an increase in heart rate.

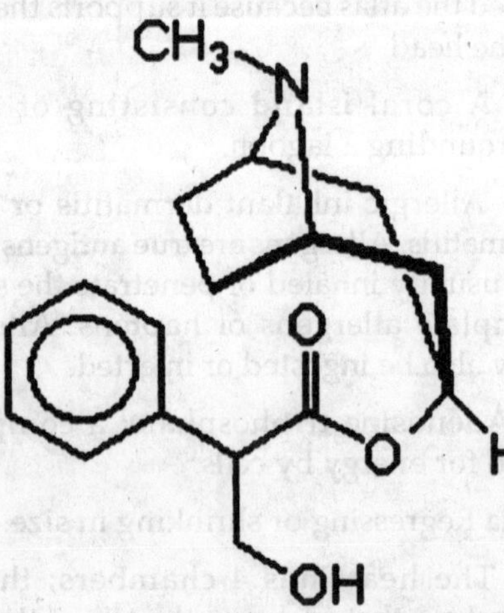

Fig. Atropine

Attack rate The proportion of a defined population affected during an outbreak. Since the attack rate is based only on new cases of disease, it is comparable to incidence.

Attenuated Process used in vaccine production to modify organisms to induce immunity without causing disease.

Attenuated strain A strain of microorganism that has been altered in virulence to exhibit diminished virulence.

Attenuated vaccine A vaccine in which live viruses are weakened through chemical or physical processes in order to produce an immune response without causing the severe effects of the disease. Attenuated vaccines currently licensed in the United States include measles, mumps, rubella, polio, yellow fever and varicella. Also known as a live vaccine.

Attenuation Diminution of the virulence in a strain of an organism, obtained through selection of variants that occur naturally or through experimental means.

Attire The rider's clothes.

Auditory meatus Ear opening.

Aura A sensation or warning that a seizure is about to occur.

Auricle The auricles are resevoirs within the heart which receive blood from the veins.

Auscultate To listen for sounds produced within the body, usually with the aid of a stethoscope.

Auscultation To listen with a stethoscope. The heart and lung sounds are heard by auscultation.

Autism A chronic developmental disorder

usually diagnosed between 18 and 30 months of age. Symptoms include problems with social interaction and communication as well as repetitive interests and activities. At this time, the cause of autism is not known although many experts believe it to be a genetically based disorder that occurs before birth.

Auto disable syringe A specifically modified disposable syringe with a fixed needle, which is automatically disabled by the plunger blocking after a single use.

Autoimmune A condition in which the immune system attacks the body's own tissues. To properly function, the immune system must identify foreign substances such as bacteria, viruses, parasites, slivers, etc., and it must be able to distinguish normal body tissue from these foreign substances. If it fails to distinguish the difference, it attempts to destroy the tissue it wrongly identifies as foreign. For example, in autoimmune hemolytic anemia, the body destroys its own red blood cells. In rheumatoid arthritis it attacks the cells in the joints.

Autoimmune hemolytic anemia The body produces antibodies directed against its own red blood cells, causing their destruction. FYI: Many if not all of the autoimmune anemias have antibodies that attack related, similar blood types, donor RBC's too.

Autoimmunity The condition in which one's own tissues are subject to deleterious effects of the immune system, as in auto allergy and in autoimmune disease; specific humoral or cell mediated immune response against the body's own tissues.

Autologous Occurring naturally and normally in a certain type of tissue or in a specific structure of the body. Sometimes used to denote a neoplasm derived from cells that occur normally at that site. e.g. squamous cell carcinoma in the upper esophagus.

Automatic Detacher or Automatic Take-off A device for sensing the end of milk flow in the milking machine which shuts of the milking vacuum and releases the milking machine from the cow's udder.

Automatic take off A device for sensing the end of milk flow in the milking machine, for shutting off the milking vacuum, and for retracting the milking unit from the cow's udder.

Autoregulatory Negative Feedback Loop A physiological thermostat that dampens and regulates the response of a system to external input.

Autosomal Any of the chromosomes other than the sex pair, the 'X' or 'Y' chromosomes. benign not cancerous or malignant.

Available protein The portion of the crude protein that can be used by the animal.

Average Daily Gain (ADG) ADG is the amount of body weight change of an animal per day. For example, between the 50 and 100-day weighings:

(100 Day Weight - 50 Day Weight) ÷ 50 Days or ADG = WT change/day.

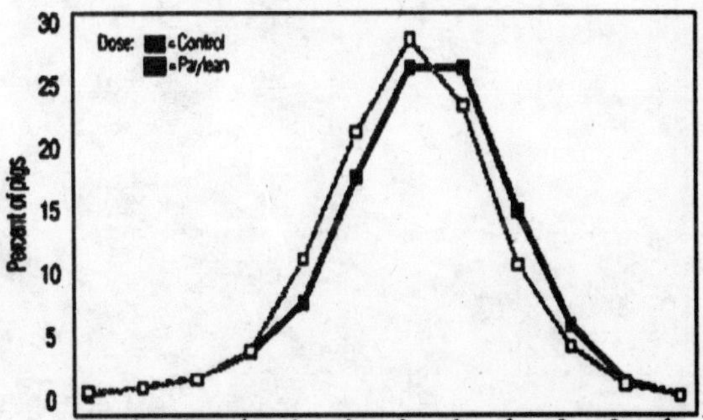

Fig. Average Daily Gain Chart

Aviculture The science of raising avian species.

Avidity The binding strength of an antibody for an antigen.

Axis In anatomy, the 2nd cervical vertebrae is called the axis. It provides the pivot for the atlas and the head.

Axon Part of a nerve cell, messages are sent along this long projection which makes contact with other neurons.

Ayurvedic medicine A form of medicine practiced in India. Health is considered to be a state of balance between the body's physical, emotional, and spiritual systems, and illness is a state of imbalance. Illness may be detected by reading of the pulse and by observation of the tongue. Nutrition, massage, natural medications, meditation, and other modalities may be used for treatment of a wide variety of ailments.

Azathioprine An immunosuppressive drug used in cancer chemotherapy and in treatment of immune mediated diseases.

Azoospermia The complete absence of sperm in the ejaculate.

Azotemia The presence of increased nitrogenous (containing nitrogen) waste products in the blood as a result of kidney malfunction.

B

B cells Small white blood cells that help the body defend itself against infection. These cells are produces in bone marrow and develop into plasma cells that produce antibodies. Also know as B-lymphocytes.

Babbler A hound that gives a sound when not on the trail.

Babcock test Traditional method of measuring the butterfat content of milk, which may be used for calibrating modern electronic testing devices.

Baby lamb Animals produced all year-round by controlled breeding and marketed at six to ten weeks of age before weaning.

Back at the knee A fault in the forelegs in which the lower limb below the knee, when viewed from the side, tends to be concave. Also known as calf-knee and buck-knee. Undesirable because the limb would be of little use in absorbing concussion.

Back The area of a dog's body extending from the withers to the croup.

Backcross Backcross is the mating of a two-breed animal back to one of the two parental breeds.

Backyard breeder A person who casually breeds purebred dogs with little or no regard to the breed standard, genetically linked defects or temperament.

Bacteremia Bacteria in the blood.

Bacteremias A bacterial population in the blood.

Bacteria Bacteria are single-celled organisms that live in and around us. Bacteria may be helpful, but in certain conditions may cause illnesses such as strep throat, most inner ear infections, and bacterial pneumonia. Pl. a unicellular prokaryotic organism that usually multiplies by cell division and has a cell wall that provides a constancy of form. They may also be aerobic or anaerobic, motile or non-motile and free-living, saprophytic, parasitic or pathogenic.

Bacterial or prokaryotes Single celled organisms without a true nucleus.

Bacterial vaccine Vaccine derived of bacteria.

Bactericide An agent or substance capable of destroying bacteria.

Bacterin A suspension of killed or attenuated bacteria (vaccine) used to increase disease resistance.

Bacteriocidal Kills bacteria.

Bacteriocide A substance that kills bacteria.

Bacteriostat A substance that inhibits or retards bacterial growth.

Bacteriostatic Describes a substance that prevents the growth of bacteria but does not kill them.

Bacterium Microscopic organisms that lack nuclei and other organelles; pathogenic species cause disease, while nonpathogenic species are harmless.

Bad Mouth Crooked teeth; when the mouth is closed, upper and lower teeth do not line up according to the standard of the breed.

Badger A grayish-brown color that may be mixed with a few dark hairs (Great Pyrenees, Sealyham Terriers). Color definitions may vary by breed. Always check the breed standard for the definitive color description.

Bag Udder, mammary gland; (v.) Enlarging the udder prior to foaling.

Balance In regard to movement, a state of equilibrium; in regard to conformation, desirable proportions. Distribution of weight between horse and rider.

Balanced ration The daily food allowance of an animal, mixed to include suitable proportions of nutrients required for normal health, growth, production, and well-being. A ration containing all the dietary requirements to meet the purpose for which it is being fed.

Balanoposthitis Inflammation of the penis (balanitis) and prepuce (posthitis).

Balb/c mice A Transgenic mouse model used in immunologic and oncologic research studies due to its genetic immuno-susceptibility.

Bald White or light color on a horse's head from poll to nose, including around the eyes.

Bale A package of wool in a standard wool pack for shipment. The common farm bale weighs between 200 and 450 lbs.

Baled hay Forage that has been compressed into a bale (round or rectangular) to save space in storage and aid in handling.

Balk To refuse or cease to move forward.

Banding This involves the use of castration rings (bands) to remove the testacles.

Bandy Legs Legs that bend outward.

Bang's disease See Brucellosis.

Bank Solid earthen ramp or wall that is used as a drop jump.

Bantam A group of breeds of chickens and ducks distinguished by their small size. Bantams typically weigh between one and three pounds. Many are miniature versions of Large Fowl breeds. A few, like the Japanese and Sebrights are only found in as bantam. Bantam ducks are made up of the Call, East Indie, and Mallard breeds.

Bantam Standard A book published by the American Bantam Association describing each of the bantam breeds recognized by that organization.

Banty or Bantie Slang term for a bantam chicken.

Bareback Riding without a saddle

Barefoot Unshod.

Barley A small grain similar to rye or wheat.

Barn Big buildings that protect animals from winter weather.

Barn Cleaner Usually a chain linked system of paddles that moved manure from gutters, up a chute, into a waiting manure spreader. Most often seen in tie-stall or stanchion barns.

Barn sour Herd-bound; a bad habit that may result in a horse bolting back to the barn or to his herdmates.

Barnsheet The prelisted sheet used in the DHI system for collection and input of DHI data and information at the farm.

Barnyard chicken A chicken of mixed breed.

Barrel A rib region that is round in cross section.

Barrel Hocks Hocks that turn out, causing the feet to toe in. Also called spread hocks.

Barren Sterile, infertile, nonbreeder, incapable, of producing offspring. Also, open or not pregnant.

Barring Striped markings.

Barrow Male pig that has been castrated or neutered when young. This is so that the meat from male pigs can be eaten. (Meat from boar pigs has a strong odor and taste that is not in meat from barrow pigs).

Bars Part of the saddle's tree that runs along each side and parallel to the horse's spine; interdental space between incisors and molars where the bit lies.

Bartering To trade goods or services for goods or services.

Basal fluid loss The basal fluid loss is the typical loss of fluids by both insensible and sensible routes. For a normal adult dog or cat, the net basal loss is about 20-30 ml/lb/day.

Basal metabolism (BM) The chemical changes that occur in the cells of an animal in the fasting or resting state when it uses just enough energy to maintain vital cellular activity, respiration, and circulation as measured by the basal metabolic rate (BMR).

Bascule The desirable arc a horse's body makes as it goes over a jump.

Base The rider's seat and weight.

Base coat The primary color of the coat.

Base excess pricing A system of pricing grade A milk whereby the quantity of milk delivered by each producer during base-forming months (usually October through December) becomes the quantity eligible for the Class I price. The excess (surplus) is paid for only at the Class II or Class III price.

Base narrow The legs are very close together when viewed from in front or behind.

Base pair One of the pairs of chemical bases in the DNA double helix that carries genetic information.

Base wide The horse has a wide space between the legs when viewed from in front or behind.

Basenji A dog of a breed originally from Africa, having a short, smooth, reddish-brown coat and characterized by the absence of a bark.

Basic A simplified, inexpensive testing plan to provide basic management information to dairy farmers. Since basic plans involve owner sampling and recording, Official DHI Rules need not be followed.

Basset Hound A smooth-haired breed of hound with short legs and long ears.

Bastard strangles Strangles that result in abscesses in internal glands.

Bat Ear An ear that stands up, with a broad base, rounded at the top, with opening facing forward.; An erect ear that is broad at the base and rounded on the top.

Batch furrow system A management system where pigs are raised in batches from piglets to market hogs and as they mature the raising area they left is cleaned, disinfected, and left vacant until the next batch of pigs is purchased.

Bay A body color ranging from tan to reddish-brown, with black mane and tail, and usually black on the lower legs.

BCG Bacille Calmette Guerin attenuated strain of Mycobacterium bovis used in the preparation of BCG vaccine that is used for immunization against tuberculosis and in the cancer chemotherapy. Named after three scientists whose names were adopted as BCG.

BCU Biomedical Communications Unit.

Beak The hard, protruding portion of a bird's mouth, consisting of an upper beak and a lower beak.

Beard The feathers (always found in association with a muff) bunched under the beaks of such breeds as Ameraucana, Faverolle, and Houdan.

Beat A single step in a gait, involving one leg or two. For example, the walk is a 4-beat gait, with each beat stepped off by a single leg, one at a time, 1-2-3-4. The trot is a 2-beat gait, stepped off by two legs landing at the same time, 1-2.

Bedded Pack Open housing in a barn that is commonly used in conjunction with an outside feeding area.

Bedding Material used to absorb moisture and provide cushion. It is easily cleaned to provide a clean, dry surface and reduce the incidence of mastitis. Possible bedding materials include: straw, sawdust, wood chips, sand, ground limestone, separated manure solids, shredded newspaper, corn stalks, bark, peanut hulls, sunflower hulls and rice hulls.

Beef bull A male animal which is part of the breeding herd for raising beef calves.

Beef cattle Generally purchased at the aged of a few days to 6 months and raised until 15 18 months old. The normal selling weight is 1,000 1,200 pounds. The purchase and sale may occur during two different years and the cost must be recovered in the year of sale.

Beefy (beefiness) A term used to designate the desirable physical conformation of a beef animal, as contrasted with a dairy animal which is trimmer (not beefy) and more angular.

Behind the bit When a horse draws his head in toward his chest to avoid contact with the bit.

Bell boots Bell-shaped rubber covering that fits over the horse's foot and hoof to protect from injury.

Belly wool That which grows on the belly of the sheep. It is often uneven, tender and shorter than wool from other parts of the body. It is often stained and seedy.

Benign Not malignant. Sometimes taken to mean noncancerous although some cancers are called benign if they do not spread to other parts of the body.

Benign prostatic hypertrophy BPH Prostatic enlargement that occurs under the influence of testosterone. The dog may be asymtomatic or have signs of infertility, urinary tract infection or straining to defecate.

Benzoyl peroxide Topical antibacterial agent svailable as a gel and shampoo.

Beta blockers Heart medications which block certain receptors in the heart called beta receptors. The beta receptors receive signals which generally increase the heart rate. If the heart rate is abnormally fast and uneven, beta blockers will help stabilize the rate and rhythm of contractions.

Beta Carotene It is one of the forms of carotene. Carotene is a yellow or red pigment from carrots, sweet potatoes, milk and body fat, egg yolk, etc. It is a chromolipoid hydrocarbon existing in several forms. Alpha-, beta- and gamma-carotene are provitamins which can be converted into vitamin A in the body by all animals except cats. Beta-carotene is the most important because of a quantitatively greater activity. Beta-carotene is an important antioxidant which may protect against some cancer types.

Beta lactamases Enzymes produced by some bacteria which inactivate certain types of penicillin, thus making the bacteria resistant to them.

Bi parietal diameter The diameter of the skull as determined using ultrasound. This diameter can be used to determine age of the fetus.

Bias Flaws in the collection, analysis or interpretation of research data that lead to incorrect conclusions.

Bib A device fastened under a horse's lower jaw to prevent it from chewing or licking itself, while still allowing it to eat and drink.

Bicarbonate precursors Bicarbonate precursors are converted by the liver to bicarbonate and include Acetate, Gluconate, Lactate, and Citrate.

Biceps The biceps are a long fusiform muscle on the front of the arm. They are used to flex the elbows.

BID Giving medication twice per day. Example 30 mg BID means that 60 mg is given a day.

Biddy Affectionate word for a hen.

Big Licked Sang term used to refer to a horse that has more than the average stride and or animation when performing its gaits.

Bight Traditionally a loop in a rope. With closed veins, such as with an English bridle, bight refers to the ends of the reins. Even though Western reins are often split, their ends are also referred to as the bight.

Bilateral Involving both sides.

Bile A liquid produced by the liver, stored in the gall bladder, and dispensed into the small intestine as needed; aids in the digestion and absorption of fats.

Bile acids Certain compounds produced by the liver, bound to amino acids, and excreted in the bile to aid in the digestion of fats.

Bilirubin A substance produced when old red blood cells are destroyed in the body. Abnormal amounts of bilirubin cause jaundice and are caused by breakdown of large numbers of red blood cells or by disease of the liver or gall bladder.

Billing out Use of the beak to scoop feed out of a feeder onto the floor.

Billy Male goat; frequently used to describe an older, adult male goat - non wether.

Biochemical oxygen demand (BOD) An indirect measure of the concentration of biodegradable substances in an aqueous solution. The degradation of organic matter uses up dissolved oxygen.

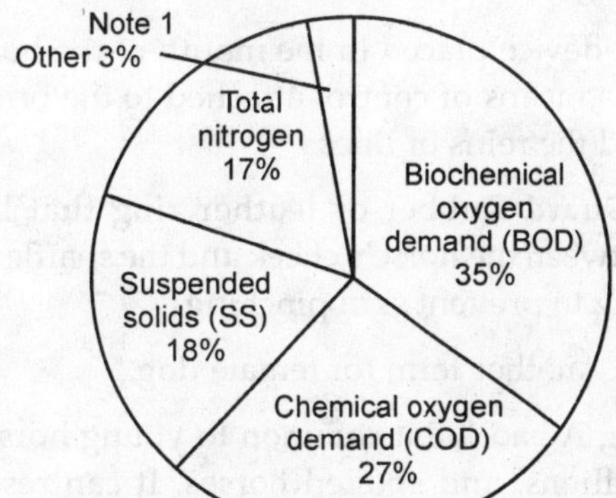

Fig. Biochemical oxygen demand

Biofeedback Therapy which uses machines to measure and display body functions and states such as heart rate, skin temperature, muscle tention, and brain activity. The patient can monitor these functions, see how and why they change through stages of rest and activity. Eventually the patient will learn to control those functions.

Bioinformatics The collection, classification, storage, and analysis of biochemical and biological information using computers, especially as applied to molecular genetics and genome sequencing.

Biological plausibility A causal association (or relationship between two factors) is consistent with existing medical knowledge.

Biopolymer Man-made microscopic structure built with organic molecules like carbon

Biopsy Obtaining a piece of tissue for analysis using a specialized needle or a scalpel balde.

Biosecurity Any of a broad range of practices enforced at a dairy farm to prevent transmittal of pathogens from other sources by feed, cattle, people, or other animals.

Biotin A member of the vitamin B complex.

Bipedal Standing on two rather than four legs.

Bird A warm blooded, egg laying, feathered vertebrate with forelimbs modified to form wings.

Bit A device placed in the mouth of the horse as a means of control attached to the bridle and the reins or lines.

Bit Guard Rubber or leather ring that lies between the horse's cheek and the snaffle bit ring to prevent skin pinching.

Bitch Another term for female dog.

Biting A bad habit common to young horses, stallions, and spoiled horses. It can result from hand-fed treats, petting, or improper training.

Black A body color that is true black over the entire body, but may have white leg and face markings.

Blackface breeds Meat breeds of sheep.

Bladder A sac that receives and holds a liquid until it is excreted, e.g., urinary bladder, gall bladder; in fish, the swim bladder holds air.

Blanch Temporarily squeeze the blood out of capillaries.

Blanket A fabric cover for a horse's body, usually made of wool or heavy material; a marking of lighter color over the rump of a dark horse. Also a term describing color pattern on an Appaloosa.

Blastocyst One of the earliest stages of an embryo.

Blaze White or light coloring on a horse's face, between the eyes from poll to nose.

Bleaching The fading of color from the beak, shanks, and vent of a yellow-skinned laying hen.

Bleat The vocal sound made by a goat.

Blemish A visible defect that does not affect serviceability. An unattractive scar or lump that does not affect the performance of the animal.

Blend price The price paid producers for market milk when classified pricing is used. The blend price is an average of class prices weighted by the quantity of milk used in each class.

Blepharitis Inflammation of the eyelids.

Blepharospasm Spasm of the eyelids often resulting in complete closure of the lids due to eye pain, such as seen with a scratch on the cornea.

Blind quarter A quarter of an udder that does not secrete milk or one that has an obstruction in the teat which prevents the removal of milk. A nonfunctional mammary gland.

Blister A thin walled structure containing fluid or air such as vesicles and bullae.

Bloat A disorder of ruminants usually characterized by an accumulation of gas in the rumen.

Block ready Lamb closely trimmed to retail specifications. This product may require cutting into portions prior to traying and overwrapping by the retailer.

Blood Blood is a body fluid that carries food and oxygen to cells.

Blood gases Gases, such as oxygen or carbon dioxide, that are in the blood.

Blood glucose A graph of blood glucose levels over time. At the time of insulin injection, and at regular intervals throughout the day, the level of glucose in the blood is determined through laboratory testing.

Blood plasma The liquid portion of blood in which the corpuscles of blood cells are suspended.

Bloodborne pathogens Infectious agents transmitted through exposure to blood or blood products.

Bloodlines The family lineage. The ancestry of an animal.

Bloodworm Usually refers to strongyles.

Bloom A term commonly used to describe the beauty and freshness of a cow in early lactation. A dairy cow in bloom has a smooth hair coat and presents evidence of milking ability (dairy character).

Blow up When a horse suddenly loses its temper.

Blowout Vent damage caused by laying an oversize egg.

Blubber Blubber is the thick coating of fat enveloping whales.

Blue The color also known as "gray" or "maltese."

Blue eye A post vaccination adverse event that had been reported by veterinarians vaccinating dogs with the modified-live canine adenovirus-1 vaccine (CAV-1).

Blue roan A body color that has a uniform mixture of black and white hairs all over the body.

Blue slip An application to register a cat of a registered litter.

Boar A male hog which is part of the breeding herd for raising feeder pigs, may weigh 1,000+ pounds.

Board To pay for facilities and care for a horse.

Body condition score BCSA score based on a scale from 1 to 5 that asseses the amount of body fat on an animal. One is emaciated, three is ideal, and five is obese.

Bolting Eating very rapidly , gulping feed without proper chewing; running away with rider.

Bolus Regurgitated food that has been chewed and is ready to be swallowed; a large pill for dosing animals.

Bone Bone is the hard skeletal part of an animal.

Bone marrow Soft tissue located within bones that produce all blood cells, including the ones that fight infection.

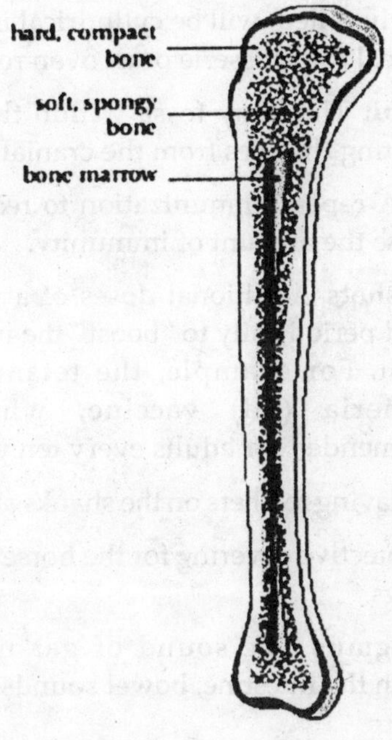

Fig. Bone marrow

Bone marrow suppression A condition in which the cells of the bone marrow which produce red blood cells, white blood cells, and platelets are inhibited. This may result from the use of certain drugs, such as anti-cancer agents.

Bone meal Animal bones that were steamed under pressure and then ground. It contains 1.5 to 2.5 percent nitrogen, 12 to 15 percent phosphorus, and 20 to 34 percent calcium. It is used as a fertilizer and as a mineral supplement for feeding farm animals.

Bone Morphogenetic Protein (BMP) A family of potent proteins involved in the promotion of bone formation. The study of these proteins and their related pathways forms a core component to the study of FOP.

Bone spavin Bony deposit on the inside and lower part of the hock which may cause the horse to drag the hind toes, or become lame

Boned, rolled and tied (BRT) A leg or shoulder completely deboned, with internal fat removed and excessive fat trimmed out. Properly rolled, will be cylindrical in shape and ideal for rotisserie or as oven roast.

Bony orbit The bony fossa within the skull separating the eyes from the cranial cavity

Booster A repeat immunization to restore or increase the amount of immunity.

Booster shots Additional doses of a vaccine needed periodically to "boost" the immune system. For example, the tetanus and diphtheria (Td) vaccine, which is recommended for adults every ten years.

Booted Having feathers on the shanks and toes.

Boots Protective covering for the horse's hoofs and legs.

Borborygmus The sound of gas moving through the intestine; bowel sounds.

Borium A hard metal spot welded to the bottom of a horseshoe to help keep a horse from slipping.

Bosal Rawhide noseband used in Western training and showing that works on the principles of balance, weight, and pressure. A hackamore type bridle that the nose piece is knotted under the chin.

Bot block A rough, porous synthetic black "stone" whose uniformly abrasive surface will remove bot eggs from the horse's hair. The block can be "sharpened" by drawing it across a hard edge.

Bot fly A fly that looks like a bee and lays eggs in a horse's hair. Flying parasite which deposits tiny white eggs on the horses legs and belly. If ingested, the larvae migrate through the tongue and/or esophagus and attach themselves to the stomach wall.

Bots Tiny larvae that crawl into nasal passages.

Bovine Pertaining to the ox or cow.

Bovine Spongiform Encephalopathy BSE is one of a group of diseases known as the Transmissible Spongiform Encephalopathies, and is often called "Mad Cow disease". It is believed to be the cause of vCJD in people.

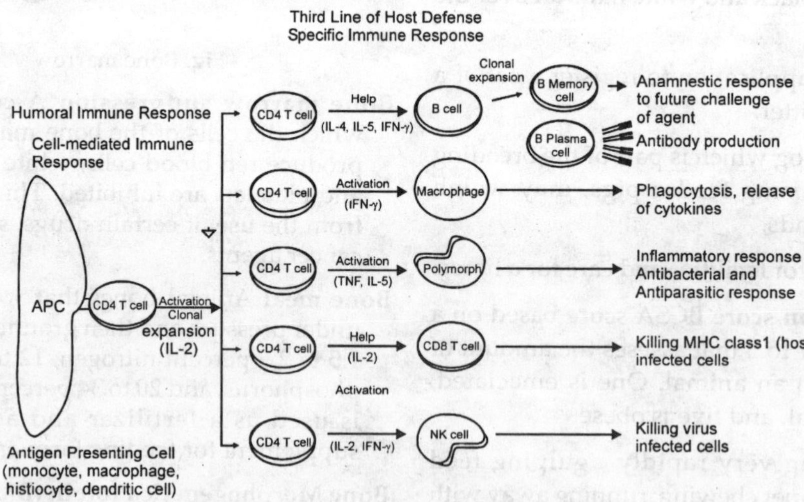

Fig. Bovine Spongiform Encephalopathy

Bow knees The front legs appear wide just above the knees when viewed from the front

Bowed hocks A weakness in which the hocks bow outwards when viewed from behind.

Bowed tendon Inflamation or damage to a tendon usually caused by overstretching due to improper conditioning, overwork, or an accident.

Bowel The bowels is a popular term for the division of the alimentary canal below the stomach, that is the intestines.

Box Boxstall, a four-sided stall to confine a horse.

Boxy feet Small, donkey-like feet

Brachial neuritis Inflammation of nerves in the arm causing muscle weakness and pain.

Brachialis The Brachialis is a muscle covering the front of the human elbow-joint. It is used to flex the elbow.

Brachiocephalic A short skull. Used to describe breeds such as Pugs, Bulldogs and Pekingnese dogs.

Bradycardia An abnormal slowing of the heart rate.

Bran The seed coat of wheat and other cereal grains which is separated from flour and used as animal food.

Break up To discourage a hen from setting.

Break wool Due to illness or lack of nutrition of the sheep at sometime during the growth of the wool, a weak area in one particular point of the staple, but still above and below the break.

Breakdown To perform the series of steps involved in skillfully cutting, boning and trimming a whole carcass into retail cuts.

Breast collar A horse collar that fits over the horse's chest instead of around its neck. A leather strap which passes around the front of the horse above his forelegs., and is attached to the cinch rings of a western saddle. Another strap passes over the horses neck just ahead of the withers. decorative yet functional in preventing the saddle from slipping back.

Bred heifer A pregnant heifer with her first unborn offspring.

Breech Area around the tail and back of hind legs.

Breech birth A birth in which the hind feet of the young are presented first.

Breechen The part of the harness that fits over the horse's rump and holds the load back or permits the horse to back it up; also called "britchen" .

Breed A population of a species that have distinct characteristics that differentiate them form other populations in that species. Individuals within that population that reproduce with another individual of the population will produce offspring that are recognizable as members of that population. Breeds can further be subdivided into varieties based on differences within the breed.

Breed association The organization that registers the birth and pedigree of a particular breed of livestock.

Breed average The average milk production of cows for a given dairy breed.

Breed character (breed type) Combination of features that identify an animal with a breed such as conformation, color and head shape.

Breed standard The ideal characteristics for the breed, as agreed upon by a group of breeders.

Breed true The characteristic of purebred chicks whereby they resemble both parents.

Breeders 1. Mature chickens from which fertile eggs are collected.

2. A person who manages chickens.

Breeding Act of copulation between a stallion and a mare.

Breeding class Conformation class.

Breeding livestock Mature male and female animals that are used to reproduce offspring. The offspring are then sold as a product of the farm.

Breeding program An ongoing program in which cats are mated together and kittens selected for breeding according to how close they come to an ideal.

Breeding quality A cat that meets its breed standard closely enough to be valuable to a breeding program, but may not be competitive as a show cat.

Breeding records Computerized or paper records that document the aspects of the reproductive life of an animal.

Breeding Season The period of time when the doe is showing estrus.

Breeding shed The building in which breeding takes place.

Breeding soundness examination BSE A series of diagnostic tests performed on a male animal in order to evaluate his capabilities as a stud. The results of the tests are typically recorded in a standardized fashion on a specific form.

Breeding value (genetic value) The genetic ability or merit of an animal for a given trait, for example, secreting milk. One-half of this genetic ability is transmitted to offspring.

Bretylium A drug which diminishes the release of norepinephrine from nerve endings with chronic oral dosing. It is used in treatment of ventricular fibrillation and ventricular tachycardia.

Bridle To maintain contact with the reins so the horse moves "in a frame" and "on the bit."

Bridle path The 4" to 6" area between the forelock and the mane that is usually clipped.

Bright wool Light appearing clean wool, such as is grown in the farming states.

Brilliance Flash or dazzle, as related to performance.

Brindle dun A dun body color with darker streaks.

Brios Spirit, used in reference to Spanish style horses. (Paso Fino)

Brisket The breast of the sheep or goat, just below the throat.

Brisket Board A raised part of the freestall platform about 6.5 feet in front of rear of the stall to keep cows positioned properly while lying. Usually made of wood or plastic, but occasionally concrete.

Britch or breech The back portion of the sheep down the hind leg, the buttocks.

Britch or breech wool Wool from the hindquarters of the sheep, usually the coarsest on the body, often approaching hair in its characterisics.

British breeds Those native to Great Britain, such as Hereford, Angus, and Shorthorn.

Broad spectrum antibiotic An antibiotic that is active against a large number of microbial species.

Brockle face or smutt-face Commercial crossbred lambs from white-faced wool breed dams and black-faced sires, i.e. Suffolk, Hampshire or Suffolk-Hampshire cross.

Broiler A young, tender meat chicken; also called a "fryer."

Broiler house Building that broiler type chicken are raised in.

Broke Trained and reliable.

Broken mouth An animal is described as "broken mouthed" when some of the incisor teeth have fallen out or have become badly worn and irregular, usually the result of old age or hard grazing.

Broken udder A term sometimes used to indicate an udder that is pendulous and loosely attached.

Bronchi (bronchiole) Small tubular structures that lead from the trachea to the microscopic sac-like structures, alveoli, in the lungs.

Bronchodilator Medication which opens up the main air passages to the lungs.

Bronchoscope A tool designed to facilitate inspection of the trachea and bronchi; used in both diagnostic and therapeutic procedures.

Bronchoscopy The internal inspection of the trachea and bronchi using a bronchoscope.

Bronchospasm A condition in which the muscles surrounding the air passages to the lungs contract, narrowing the passages.

Bronopol A noncorrosive milk preservative.

Brood 1. To care for a batch of chicks.

2. The chicks themselves.

Brood cow A female cow which is part of the breeding herd for raising beef cattle.

Brood Doe A doe kept for the purpose of continuing a desireable bloodline and genetics in her offspring.

Brooder A heated enclosure used to imitate the warmth and protection a mother hen gives her chicks.

Brooding period The time between when chicks are one day old until they can be on their own without any heat.

Broodmare A mare used for breeding.

Broody A hen that covers eggs to warm and hatch them. Sometimes refers to a hen that stays in the nest for an extended period without producing eggs.

Browband The topmost horizontal leather strap of the bridle which fits under the forelock.

Brown A body color with mixed brown and black hair, with black mane, tail, and legs.

Browse Small, woody plants with fedder shoots used as feed by goats, sheep, and cattle.

Brucellosis Infection with bacteria of the Brucella group, frequently causing abortions in animals and remittent fever in man. Also called Undulant fever, Malta fever, or Mediterranean fever.

BST (bovine somatotropin) A complex, biologically active protein secreted by the pituitary gland. It stimulates body cell growth and milk production available as a synthetically produced product for use in cattle. Sometimes called "growth hormone" or BGH.

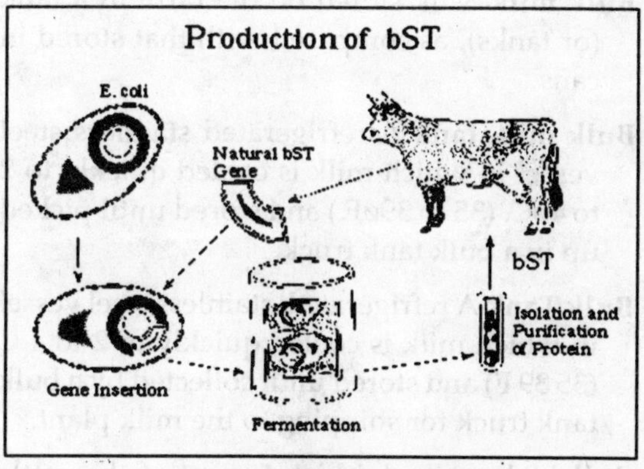

Fig. Bovine Somatotropin

Buck A male goat used for breeding. In the United States, this term is sometimes used to refer to a male sheep.

Bucket Milking System A system in which the milk coming from the cow is drawn into a bucket or pail and manually transferred to a collection area or the milk house.

Buck kneed With knees bent slightly forward.

Buckling Baby male goat.

Buckskin A body color that is tan, yellow, or gold with black mane, tail, and lower legs.

Buckstitching The decorative wide, white stitching used on western saddles and bridles.

Buffer A substance used in livestock rations to help resist changes in the acidity of the digestive tract. Examples: sodium bicarbonate, bentonite.

Buggy trot Slang used when referring to the gait of a horse that is long trotting or square trotting.

Bulb of heel The rounded portion of the horse's foot just behind the hoof.

Bulbourethral glands An accessory sex gland of the male.

Bulbus glandis The rounded base of the penis.

Bulk Indigestible fiber found in feed.

Bulk milk Milk stored on the farm in a tank (or tanks), as compared with that stored in cans.

Bulk milk tank A refrigerated stainless steel vessel in which milk is cooled quickly to 2 to 4øC. (35 to 39øF.) and stored until picked up in a bulk tank truck.

Bulk Tank A refrigerated, stainless steel vessel in which milk is cooled quickly to 2 to 4 C (35 39 F) and stored until collected by a bulk tank truck for shipping to the milk plant.

Bull Male animal which is part of the cattle breeding herd.

Bull pen A training corral, also called a "round" pen.

Bulling A cow in heat (estrus).

Bullous pemphigoid An immune mediated skin disease in which autoantibodies are directed against antigens in basement membrane zone.

Bullous retinal detachment The retina has detached from all points of contact except for around the periphery and at the optic disk.

Bump To pull and release the reins for a brief contact with the horse's mouth.

BUN Short for 'blood urea nitrogen,' a blood test that estimates kidney function.

Bunk A feed trough or feeding station for cattle.

Bunker (Sometimes called Bunker Silo) A flat rectangular structure with concrete floors and walls used to ensile and store forages.

Buphthalmos Enlarged eye caused by glaucoma.

Burden of disease The health and socio-economic cost of a given medical condition of society.

Burdizzo tool Used to castrate lambs by severing the cord without breaking the skin of the scrotum.

Buretrol Buretrols are small plastic cylinders that are filled from a stock bottle, or bag, of fluids. It is much easier to see the residual volume of fluid in a rigid sided container than a flexible container.

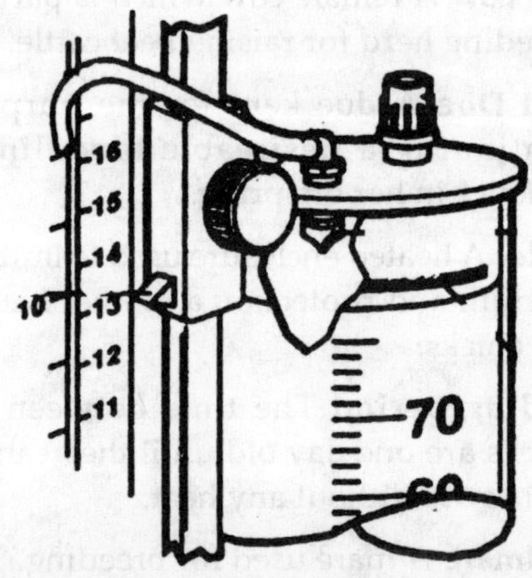

Fig. Buretrol

Burner A rawhide section on a rope, covering the eye of the hondo to protect the rope from wear.

Butcher hogs Farrowed or purchased as "feeder pigs" at a weight of 40 50 pounds and raised until 5 6 months old. Their normal selling weight is 200 280 pounds. Purchase and sale may or may not take place in the same year. Cost must be recovered in year of sale, also market hogs.

Bute Phynalbutazone, a drug which reduces pain.

Butterfat See milk fat.

Butterflied leg of lamb A leg completely boned and removed of all excess fat for broiling or outdoor cooking. When spread flat on the cooking surface, it resembles a butterfly.

Butterfly catheter A style of catheter that has a rigid needle attached to a plastic finger grip that looks like "wings" and then attached to a short piece of flexible tubing.

Buttermilks There are two kinds of buttermilk. Natural buttermilk is the by-product of churning cream into butter. Cultured buttermilk is usually made from skim milk by adding a starter culture and incubating until lactic acid develops to about 0.8 percent. Salt is usually added to accentuate the flavor.

Butting Method of fighting among goats (especially bucks) by the striking of the head and horns.

Byproduct Feeds produced as a result of industrial manufacturing, plant or animal processing. Examples: distillers grains, beet pulp, meat and bone meal, fish meal.

C

C Candle To examine the contents of an intact egg with a strong light source.

CAB A new order of CPR in which chest compressions are first applied to cause circulation of blood, the an airway for breathing is established. Used more commonly in humans and originated due to concerns of transmission of infectious diseases. In animals consider this order if the arrest is witnessed and it is known that the patient does not have underlying respiratory disease.

Cachexia Very thin, a synonym for emaciation.

Cadence The rhythmic clarity of a gait.

CAE Caprine Arthritic Encephalitis, a goat virus alot like AIDS in humans.

Caeca Plural of caecum.

Caecum A diverticulum on each side of the gut at junction of small and large intestines, for additional digestion.

Caesarian section C-section Performing abdominal surgery to remove a fetus from the mother.

Cairn Terrier A small dog of a breed developed in Scotland, having a broad head and a rough shaggy coat.

Calcaneum In human anatomy, the calcaneum is the largest and strongest of the tarsal bones. It projects backwards beyond the bones of the leg to provide a lever for the muscles of the calf.

Calcified The hardening of tissue through the influx of calcium, usually as a result of chronic inflammation.

Calcinosis circumscripta Deposits of calcium found in small lumps under the skin, in the tongue, or attached to tendons or in joint capsules.

Calcinosis cutis Hard crusts or white plaques in the skin of some patients with hyperadrenocorticism.

Calcitriol The active form of 1, 25 dihydroxycholecalciferol (vitamin D). Can be exogenously administered to patients with chronic renal failure to suppress PTH secretion by the parathyroid glands with reversal of some of the clinical manifestations and possibly a resultant slowing of the rate of progression of renal dysfunction.

Calcium channel blocker These drugs inhibit the movement of calcium ion across cell membranes. Calcium channel blockers are used in the treatment of certain heart conditions. In CPR, they may be used after resusitation to protect the heart from the effects of calcium administered during CPR.

Calcium phosphorus ratio The amount of calcium compared to the amount of phosphorus in the diet. A ratio of somewhere between 1:1 or 2:1 is conductive to proper bone development.

Calculi Describing a variety of stones that are found in the urinary system. These include kidney and bladder stones.

Calculus Abnormal stone-like structure(s) usually composed of mineral salts, e.g., a bladder calculus is the same thing as a bladder stone.

Calf A young male or female bovine. Usually referred to as calves until reaching sexual maturity.

Calf Hutch Individual housing unit for young calves, assists in blocking transmission of disease.

Calf starter Grain based mixes fed to young calves.

Calf kneed With knees bent slightly backward.

California Mastitis Test or Wisconsin Mastitis Test CMT/WMTCMT is a cowside test that crudely measures the milk somatic cell count as a screen for subclinical mastitis. The WMT is a laboratory procedure which is a more precise measure of somatic cell count, although it is not as precise as a direct count.

Calipers A device used to measure the diameter of the testes.

Calk A pointed projection on a horseshoe to prevent slipping; (v.) To injure with the calk on a shoe.

Calked shoes Shoes having projections downward from the toe or heel to provide better traction.

Call name The name that a cat is called. Often a shortened form of the cat's registered name. For example, "Ashley" is the call name for the cat registered as "CH Sheenah's Ashley of Ashmanor, DM."

Calling The characteristic vocalizations (typically yowling, howling, or screaming) made by a queen in heat.

Callus Hypertrophy of the stratum corneum especially over pressure points such as the elbow.

Calorie The unit of measurement of energy derived from digested food. Fat contains about twice as many calories per gram as protein or carbohydrate.

Calving interval The time between one calving and the next. Should not exceed 13 months.

Camel Back An arched back.

Camelids Camelids are a large family including Old World camelids: camels and the bactrians, which are two-humped camels, and the New World camelids, llamas and alpacs.

Camouflage Concealment by appearing to be part of the natural surroundings.

Can milk That milk placed in 10-gallon cans on the farm for cooling and transportation to a dairy product manufacturing plant.

Cancer A group of diseases caused by transformation of normal cells into malignant ones. When these cells shed and travel to other areas of the body, the cancer is said to metastasize. As the cancerous growth draws nutrients, and the general lack of well-being diminishes the appetite, the resultant emaciation is called cancer cachexia.

Candida A certain genus of yeast which can cause disease in humans and animals; an infection with Candida is called candidiasis.

Candidate gene A gene that is suspected of being involved in a disease. Candidate genes may be identified by their location in a chromosomal region that has been linked to the disease and/or by what is known about the cellular function of the protein product encoded by the gene (often of the same name).

Candle Flame Ears A type of dog-ear that is large and erect with uneven edges.

Candler A device which uses strong light to examine the contents of the egg.

Candling Shining a light behind eggs to check for cracks and other problems.

Canid A family (Canidae) of carnivorous animals including dogs, wolves, coyotes, foxes, and jackals.

Canine adenovirus 2 CAV-2 One of the agents causing "kennel cough". Also protects against CAV-1 (infectious canine hepatitis) when included in vaccines.

Canine Distemper The most important viral infectious disease in dogs, caused by canine distemper virus and characterized by acute upper respiratory disease symptoms and fever and later by more serious respiratory symptoms as well as fever, vomiting, diarrhea and neurological signs.

Canine eosinophilic granuloma Possibly a hypersensitivity reaction resulting in oral lesions in young, Siberian Husky dogs.

Canine Pertaining to dogs.

Canine Teeth The large, sharp, curved teeth that are located on each side of the mouth. Also referred to as eye teeth.

Cannibalism The bad habit chickens have of eating each other's flesh, feathers, or eggs.

Cannon The area between the knee on the front leg, or hock on the rear leg, and the fetlock.

Cannula A special tube designed for placing drugs into the udder through the teat end and streak canal.

Canter A gait with three beats to each stride, two legs moving separately and two as a diagonal pair. Slower than the gallop and not as tiring.

Canthus Corner of the eye (medial and lateral).

Cantle The back of the seat of the saddle. The part of the saddle which projects upwards toward the rear.

Cap Darkly shaded color pattern on the skull of some breeds.

Capacity (internal volume) Internal body dimensions.

Cape The narrow feathers between a chicken's neck and back.

Capillary A capillary is a fine blood vessel which carries blood to cells.

Capitate bone The capitate bone is the largest bone in the human wrist.

Capon A "fixed" male Rooster - the equivalent of a chicken steer.

Capping If the rear foot of a horse sets down squarely on the track of the same side front foot as it is set down, the horse is said to be capping.

Capriculture The study of goat keeping.

Caprine arthritis encephalitis CAEA disease characterized by the development of chronic arthritis and debility.

Carapace The upper shell of a turtle or tortoise.

Carbohydrate Compounds made up of chains of sugar units. Simple carbohydrates include table sugar (sucrose), milk sugar (lactose), and fruit sugar (fructose). Complex carbohydrates are very long chains held together by bonds that may not be digestible in the stomach and intestine of a carnivore. Starch is a digestible complex carbohydrate. Seed hulls such as oat bran are digestible by ruminants and horses, but not carnivores.

Carbonic anhydrase An enzyme located in the eye and in the kidney tubules that is important in reabsorbing bicarbonate (kidney) and in the active secretion of aqueous in the eye.

Carbonic anhydrase inhibitor A drug that interfers with the action of the enzyme carbonic anhydrase. e.g. acetozolamide, dorzolamide (Truceopt). These drugs are used to reduce aqueous production in animals with glaucoma.

Carbuncle Multiple cutaneous abscesses that are connected by sinuses.

Carcass Animal after the hide, head, hooves, and internal organs are removed when being made ready for the supermarket.

Carcinoembryonic antigen (CEA) A glycoprotein constituent of the glycocalyx of the embryonic endodermal epithelium, generally absent from adult cells with the exception of some carcinomas. It may also be detected in the serum of patients with colon cancer.

Carcinogen A substance which causes cancer.

Carcinoma A type of cancer originating from epithelial cells. Example squamous cell carcinoma originates from cells of the skin and mouth, transitional cell carcinoma originates from the cells of the bladder.

Cardiac A synonym for heart.

Cardiac pump theory In CPR, when the chest is compressed the heart underneath the chest wall is directly compressed as well, squeezing blood out into the major blood vessels so it can return to the heart and then go to the brain. CPR in animals weighing less than 7 kg is probably using the cardiac pump theory.

Cardiomyopathy Diseases of the heart muscle; does not include diseases of the valves of the heart or congenital defects.

Cardiopulmonary Relating to the heart and lungs.

Cardiopulmonary resuscitation CPRA life saving procedure that includes the external compression of the chest wall to stimulate blood flow and breathing (by mouth to mouth or other methods) to provide oxygen.

Cardiovascular The organ system that includes the heart and blood vessels.

Carnivore An animal whose natural diet includes meat.

Carotene A substance that is converted to vitamin A in the animals body that is found in green and yellow feeds.

Carpus The carpus are the bones of the human wrist.

Carrier An animal which harbors an infectious organism, such as a virus, bacteria, or parasite. The animal does not appear ill, but can still transmit the organism to other animals by direct contact or releasing the organisms (bacteria, protozoa, viruses) into the environment in the stool, urine, respiratory secretions, or vaginal discharges.

Carrying capacity The number of animals that a pasture can properly carry with feed for a certain period of time.

Cartilage Cartilage or cartilaginous tissue covers the ends of the bones where they come together to make a joint. It enables the bones to move easily.

Cartilaginous joint In anatomy, a cartilaginous joint is an articulation where the bones are joined by cartilage, and a limited amount of movement is possible.

Casein The major protein of milk and cheese.

Cash market Market for immediate delivery of commodities against payment.

Cash price Price in the cash market for actual or spot commodities with delivery through customary market channels.

Caslick The surgical technique in which the vulvar lips of the mare are cut and sutured so that they grow together making the vulvar opening smaller.

Cast Condition where full wooled sheep gets on its back and is unable to rise. Cast ewes are old ewes that are culled from the flock.

Castration The removal of the sex organs making the animal incapable of reproduction; the correct use of the word can be used to describe both male and female animals, but it is commonly used to describe only males.

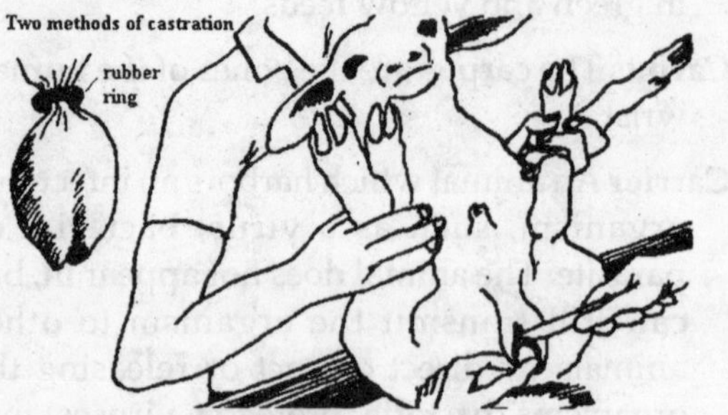

Fig. Castration

Cat fancy The overall group of individuals, clubs, and registering associations involved with breeding and showing cats.

Cat's Claw The plant, Uncaria tomentosa, derives its name from the pattern of thorns found on the vines. It grows in the Peruvian rain forest and was traditionaly used by the indigenous people to treat cancer and arthritis. It contains immune-enhancing substances, including several antioxidant compounds, which may account for the antitumor properties reported for cat's claw.

Catagen The transition phase of the hair cycle between growth (anagen) and cessation of growth (telogen).

Cataract A cloudiness of the lens of the eye, reducing vision and giving the eye a pearly appearance.

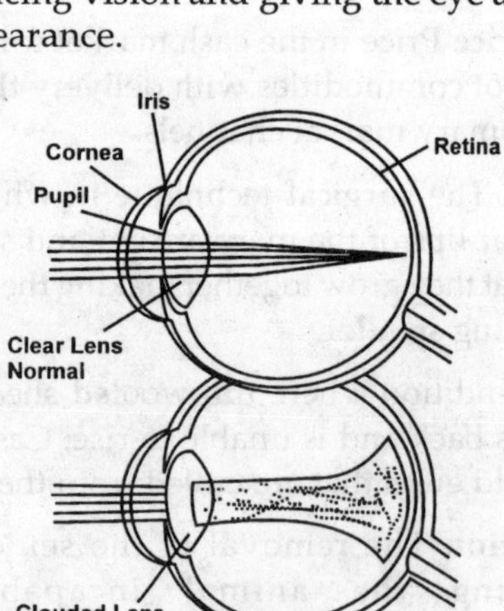

Fig. Cataract

Catheter tip dose syringe A large hypodermic syringe with a blunt nozzle tip.

Cattery name A name registered with a cat registering association, used to identify cats bred by a particular breeder. A registered cattery name always appears a prefix on the names of cats bred by that breeder. It may be added as a suffix to the names of cats owned, but not bred by, that breeder.

Cattle 1. A cow usually has a single calf every 12 months. This will be. true of both dairy and beef cattle. The young heifer added to the herd will usually be bred for the first time at the age of 16 months.

2. On a dairy farm, the calf is usually sold within a very short time after birth, less than 30 days, unless it is a heifer which may be kept for the dairy herd. The cattle rancher will not sell his calves until they are 6-8 months old. He may also keep some of the better heifers for breeding purposes.

3. Feeder calves (heifers or steers) are usually placed in the feedlot at a weight of 500 700 lbs, or around 6 9 months old. The calves are in the feedlot from 4 6 months or to a weight of 1,000 1,200 pounds before being sold to packing plants.

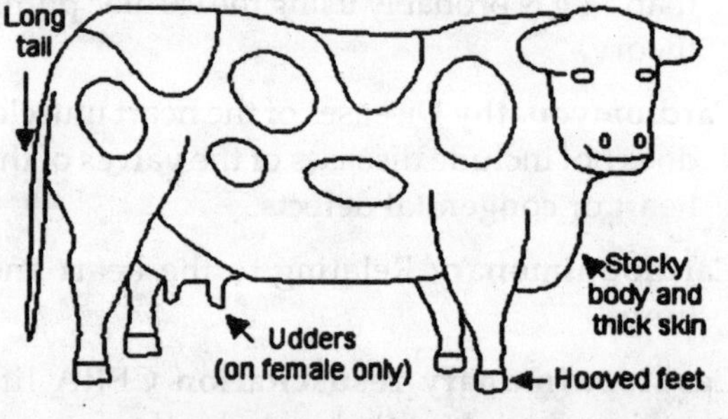

Fig. Cattle

Cattle tracing system A computer database which registers all cattle and their movements. Owners of cattle must report all births and imports of cattle, their subsequent movements and eventual death or slaughter.

Caudal Refers to the rear or in a direction toward the rear of the animal. For example the abdomen is more caudal than the chest. The opposite term is cranial meaning closer to the head of the animal.

Causal association The presence or absence of a variable (e.g. smoking) is responsible for an increase or decrease in another variable (e.g. cancer). A change in exposure leads to a change in the outcome of interest.

Caval syndrome Disease caused by large numbers of worms in the right side of the heart and vena cava, which results in blood circulation problems in the liver leading to the breakdown of red blood cells, anemia, weakness, and collapse.

Cavalletti Ground rail suspended between two wooden Xs designed to provide three different heights for working horses. A very small jump.

Cavesson Leather noseband (customarily used with the English snaffle bridle) which encourages the horse to keep its mouth closed; a longeing cavesson is a leather or nylon headstall with a weighted noseband that has metal rings for various attachments of the longe line. Part of the bridle that goes over the nose and under the horse's jaw.

CC (cubic centimeter) A volume measurement identical to mL.

CD Abbreviation for clusters of differentiation. Groups of monoclonal antibodies that identify the same surface molecule. The cell surface molecule is designated CD followed by a number (e.g. CD4 and CD8)

CD4 The cell surface protein CD4 is important for recognition by the T cell receptor of antigenic peptides bound to MHC class II molecules. It acts as a co-receptor by binding to the lateral face of MHC class II molecules.

CD8 The cell surface protein CD8 is important for recognition by the T-cell receptor of antigenic peptides bound to MHC class I molecules. It acts as a co-receptor by binding to the lateral face of MHC class I molecules.

Cean wool Wool after it has been "scoured" to remove the extra materials.

Cear media Includes the aqueous, lens and vitreous of optic system.

Cecum (caecum) The blind gut; in the horse it is huge compared to other animals, holding five to ten gallons of ingesta. Large, sock-shaped pouch between the small and large intestines of a horse. Important in the digestion of cellulose.

Cecum A blind pouch at the juncture of the small and large intestine (resembles the human appendix); plural: ceca.

Cell A cell, in biological terms, is the material unit of all living things.

Cell adhesion molecules (CAMS) Are cell-surface proteins that are involved in binding cells together in tissues and also in less permanent cell-cell interactions.

Cell mediated immunity The immunity that is the result of either special lymphocytes directly killing the foreign invader, or lymphocytes (T cells) releasing special chemicals which activate macrophages to kill the invader. Compare with 'humoral immunity.'

Cellular immunity Immunity due to macrophages and natural killer cells attacking any antigen. It is not specific to one antigen.

Cellulose The principal carbohydrate constituent of plant cell membranes. It is made available to ruminants through the action of cellulolytic bacteria in the rumen.

Cemastine avist an over the counter antihistamine.

Census A survey to count or estimate the number of subjects (for instance, animals or farms) in a population.

Central Test A central testing location where animals from different flocks are gathered to evaluate differences in performance traits under uniform management and environmental conditions.

Central venous catheter A long catheter with its tip placed in a large diameter vein such as jugular catheter, or a long, lateral saphenous catheter.

Central venous pressure Central venous pressure measures the ability of the right heart to accommodate the fluid load presented to it. Normal animals have a central venous pressure of less than 5 cm of water. Assuming there are no clots in the IV catheter, central venous pressures repeatedly above 10 cm of water are indicative of impending onset of edema and fluid overload. Measurement of central venous pressure requires a central catheter (jugular catheter) be in place. CVP readings can be influenced by catheter position and patency.

Centrifugal separation Removal of one substance from another mechanically by centrifugal force, as with cream which is less dense than skim milk.

Centrifuge A machine that rapidly spins liquid samples and separates out the particles by their density.

Cephalic Cephalic is a classification of human skull. It refers to the shape of skull posessed by Kaffirs and Native Australians.

Cere Fleshy area at bill base enclosing nostrils.

Cerebellar degeneration Degeneration of the cerebellar portion of the brain.

Cerebellum The cerebellum is the lower part of the brain, it controls muscular movements and postural equilibrium.

Cerebral Relating to the part of the brain known as the cerebrum.

Cerebrum The largest portion of the brain that performs all higher cognitive functions and is situated in the front part of the cranial cavity.

Certificate In European associations like fife, cats are awarded certificates at shows, which are accumulated towards titles much in the way that points are accumulated in North American associations.

Certified milk Milk produced and distributed under conditions which conform with high standards for cleanliness and quality set forth by the American Association of Medical Milk Commissions.

Certified pedigree A pedigree officially issued by a cat registering association.

Cerumen Waxy secretion of the apocrine glands of the ear.

Ceruminolytic agents Agents that loosen and dissolve ear wax. Includes dioctyl sodium sulfosuccinate, squalene, propylene glycol, carbamide peroxide, and others.

Cervical vertebrae The cervical vertebrae are the 7 vertebrae closest to the skull.

Cervical vertebral instability (wobblers) Compression of the cervical (neck) spinal cord caused by instability or malformation of the cervical vertebrae. Dogs show lack of muscle coordination in the back legs and possibly neck.

Cervicitis Inflammation of the cervix.

Cervix Part of the female reproductive tract located between the vagina and uterus.

Cestodes Tape worms.

Chaff Husks or other seed coverings and other plant parts separated from seed during harvest or processing.

Chalazae Two white cords on each side of a yolk that keep the yolk properly positioned within the egg white; singular: chalaza.

Chalk Sticks Used to mark treated, fresh, or special-needs cows.

Challenge In vaccine experiments, the deliberate exposure of an immunized animal or person to the infectious agent.

Chamomile Herbal remedy from the chamomile plant. The most popular is German chamomile. The oil of the chamomile flower appears to calm the central nervous system, relax the digestive tract, and speed the healing process.

Championship The championship class at a North American show is open to whole adult cats that are purebred and registered and meet the standard for their breed. Altered cats compete in the premiership class.

Change of leg or lead Change of the leading legs at the canter or lope.

Check offs The practice of deducting a portion of the payment to a farmer for his or her produce.

Check rein A strap that fastens to the bit to keep the horse's head up.

Chediak Higashi syndromeA macrophage deficiency.

Cheese A solid food made from milk.

Cheese Curd The clumps of casein and other milk components that are formed during the cheese making process. These curds are then pressed into blocks or barrels for proper aging and curing of the cheese.

Chelation Binding of a substance to a metal, thus helping the body to remove it.

Cheloid A type of hypertrophied scar.

Chemical defibrillator In the absence of an electrical defibrillator machine, certain drugs may be used in an attempt to reverse the cardiac arrhythmia of atrial fibrillation.

Chemokines A group of specific chemotactic polypeptides all of which have a similar structure (4-cystein structure), involved in the migration and activation of cells, especially phagocytic cells and lymphocytes. They have a central role in inflammatory responses.

Chemosis Edema of the conjunctiva.

Chemotherapy Treatment of a disease with chemical agents (drugs); the term is most commonly used to describe the treatment of cancer with medication.

Cherry eye Prolapse of the third eyelid gland.

Chestnut A color in which the body, mane, and tail are various shades of brown.

Cheviot A breed of sheep.

Chevon Goat meat.

Cheyenne roll A style of cantle where the edge bends downward to form a rim or lip.

Chi In traditional Chinese medicine, it is the vital force or energy of the body. Disease is an imbalance in this flow of energy in and around the body.

Chick The young of birds, particularly chickens and gamebirds.

Chicken A member of the Pheasant family, chickens probably descended from the Jungle Fowl of Ceylon. Chickens have been domesticated for thousands of years and have been developed into many different breeds and varieties by man. They are an efficient source of protein, producing both meat and eggs. They are one of the most prevalent forms of livestock bred around the world today.

Chiggers Common name for Trombiculidiasis.

Chiropractic A system of healing which is based on the idea that the body has an innate self-healing ability and seeks homeostasis. However, subluxations in the joints interfere with the body's ability to maintain optimal health. Through manipulation of the spine and other joints and muscles, the body is brought back into balance and the neuromusculoskeletal system can function smoothly.

Chlamydia Small organisms associated with pneumonia, abortion, diarrhea, conjunctivitis, arthritis and encephalitis.

Chlamydiosis Type of infectious abortion. The most common abortion disease experienced by the sheep industry.

Chlorhexidine Novalsan. Antibacterial, antifungal, and viricidal. Use primarily as soaks or in conjunction with whirlpool therapy.

Chlorpheniramine An antihistamine.

Choana (Plural choanae) An opening between the nasal cavity and oropharynx (mouth) in birds and reptiles.

Choanal atresia A failure of a seperation to form between the nasal cavity and the nasopharynx. A common birth defect in the crias.

Cholangiohepatitis Inflammation of the gall bladder, bile ducts, and liver

Cholangitis Inflammation of a bile duct; see cholecystitis.

Cholecystitis Inflammation of the gallbladder; see cholangitis.

Cholesterol A white, fat-soluble substance found in animal fats and oils, in bile, blood, brain tissue,, nervous tissue, the liver, kidneys, and adrenal glands. It is important in metabolism and is a precursor of certain hormones.

Choline A quaternary amine which occurs in the phospholipid phosphatidylcholine and the neurotransmitter acetylcholine. It is an important methyl donor in intermediary metabolism. It was formerly considered to be a B vitamin.

Chondroitin Decreases the activity of enzymes which break down cartilage in a joint.

Chondroprotective agent A nutritional supplement that protects cartilage.

Chooks Popular term for chickens.

Chorioditis Inflammation of the choroid.

Chorioretinitis Inflammation affecting the choroid and retina causing choroidal, +/- retinal, blood vessels to become leaky and either transudative fluid or exudative fluid and cells to leak into the space between the choroid and retina, elevating the retina.

Choroids The posterior uvea lying between the sclera and retina, and joining the ciliary body anteriorly. The choroid provides nutrition to the outer layers of the retina and contains the tapetum.

Chrome Flashy white markings.

Chromosome One of the DNA-containing structures of the cell that contain most or all of the genes of the individual.

Chronic Exposure to the poison occurs over a period of weeks, months, or years; onset of signs may be sudden and dramatic, or can be insidious like a slow loss in body condition or reduced productivity.

Chronic health condition A health related state that lasts for a long period of time (e.g. cancer, asthma).

Chronic superficial keratitis A chronic condition of the eye in which blood vessels grow across the cornea (the clear surface of the eye). The cornea looks hazy and sometimes reddened; it may eventually take on a dark pigment. This condition is also called pannus.

Churning The process of stirring and agitating cream in the process of making butter. Churning causes the fat globules in cream to clump together and separate from the liquid.

Chute In cattle events, a fenced lane that contains a single cow behind a gate.

Cinch Band that fastens a Western saddle in place.

Cinch strap The strap of leather on the near side that is looped through the cinch to

Cinical study clinical study or clinical trial is a test of a new drug or procedure that is being evaluated for effectiveness in animals with naturally occurring disease. In some cases the effectiveness of the new drug or procedure is compared with currently available treatments.

Cleaned in place(CIP) Most milk-handling equipment are cleaned by circulating washing solutions through them without disassembly.

Cirrhosis A liver disease caused by the replacement of damaged cells with connective tissue; severe scarring can eventually cause liver failure.

Cis platin A chemotherapeutic drug that is based on a metallic element (platinum complex). Its greatest impact has been on testicular and ovarian cancers but its limitations are the often severe nephro- and neurotoxicity.

Caseous Lymphadenitis(CL) An abscess disease of goats that is highly contagious.

Clarification The process of removing suspended material; in milk processing, clarification is achieved by centrifugal treatment which removes sediment (extraneous matter) and somatic cells.

Class I Base plan The system used in some Federal Milk Marketing Orders whereby a producer is allowed to deliver a specific quantity of milk based on production during the lowest production period of the previous year, at one price, but receives a lower price for remaining deliveries.

Class I, II, III, IV medications Drugs are classified by the Drug Enforcement Administration of the Department of Justice depending upon such criteria as the potential for human abuse.

Classification An appraisal program offered by a breed association to evaluate each animal's resemblance to the breed's ideal. A numerical score is assigned to each animal.

Classified pricing A pricing plan by which handlers are charged for market milk according to the products in which it is used, hence the term use classification. Class I milk goes into fluid products and demands the highest price. Prices of surplus milk, Class II or III, depending on the Federal

Milk Marketing Order, are about the price of manufacturing milk.

Classing 1. The process of culling and selection applied to a flock/herd of animals.

2. A term applied to the grading of males according to sale value.

3. The division of a flock/herd of females into various groups prior to mating.

Clathrin The major component protein of a cage-like structure that is important in brining proteins from the outside to the inside of a cell.

Clavicle In human anatomy, the clavicle is a long bone which lies almost horizontally at the root of the neck. It serves 2 main functions; to act as a prop which braces back the shoulder and enables the limb to swing clear of the trunk. And to transmit part of the weight of the limb to the axial skeleton.

Cld hemagglutination disease CHDA form of autoimmune hemolytic anemia in which there is formation of cold acting anti-erythrocyte antibodies (IgM)resulting in agglutination of red cells in areas exposed to cold surface temperatures such as the extremities, ear margins and nose.

Cld nursery nursery where piglets older than four weeks old are kept and the ambient temperature is around 65F.

Clean A lay term commonly used by cattle breeders to mean that a cow has shed her afterbirth. Also refers to the natural, wholesome flavor of dairy products.

Clean legged Having no feathers growing down the shanks.

Cleats (clays, claws, clees) the two halves of the sheep's foot.

Cleft palate A congenital split involving the hard or soft palate in the mouth. May cause nasal regurgitation in newborns. Known to be inherited in some breeds, may also be caused by environmental factors.

Clia Eyelashes.

Cliary body H section of uvea between the iris and choroid. It functions to produce aqueous and is the site of attachment for the lens zonules. Contraction of the ciliary body muscle results in lens accommodation for focusing.

Clic Abdominal pain not necessarily associated with the digestive system; any painful abdominal stucture can cause colic.

Click Breeding term for situation where certain blood lines, if crossed, produce exceptional offspring.

Clinches The folded-over ends of horseshoe nails on the outside of a shod horse's hooves.

Clinical Having disease signs or symptoms that can be readily observed.

Clinical study A planned examination of the effectiveness of a new drug or treatment for a disease as compared to a control group not receiving the treatment; also called a clinical trial.

Clinical trial A scientifically controlled study carried out under specific conditions, usually to test the effectiveness of a new treatment.

Clinimix™ pre-made solution used in partial parenteral solution.

Clisepticemic E. coli E. coli that spreads from the gut through the calf's body and causes abscessed in the brain, eyes, kidneys, and joints. This occurs when the newborn calf ingests it in manure, mud, or other material before or along with getting colostrum.

Clitoris Sensitive mound of erectile tissue in the lower portion of a mare's vulva.

Cloaca A common tube-like structure through which feces, urine, and reproductive fluids/eggs pass in birds, turtles, and other lower vertebrates.

Clone A clone is a population of cells all derived from a single progenitor cells.

Clonic Movements during a generalized seizure which includes paddling and/or chewing.

Cloning The production of genes or individuals which are genetically the same as the donor.

Close breeding A form of inbreeding, such as mating brothers to sisters, sire to daughter, and son to dam.

Closed Flock An existing flock that does not introduce any outside breeding stock.

Close up Cow A pregnant cow within 10 to 16 days of calving.

Closing option transaction Cancels a previously established longor short-option position.

Clostridial Organisms Anaerobic bacteria that produce spores under certain conditions.

Clotting factors Protein components in the blood which help it to clot. Clotting is a complex mechanism. In addition to platelets, clot formation is the result of a long chain of chemical reactions carried out by individual molecules called 'clotting factors.' Each factor is numbered such that factor I leads to a reaction with factor II forming a new substance. This then reacts with factor III and so on to factor XII.

Clover A legume used for hay and pasture.

Cluster Seizures More than 1 seizure in a 24 hour period.

Clutch 1. A batch of eggs that are hatched together, either in a nest or in an incubator (from the Old Norse word "klekja," meaning to hatch), also called a "setting".

2. All the eggs laid by a hen on consecutive days, before she skips a day and starts a new laying cycle.

Clutch The egg laying cycle. The hen lays one egg each day for several days in a row and then does not lay for one or two days.

CNS Central nervous system. Includes the brain, spinal cord, and the nerves leading from them.

Coagulation The process of clotting.

Coagulopathy A condition affecting the blood's ability to form a clot.

Coarse A horse lacking refinement, breeding, and quality. A course feed has a high

Coat A cat's fur.

Cob A small horse.

Cocci An oxycyt that destroys the lining of the small intestine causing diarrhea and death; (also known as coccidiosis)

Coccidia A one-celled parasite in the category of protozoa. In dogs and cats, coccidia are generally parasites of the intestinal tract.

Coccidiasis Infection with coccidial protozoa without showing any signs.

Coccidiosis An oxycyt that destroys the lining of the small intestine causing diarrhea and death; (also known as cocci)

Coccidiostat A drug used to keep chickens from getting coccidiosis.

Coccyx In human anatomy, the coccyx is the bone at the apex of the sacrum. It is usually comprised of 4 vertebrae fused together.

Cock A male chicken; also called a "rooster."

Cockerel A male chicken (sometimes applied to other species) under 1 year of age.

Chemical oxygen demand(COD) An indirect measure of the biochemical load exerted on the oxygen of a body of water when organic wastes are introduced into the water. If wastes are readily biodegradable, COD and BOD are nearly the same.

Coenzyme Q A natural substance that assists in oxidative metabolism. It may improve the utilization of oxygen at the cellular level.

Coffin joint The joint within the hoof of the horse between its short pastern bone (second phalanx) and the coffin bone (third phalanx) also including the navicular bone.

Coggins certificate A veterinarian's document that certifies the horse free of the disease, equine infectious anemia.

Coggins test A laboratory blood test used to detect previous exposure to equine infectious anemia or swamp fever, developed by Dr. Leroy Coggins.

Cognitive dysfunction A common medical condition in older dogs that results from abnormal brain function, causing certain behavior changes such as disorientation, housebreaking problems, and changes in sleeping patterns and interactions with others.

Cold blooded Refers to horses having ancestors that trace to heavy war horses and draft breeds. Characteristics might include more substance of bone, thick skin, heavy hair coat, shaggy fetlocks, and blood that makes it suitable for slow, hard work.

Colic Spasmodic pain in the horse, usually caused by spasm of the intestine; (v.) The reaction of a horse to abdominal pain, kicking, rolling, sweating.

Coliform bacteria Bacteria from the intestinal tract of warmblooded animals. Presence is considered indicative of fecal contamination.

Colitis Inflammation of the large intestine (colon).

Collagenases Enzymes secreted by certain bacteria that break down collagen and inhibit wound healing.

Collateral Relatives Relatives that are not progeny or parents (descendants or ascendants). For example, brothers.

Collect To coordinate the horse's moving forward with impulsion while shortening the frame for slow motion.

Collection Gathered together; a state of organized movement; a degree of equilibrium in which the horse's energized response to the aids is characterized by elevated head and neck, rounded back, "dropped croup," engaged hindquarters, and flexed abdominals. The horse remains on the bit, is light and mobile, and is ready to respond to the requests of the trainer. Shortened and raised strides in any gait (walk, trot, gait, canter). The speed is slower because the stride is shortened, the joints of the fore and hind legs are more active, the head and neck are raised, with the head approaching the vertical position.

Colloid Microscopic particles suspended in a solution. The particles in a colloidal solution are large in molecular weight and can pull fluid into the intravascular space. Because the particles are large they stay in the vascular space longer than crystalloids and therefore exert their effect for a longer time.

Colloidal solutions Colloidal solutions are solutions that contain large particles. These large particles are either proteins or complex sugars, such as dextrans or hetastarches. Colloidal solutions because they are physically large molecules, will stay in the bloodstream and hold water in the bloodstream by their oncotic effect.

Colon A part of the digestive tract, specifically the part of large intestine that extends from the cecum to the rectum.

Color Description or class in which body coat color and pattern, not conformation is a deciding factor (e.g., Palomino, Dun Factor, etc.).

Colostrum First fluid secreted by the udder for a few days pre- and postpartum. High in antibodies, this milk protects newborn lambs or kids against disease.

Table
Composition of Colostrum and Milk

	(milking postpartum)			
	1	2	3	Whole
	Colostrum	Transition Milk		Milk
Total Solids, %	23.9	17.9	14.1	12.5
Fat, %	6.7	5.4	3.9	3.6
Solids Non-Fat, %	16.7	12.2	9.8	8.6
Total Protein, %	14.0	8.4	5.1	3.2
Immunoglobulin, %	6.0	4.2	2.4	0.09
IgG (g/100 ml)	3.2	2.5	1.5	0.06

Fig. compostion of Colostrum

Colostrum The accumulated secretions of the mammary gland over the last few weeks of pregnancy. It is rich in IgG (65-90%) with variable levels of IgA and IgM. Form of passively acquired immunity (short-lived).

Colt Name for a young male horse up to 5 years of age.

Comb Red crest on top of the head of most chickens. Roosters have large combs.

Combination Series of two or more fences within 39 feet 4 inches of each other that must be taken as a pair, an in-and-out.

Combination vaccine A vaccine that combines several antigens to induce protection against disease.

Comedo (comedomes) Keratin and dried sebum plugging a hair follicle.

Commensal A relationship where one party gains but at no cost to the other.

Commensalism A Parasitic state in which the parasite lives with the animal without causing disease. Be cautious with this type of parasite.

Commissure Line formed by meeting of maxilla and mandible.

Commodity feed A feed that has high energy, and often a high protein content.

Commodity Storage Usually a steel framed shed that provides storage for commodity feeds, such as cottonseed, brewers grains, chopped hay, etc.

Common An ordinary. plain-appearing horse.

Communicable Capable of spreading disease. Also known as infectious.

Community immunity Having a large percentage of the population vaccinated in order to prevent the spread of certain infectious diseases. Even individuals not vaccinated (such as newborns and those with chronic illnesses) are offered some protection because the disease has little opportunity to spread within the community. Also known as herd immunity.

Compaction Closely packed feed in the stomach and intestines of an animal causing constipation and/or digestive disturbances.

Complement A protein complex consisting of enzymes that facilitate the reaction of antibody with antigen resulting in destruction of cells or invading bacteria.

Complete blood count A count of the total number of cells in a given amount of blood, including the red and white blood cells; often referred to as a 'CBC,' it is one of the most common tests done to check for abnormalities of the blood.

Complete feed A thoroughly blended mixture of different feed ingredients formulated to meet specific nutrient requirements.

Complete ration A blend of all feedstuffs (forages and grains) in one feed. A complete ration fits well into mechanized feeding and the use of computers to formulate least-cost rations. Sometimes called total mixed ration or TMR.

Complex Partial Seizure Seizures that are associated with bizarre or complex behaviors that are repeated during each seizure. These behaviors can last for minutes or hours and can also be followed by a generalized seizure. Thought to be associated with Secondary Epilepsy.

Components The nutritional solids in milk other than water, like fat, protein, lactose, and minerals.

Composting Pad A concrete or hard packed surface that provides an area on which manure and discarded feed may be composted with ready access to aerate the composting materials.

Compound To mix components following a "recipe" or protocol.

Compounding To create a medication by combining parts or to change the formulation of a drug, for example from tablet to liquid.

Compressed Flattened from side to side.

Computerized tomography scan (CT scan) A radiological imaging procedure that uses x-ray pictures to produce "slices" through a patient's body; also called a computerized axial tomography (CAT).

Concentrate A feed high in nitrogen-free-extract (NFE) and total digestible nutrients (TDN) and low in crude fiber (less than 18 percent). Included are cereal grains, soybean oil meal, cottonseed meal, and by-products of the milling industry such as corn gluten and wheat bran. A concentrate may be low or rich in protein.

Concentrated milks Milk, skim milk, and components of these that have been concentrated by removing varying amounts of water under carefully controlled conditions of heat and/or vacuum. Concentrated milks may be reconstituted by adding appropriate quantities of water.

Conception Fertilization or penetration of the ovum by a sperm cell.

Conception Rate The number of ewes that lamb compared to the number of ewes exposed for breeding. This is usually expressed as a percentage.

Conchas The decorative round leather, metal, or silver discs through which pass the saddle strings.

Condition Refers to the amount of flesh (body weight), quality of hair coat, and general health of animals. Also called body condition.

Conditioning The art and science of preparing a horse mentally and physically for a particular use such as pleasure riding, competitive trail riding, or showing.

Cone A red vinyl traffic cone, used as a marker.

Confidence range (CR) Indicates the accuracy in the estimation of a sire's genetic merit in a sire proof by giving a probable range for future summaries.

Confinement Livestock kept in corrals or housing for maximum year-round production. Facilities may be partial or complete, usually with a solid floor and enclosed, or covered.

Confirmed sire One that has been used for breeding before and has known good fertility.

Conformation The body form or physical traits of an animal; its shape and arrangement of parts.

Conjunctiva The tissue covering the anterior portion of an eyeball.

Congenital A characteristic of an animal that is present at birth. It may be inherited or induced by events that occur during pregnancy.

Conjugate Joined or paired.

Conjugate vaccines Vaccines made from capsular polysaccharides bound to proteins of known immunogenicty, such as tetanus toxoid.

Conjunctiva The thin, moist, mucus membrane that lines the inside of the eyelids (palpebral conjunctiva) and curves around at the fornix to cover the eyeball up to the cornea (bulbar conjunctiva) ventrally it also covers both sides of the nictitans

Conjunctivitis An inflammation of the lining of the eyelids; may cause pain, redness. itching, and a discharge.

Connective tissue Connective tissue is derived from the mesenchyme and includes a number of tissues which have a passive, binding function. In a connective tissue the parent cells are separated more or less widely from one another by a homogeneous matrix or ground substance, in which fibres may or may not be present.

Consignor The person who consigns a horse for sale or puts it up for auction.

Constipation A condition in which the contents of the large intestines (bowels) are discharged at abnormally long intervals or with difficulty.

Contact The horse's stretching forward into the bit and accepting the ein as a means of communication with the rider.

Contact dermatitis Inflammation of the skinfrom contact with an irritant.

Contagious An infection capable of spread amongst animals by direct contact, e.g. Pasteurella spp. in nasal droplets.

Contagious disease A disease that is capable of being spread amongst animals by direct contact, e.g. Pasteurella spp. in nasal droplets.

Contagious mastitis Mastitis that is caused by coagulate negative Staphylococci.

Containment of antimicrobial resistance Infectious disease control measures that minimize the emergence and spread of antimicrobial-resistant microorganisms.

Contemporaries Cows of the same breed that were born and raised, and initiated their lactations during similar periods. Usually separated into two lactation groups for comparison—first lactation and all other lactations.

Contemporary comparison Method for estimating the transmitting ability of bulls and cows using information on contemporaries.

Contemporary Group A genetically similar group of sheep born in a particular time period and raised under the same management and environmental conditions.

Contracted heels Heels are pulled close together due to the frog shriveling. caused by lack of use or disease.

Contraindication A condition in a recipient, which is likely to result in a life-threatening problem if a vaccine were given.

Contrast A dye given by mouth or in the vein that will make some organs more visible on an x-ray (radiograph).

Contrast agents A substance given orally or injected into a patient that makes the affected tissue easier to identify on an x-ray.

Controlled breeding Also called a timed breeding technique. Modification of the physiology of the ovaries in such a way that one can predict exactly when that female is going to be ready and breed her only once.

Contusion An injury to underlying tissues without breaking the skin; a bruise.

Conventional Early maturing.

Coop The house or cage in which a chicken lives.

Cooperative A form of business owned and controlled by the people who use its services, such as a milk marketing or processing cooperative.

Cooperative An enterprise owned by and operated for the benefit of those using its services.

Cooperative Extension Service (CES) The state, university and county educational outreach service of each state land-grant institution. This service extends the research results and educational programs of land-grant institutions to all the people in the state.

Coprophagia Eating dung or fecal matter; normal behavior in some animals, such as rabbits.

Copulation Insertion of the penis into the female reproductive tract.

Coracobrachialis The Coracobrachialis is a human muscle used to draw the arm forwards and prevent side-sway when the arm is raised by the Deltoid.

Coracoid Bone In birds, the Coracoid Bone is the bone joining the sternum to the shoulder and supporting the wing. In mammals it is represented by the coracoid process of the scapula.

Core vaccine Vaccine which should be given to all animals of certain species, example, parvovirus vaccine in dogs or panleukopenia in cats.

Cornea The clear part of the front of the eye which allows light in.

Corneal degeneration After certain corneal or scleral injuries, lipid or cholesterol can be deposited in the cornea.

Corneal reflex Used to assess corneal sensation.

Corneal sequestrum A focal area of collagen degeneration in the cornea with brown to black discoloration.

Corneoscleral transposition A surgical technique used to patch conjunctiva over a corneal ulcer.

Cornification The angular appearance of epithelial cells during estrus under the influence of estrogen.

Cornified With a keratinous (horny) covering.

Corona A fancy western saddle pad featuring a border of alternating colored thick fabric.

Coronary band The top of the hoof between hair-covered skin and hoof where growth takes place.

Coronavirus A single stranded RNA virus.

Coronet Coronary band. All growth occurs here. Soft tissue is turned into the hardened horn of the hoof wall.

Corpora nigra Structures present mainly on the upper pupil margin in horses, upper and lower margins in the lamb. Quite obvious and elaborate on llamas and alpacas. Their function is not really known.

Corpus hemorrhagicum Also called a hemorrhagic follicle. A follicle that has been present on the ovary and has not been given the chance to ovulate so it will continue growing and becomes large and cyst-like and bleeds inside.

Corpus luteum A ductless gland developed within the ovary by the reorganization of a Graafian follicle following ovulation. Also known as an extract of this gland of the hog or cow, the chief principle of which is progesterone. plural = corpora lutea.

Corral A pen or enclosure for confining livestock.

Correlation A measure of how two traits relate to each other. Correlation coefficients are expressed in the range –1.00 to +1.00.

Traits which are negatively correlated act opposite, as one trait increases the other decreases. Positively correlated traits, both traits increase or decrease together. A zero correlation means as one trait changes, there is no consistent response of the other trait.

Corriedale A New Zealand breed of sheep. A Lincoln-Merino cross, also used in Australia and South America.

Cortex Part of the brain involved in higher order thought processing.

Corticospinal tract A bundle of axons going from the brain through the spinal cord that, in humans, carries information on movement; has a specific location in the spinal cord

Corticosteroid Hormones produced by the adrenal gland which are important to almost every function of cells and organs. They are divided into two groups: glucocorticoids and mineralocorticoids. Glucocorticoids regulate protein, carbohydrate, and fat metabolism. Mineralocorticoids regulate electrolyte balances.

Cortisol A hormone produced by the adrenal gland that affects the function of most organs in the body. Some primary functions are to increase blood sugar and to reduce inflammation.

Cost effectiveness Ratio comparing the results of a healthcare program or procedure to the direct and indirect net costs of this program or procedure.

Costal Cartilages In human anatomy, the costal cartilages are bars of hyaline cartilage which extend forwards from the anterior ends of the ribs and contribute to the elasticity of the thorax.

Costridium A group of bacteria that produce spores. One type of clostridium causes tetanus.

Cotyledonary type of placenta A type of placenta where the connection between the placenta and the fetus is based on buttons of tissue. Cattle and sheep have this type of placentation.

Coumestan Estrogen-like substance produced by certain plants such as alfalfa; types of phytoestrogen.

Coumestral Estrogen-like substances produced by certain plants such as alfalfa; types of phytoestrogen.

Countercanter Deliberately asking the horse to canter on the lead opposite the direction of movement. For example, in a circle to the right, requesting a countercanter would result in a canter left lead.

Cover To breed a mare.

Coverall A brand name, but commonly referring to any of a group of hoop type barns with opaque or mylar fabric covers over a tubular steel frame.

Coverts Smaller feathers covering large wing and tail feathers.

Cow A mature female bovine. Usually referring to any dairy females that have borne a calf. Some may consider females having given birth only once as "first-calf heifers" until they have a second calf.

Cow hocked A condition of a cow in which the hocks are close together and the fetlocks (located just above the hoof) wide apart.

Cow Trainer A tin or wire structure supported a few inches above a cow to prevent her from soiling the platform of her stall by administering a gentle electric shock if she arches her back to urinate or defecate while too far forward in the stall.

Cow trot Term used to refer to method of moving the back end of a horse when trotting. A cow trotting horse is stiff in the rear joints, and uses the hips for most of the forward movement. A cow trotting horse will swing its tail side to side and its feet out in an arc as it moves them forward. A cow trotting horse will not break over in the hocks, but will swing them side to side in a stiff motion. A cow trotting horse may also be either long trotting or square trotting.

Cow hocked Hocks closer together than feet, hocks bend in as viewed from the rear.

COX inhibitor Drugs that block cyclooxygenase and that are intended to relieve pain and inflammation.

Cradle A device put on a horse's neck so it can't reach to bite or lick its sides or legs.

Crampiness A condition among cattle, especially bulls in confinement, in which involuntary contractions of muscles of the hind legs result in pain and discomfort. Affected animals shift from foot to foot.

Cranial Refers to the head or in a direction toward the front of the animal. For example the chest is more cranial than the abdomen. The opposite term is caudal meaning closer to the rear of the animal.

Crate An elevated stall for a calf in an indoor facility.

Creamery A butter factory or, more commonly, a milk processing plant.

Creep An enclosure into which young (small) animals may enter but larger animals cannot. Any feeders in this area or in farrowing crates or parturition pen that are only accessible to the young are called creep feeders.

Creep area An area where new born piglets crawl to, to keep warm and avoid being accidentally crushed by their mother.

Crest A puff of feathers on the heads of breeds such, as Houdan, Silkie, or Polish; also called a "topknot."

Creutzfeld Jacob disease A disease of people which causes progressive degeneration of the brain. It is the commonest human Transmissible Spongiform Encephalopathy, and occurs naturally in about one person in every million.

Cria The term describing a llama from the age of birth to weanling (4-6 months).

Cribbing A vice whereby a horse anchors its teeth onto an object, arches its neck, pulls backward, and swallows air. It can cause the horse to lose weight, suffer tooth damage, and other physical disturbances.

Cricket A copper attachment to a bit's port which will spin in the horse's mouth as he moves his tongue. By having such a thing to play with the horses mouth will stay moist and it helps pacify the horse.

Crimp The "wave" in the staple of wool

Crimped Rolled with corrugated rollers. The grain to which this term refers may be tempered or conditioned before crimping, and may be cooled afterward.

Critical Temperature Maximum or minimum environmental temperature tolerated by the animal before additional dietary energy is required to maintain normal body temperature.

Crohn's disease A chronic medical condition characterized by inflammation of the bowel. Symptoms include abdominal pain, diarrhea, fever, loss of appetite and weight loss. The cause of Crohn's disease is not yet known, but genetic, dietary and infectious factors may play a part.

Cronic interstital nephritis CIN Chronic interstitial nephritis (CIN) is similar to the term end stage renal disease (ESRD) in that it is a non specific histologic finding on renal biopsy and may be the end result of renal disease of any etiology.

Cronic renal disease CRD Irreversible renal disease caused by damage to a large part of both kidneys. Two thirds of both kidneys must be damaged before the animal loses the ability to concentrate and dilute urine and 75% of both kidneys must be destroyed before azotemia is observed.

Cronological records ecords that are organized by arranging all the data in the record in the order in which it was collected.

Crop 1. A pouch at the base of a chicken's neck that bulges after the bird has eaten.

2. To trim a bird's wattles.

Cross firing A horse is cross firing when the inside rear foot hits first, and the inside front foot hits last when the horse is in the canter or lope.

Crossbreed The mating of cats of two different breeds. The offspring of such a mating is considered a hybrid.

Crossbreeding Mating of animals from two distinct breeds to produce a half-bred.

Crossing Breeding horses of different pedigrees.

Cross priming A phenomenon whereby virus like particles act as an adjuvant by carrying peptide sequences inside the antigen presenting cell and feeding peptides into the endogenous processing pathway.

Cross tie A means of tying a horse in which a chain or rope from each side of an aisle is attached to the side rings of the horse's halter.

Crowd Gate A motorized or manual gate at the end of the holding pen that may be moved forward to guide cows toward the entrance to the milking parlor.

Crown roast Made by adjoining two Frenched eight-rib racks with twine and bending them to form a circle. The joined ends are secured by twine.

Cruciate Shaped like a cross. Cruciate ligaments are found on the front (cranial or anterior) and the back (caudal or posterior) of the stifle ('knee') joint.

Crude fiber (CF) That portion of feedstuffs composed of cellulose, hemicellulose, lignin and other polysaccharides which serve as structural and protective parts of plants (high in forages and low in grains). Not soluble in acid or alkali detergents.

Crude protein (CP) Total protein in a feed. To calculate the protein percentage, a feed is first chemically analyzed for nitrogen content. Since proteins average about 16 percent (100 ö 6.25) nitrogen, the percentage of nitrogen in the analysis is multiplied by 6.25 to give the CP percentage.

Crupper A leather loop which passes under the horse's tail and is attached to the saddle to prevent it from slipping forward. Also used in a biting rig or harness.

Crust Area of dried fluid or cells on the skin. The fluid may have been blood, serum, pus, or medication.

Crutching or tagging The act of shearing wool from the breech area and hind legs and sometimes the belly.

Cryoprotectant A substance such as glycerol which is added to semen to protect the sperm membrane from injury. by ice crystals formed during the freezing and thawing process.

Cryptorchid An adult male cat whose testicles have not descended into the scrotal sac. This is a disqualification in all associations.

Cryptorchidism The failure of one or both testicles to descend into the scrotum.

Cryptosporidiosis An organism that proliferates in the small intestine.

Crysotherapy Gold salt therapy used in treatment of immune mediated disorders.

Crystallography A science that deals with the forms and structures of crystals. A molecule forms a three-dimensional structure and this is the study of that specific structure and how it relates to cellular processes.

Crystalloids Crystalloid solutions are solutions that contain small particles, particles with molecular weights of less than a few 100 molecular weight units. Examples of crystalloid solutions are lactated Ringer's solution, Ringer's, and the dextrose and saline containing solutions.

Cud Cattle eat grass and grain, and they chew their food two separate times to digest it. After they chew and shallow the food, they bring it up from one stomach and chew it again.

Cue A single signal, often made up of several aids, from the rider or handler that tells a horse what to do. Often used in performing tricks.

Cull cow Cow removed from a herd due to poor profitability. Generally due to poor production, reproduction, or mastitis.

Culling The process of eliminating nonproductive or undesirable animals. The removal of cows from a herd as a result of low production or other factors that reduce the profitability of the cow.

Culls Goats which are below a required standard.

Culmen Upper ridge of maxilla.

Cultivator Used to smooth the rough, plowed soil or used to dig up weeds and loosen soil while crops are growing.

Culture In microbiology, a population of microorganisms in a growth medium or the act of growing bacteria in media for identification. A pure culture contains only organisms that initially arose from a single cell. Cultures are used in manufacturing cultured dairy products and most cheeses.

Cuneiform bones The cuneiform bones are three bones in the human foot behind the first three metatarsal bones.

Curb A type of leverage bit with shanks and generally a hump in the middle called the port.

Curb chain The chain attached to the bit passing under the horse's chin.

Curb strap The leather strap on the bit passing under the horse's chin.

Curd The coagulated or thickened part of milk. Curd from whole milk consists of casein, fat, and whey, whereas curd from skim milk contains casein and whey but only traces of fat.

Cured Hay Hay that has been dried to allow safe storage, without molding.

Curry comb A metal, plastic, or rubber device with many small teeth for cleaning hard-packed filth off a horse or cow.

Cush The laying down position of the female camelid during mating.

Cushing's Disease A disease of the adrenal gland that produces too much of the hormone cortisol. Too much cortisol causes signs including drinking, eating and urinating increased amounts and loss of hair on the body. Also called hyperadrenocorticism.

Custom Feeding The practice of having livestock fed and managed for the livestock owner in another facility for a fee.

Cut To castrate.

Cutability The percent of trimmed retail cuts, ready for purchase by the customer.

Cutaneous lupus erythematosus CLEDiscoid lupus. A form of systemic lupus erythematosus which only onvolves the skin.

Cutaneous Relating to the skin.

Cutaneous vasculitis Skin lesions caused by deposition and subsequent activation of soluble immune complexes along the basement membrane of blood vessels.

Cuticle The cuticle is the horny outside layer of skin.

Cutting loss The actual weight lost from the carcass after processing (cutting, boning, and trimming).

Cwt Hundredweight or 100 pounds of milk

Cyanosis Bluish or grayish color to the skin and gums which occurs when the animal has insufficient oxygen.

Cycle Events that happen in the female such as ovulation, hormone production, receptivity, etc. In camelids the cycle does not follow regular time periods as it does in horses or cattle.

Cyclitis Inflammation of the ciliary body.

Cyclo 0xygenase (COX) An enzyme involved in the production of prostaglandins from arachidonic acid in cell membranes. There are 2 forms, COX 1 & COX 2. COX 2 plays a greater role in inflammation.

Cyclocryotherapy A freezing probe is applied to sclera to destroy the underlying ciliary body in treatment of glaucoma.

Cyclooxygenase 2 (cox 2) Inhibitors Any of a class of drugs (as celecoxib or rofecoxib) that selectively block the COX-2 enzyme but not the COX-1 enzyme. These drugs are intended to relieve pain and inflammation while minimizing gastrointestinal side effects – called also COX-2 blockers .

Cyclophosphamide A chemotherapy drug also used in the treatment of immune mediated diseases.

Cycloplegic A drug that paralyses the ciliary muscle and helps reduce pain.

Cygnet A baby swan.

Cyst An abnormal sac-like structure that is lined with cells which produce a liquid or thick material.

Cystic endometrial hyperplasia CEHMorphological changes occurring in the uterus under the influence progesterone secreted from the corpus lutei (CLs) of the ovaries during diestrus.

Cysticercosis The condition where a larval form of a tapeworm has encysted or embedded itself in the tissue of its host.

Cystitis Inflammation of the bladder.

Cystocercus The larval stage of a tapeworm encysted in muscle.

Cythioate an oral organophosphate.

Cytokines Hormone-like low molecular weight proteins secreted by many different cell types, which regulate the intensity and duration of immune responses. Cytokines amplify some parts of the immune system and suppress other parts. Many cytokines have been identified such as interferon-a,b, tumor necrosis factor (TNF) and granulocyte colony stimulating factor (G-CSF). Cytokines made by lymphocytes are often called lymphokines or interleukins (abbreviated IL).

Cytology The study of cells; often refers to the microscopic examination of a sample taken from the skin or lesion to look for the cause of a condition.

Cytoplasm The living matter within a cell (excluding the nucleus) that is responsible for the function of the cell (for example, protein synthesis).

Cytoplasmic droplet A round drop of cytoplasm that moves from the neck of the sperm down it's tail and is gone by the time normal sperm are ejaculated.

Cytotoxic T cells T cells that can kill other cells. Most cytotoxic cells are MHC class I-restricted CD8 cells, but CD4 T cells can also kill in some cases. Cytotoxic T cells are important in host defense against cytosolic pathogens.

Cytotoxicity Degree to which a substance is poisonous to cells.

D

D.M.S.O. Dimethyl sulfoxide, a solvent whichis an organic chemical that readily passes through the skin. Anti-inflammatory, antibacterial and analgesic.

Dachshund A small dog of a breed developed in Germany for hunting badgers and having a long body, a usually shorthaired brown or black and brown coat, drooping ears, and very short legs.

Dacryocystitis Inflammation of the lacrimal sac usually as a result of infection.

Dacryocystorhinography A technique in which radiopaque contrast material is injected into the punctum and flushed through the nasolacrimal duct, followed by lateral and VD radiographic views of the skull, to evaluate the nasolacrimal system and surrounding bony structures.

Dags Breech wool that is coated with feces. "To dag" the sheep means to remove this wool by selective shearing or clipping with dagging shears.

Dairy bull A male dairy animal which has been used in the dairy herd for breeding.

Dairy cattle Produce milk and cream from which many products, such as butter, cheese, and ice cream are made.

Dairy cattle breed Group of dairy cattle having a common origin and identifiable traits (frequently color). The major U.S. breeds are Ayrshire, Brown Swiss, Guernsey, Holstein, Jersey and Milking Shorthorn.

Dairy character Physical traits that suggest high milking ability. Important indications of this include an alert, feminine head; long thin neck; openness and sharpness throughout; prominent hips and pins; sharp withers; thin thighs; flat flinty bone; and thin, pliable hide with a soft silky hair coat.

Dairy Cow A bovine from which milk production is intended for human consumption, or is kept for raising replacement dairy heifers.

Dairy farm Where cows are kept to produce milk.

Dairy goat Any goat from which milk production is intended for human consumption, or is kept for raising replacement dairy kids.

Dairy goat breed Group of dairy goats having a common origin and identifiable traits (frequently color). The major U.S. breeds are Alpine, LaMancha, Nubian, Oberhasli, Saanen and Toggenberg.

Dairy Herd Improvement (DHI) Official DHI type of testing plan that requires supervision and compliance with all Official DHI Rules (DHI abbreviation is used commonly to designate the testing plans).

Dairy Herd Improvement Association (DHIA) An organization with programs and objectives intended to improve production of dairy cattle and profitability of dairy farming and especially to aid dairy farmers in keeping milk production and management records.

Dairy Herd Improvement Registry (DHIR) A modification of the DHIA program to make milk production records acceptable by dairy breed associations. An official production record program. Abbreviation used to designate Official DHIR type of testing plan for registered cows. Record supervision and verification are required in compliance with Official DHI and DHIR rules.

Dairy producer Farmer who owns or runs a dairy farm.

Dairy Records Processing Center (DRPC) A computing facility where information from the periodic tests in NCDHIP herds is summarized and analyzed and where information to be used in future management decisions is prepared for the dairy producer.

Dairy Steer A neutered male of any of the dairy cattle breeds. The "dairy steers" are raised for meat production and usually managed like beef cattle.

Dally To wind the rope end around the saddle horn.

Dalmatian A dog of a breed believed to have originated in Dalmatia, having a short, smooth white coat covered with black or dark brown spots.

Daltons A term used to indicate a unit of mass equal to 1/12 the mass of a carbon-12 atom.

Dam The female parent of any dairy animal.

Dam family Sibling chickens that all have the same dam as well as sire.

DAMN IT acronym A method of looking at possible causes for a problem.

D= degenerative

A = anomalies or autoimmune

M= metabolic

N = neoplasia or nutritional

I = inflammation or infectious or immune mediated or iatrogenic

T= toxic or traumatic idiopathic

Dander Small scales from the skin, hair, or feathers of an animal, often causing an allergic reaction in sensitive individuals.

Dandie Dinmont Terrier A breed of small terrier with long wiry coat and drooping ears.

Dandy A medium-hard brush for grooming to remove loose hair and dirt.

Dapple A mottled or variegated coat color pattern. Single dapple is expressed as lighter color areas contrasting with the darker base color, which may be acceptable color. Looks like the merle effect in Shelties, Collies, etc., except that it is found in Dachshunds. Color definitions may vary by breed. Always check the breed standard for the definitive color description.

Dappled Rings or spots of different-colored hair on the coat of a horse.

Dapsone Diaminodiphenylsulfon. Used in the treatment of subcorneal pustular dermatosis.

Data base The data base is information that is collected by the user of the medical record, either the veterinarian or a technician. In order to collect a similar amount of baseline information about all patients, and to avoid omissions, the minimum data base should be defined in advance and should always be collected. The data base may include laboratory tests, radiographs, or other diagnostic tests.

Data confidentiality The protected storage, communication or exchange of data which is considered private, normally for ethical or legal reasons. Most modern computer systems normally provide services which ensure that confidential information can only be accessed and read by authorised users or programs. Some data may have a higher degree of confidentiality than others e.g. disease data which can be traced back to an individual.

Data sharing protocol A formal agreement between organisations that are sharing data. The agreement sets out the purpose, principles and commitments that organisations should adopt when they share data.

Date of Whelping Date of birth.

Daughter herd mate comparison Amount by which a daughter of a bull differs in yield or other traits from the average of cows of other bulls' daughters of the same breed in the same herd during the same period.

Days dry As used in DHIA records, this is the number of days dry prior to calving at the start of the production record listed.

Days in milk (DIM) The number of days during the present lactation that the cow has been milking, beginning with the last date of calving to the current test date.

Days open The number of days between calving (parturition) and conception. Should be less than 120 days.

Dead end host It can not be transmitted from human to human. Example: brucellosis.

Deadgrass Tan or dull straw color. Color definitions may vary by breed. Always check the breed standard for the definitive color description.

Debeak To remove a portion of a bird's top beak to prevent cannibalism or self-pecking.

Debilitated A weakened or sick condition.

Debride To clean out dead or dying tissue from a wound.

Deciduous teeth Non-permanent teeth(baby teeth)that will be shed and replaced with permanent adult teeth.

Decontaminate Remove injurious material.

Decubital ulcers Pressure sores, usually seen over bony prominances.

Decurved Curved downward toward tip.

Deep mycoses Diseases incluing Histoplasmosis, Blastomycosis, Coccidioidomycosis and Cryptococcosis.

Deep Chested Term describing the rib cage structure of dogs like German Shepherds, Great Danes and Irish Setters. Deep-chested dogs have a greater tendency to develop stomach dilatation, also referred to as bloat.

Defecation The elimination of feces from the rectum.

Definitive host Where sexual reproduction takes place.

Degradable intake protein DIPPortion of intake protein that is degraded (broken down) by rumen microbes to ammonia and amino acids. DIP is used for microbial synthesis.

Degraded intake protein See DIP.

Dehorn To remove horns from animals or to treat young animals so horns will not develop.

Dehorning Procedure to remove horn or terminate horn growth permanently.

Dehydrate The loss of body fluids by fever, virus or heat.

Dehydration An inadequate amount of fluid in the body. The minimum amout of dehydration that can be detected is about 5% loss of total body weight as fluid loss.

Delayed wound closure This is a wound you will suture but not immediately; first you debride the wound several times through bandage changes to make it more amenable to closing.

Deltoid The deltoid muscle is a triangular muscle in the shoulder used to lift the upper arm.

Demodectic mange Skin disease characterized by hair loss particularly on the head, face, neck, shoulders and the front of the forelegs. Caused by the demodex mite which is normally found on the skin of most dogs, but due to an abnormality of the immune system, the body overreacts to its presence. It can be treated, but it is occasionally resistant to treatment.

Demodex A mite that causes mange.

Demodicosis generalized Also called the pustular form. Many small focal areas of involvement or a diffuse generalized distribution. Lesions include generalized erythema, crusting, scaling and patchy to diffuse alopecia.

Demodicosis localized Also called squamous. One or more well circumscribed areas of alopecia with mild scaling and erythema usually located on the forelimbs, face and on periocular skin.

Demyelinating disorders A medical condition where the myelin sheath is damaged. The myelin sheath surrounds nerves and is responsible for the transmission of impulses to the brain. Damage to the myelin sheath results in muscle weakness, poor coordination and possible paralysis. Examples of demyelinating disorders include Multiple Sclerosis (MS), optic neuritis, transverse neuritis and Guillain-Barre Syndrome (GBS).

Dendrite Projections from a nerves cell's body that receive information from other cells

Dendritic cell Also known as interdigitating reticular cells, are found in T cell areas of lymphoid tissues. They have a branched or dendritic morphology and are the most potent stimulators of T cell response. Non-lymphoid tissues also contain dendritic cells but these do not seem to stimulate T cell responses until they are activated and migrate to lymphoid tissues. The dendritic cell derives from bone marrow precursors. It is distinct from the follicular dendritic cell that presents antigen to be cells.

Denitrification The chemical or biological reduction of nitrate or nitrite to gaseous nitrogen, either as molecular nitrogen (N2) or as an oxide of nitrogen (N_2O).

Dentition Forty-two adult teeth, including incisors, canines, premolars, and molars.

Denver ribs Generally eight breast of lamb ribs, not less than three inches wide. This includes the area four inches below the eye of the rack of lamb to the cartilage bone. It is trimmed free of fell, fat and connective tissue.

Deoxyribonucleic acid (DNA) The chemical substance that is the principal nuclear material of cells. The structure of DNA determines the structure of ribonucleic acid which, in turn, determines the structure of proteins of the cell.

Department for Environment, Food and Rural Affairs The Government Department whose responsibilities include animal disease surveillance. Defra's overall aim is sustainable development.

Depressed Flattened from top to bottom.

Depth of Chest An indication of the volume of space for heart and lungs, and commonly referenced to the elbow (i.e., above, at the level of, or below).

Dermal Relating to the skin.

Dermatitis Inflammation of the dermal layer (outer layer) of the skin.

Dermatitis herpetiformis A pruritic, vesiculoulcerative dermatitis which is poorly documented in veterinary medicine and is associated with IgA deposition and gluten enteropathies in man.

Dermatologic examination The dermatologic exam should include examination of the entire hair coat, careful palpation of the skin, careful examination of the skin surface over several areas of the body, visual examination (otoscopic) of the external ear canals, and inspection of the foot pads. In many cases it is helpful to clip hair from the patient so that specific lesions may be seen more clearly. It is also helpful to have a form for the medical record, on which lesions may be drawn and recorded, as well as other information.

Dermatomyositis A immune-mediated, familial dermatopathy suggested to be a primary vasculopathy with secondary dermatitis and myositis. Breed predilection includes Collies and Shetland Sheepdogs.

Dermatophilosis Pyoderma caused by the aerobic and facultative anaerobic actinomycete: Dermatophilus congolensis. Also called Streptotricosis, rain scald, and streptothricosis (horses)

Dermatophyte Fungus that causes ringworm; include Trichophyton, Microsporum, and Epidermophyton.

Dermatophyte test medium DTM Agar for growing fungi. Dermatophyte test media (DTM) contains phenol red as a pH indicator and substances to inhibit growth of saprophytic fungi and bacteria.

Dermatophytosis Ringworm. Dermatophytes live and grow only on non-viable keratinized tissue (skin, hair, nails). They will not grow in living cells.

Dermis The dermal layer of the skin that contains blood vessels, hair follicles, sebaceous glands, erector pili muscles, and apocrine sweat glands.

Dermoid A piece of skin growing on the cornea.

Descemet's membrane A clear membrane forming the inner boundary of the cornea.

Descemetocele Very deep ulcers right down to decemets membrane.

Descenting The removal of the anal sacs of a carnivore to prevent the animal from releasing the very strong-smelling secretion.

Desmology Desmology is the branch of anatomy dealing with ligaments and sinews.

Deviation The difference between the average performance of the group and the performance of an individual in the group.

Dewclaw An extra claw on the inside of the leg; a rudimentary fifth toe, removed on most breeds.

Dewlap Loose, pendulous skin under the throat and neck.

Dextran High molecular weight polysaccharides used to expand blood volume. A colloid. Dextrans have an average molecular weight of 40,000 daltons (Dextran 40) or 75,000 daltons (Dextran 70).

Dextrose 5% D5W5% dextrose is hypotonic relative to extracellular fluid. It contains only dextrose, no electrolytes. 5% dextrose is a constituent of most maintenance solutions. It can be used a sole fluid for rehydration for animals who cannot tolerate the administration of sodium, such as those with cardiac disease. More commonly, it is used as part of the rehydration solution in these sodium intolerant animals, used in combination with lactated Ringer's or sodium chloride.

Dextrose hypertonic Hypertonic dextrose is any percentage of dextrose which has an osmolality in excess of extracellular fluid. Dextrose is available in several commercial strengths. Any concentration of dextrose can be created by adding additional dextrose to a commercial solution. The predominant use of hypertonic dextrose solutions is as a calorie source in total parenteral nutrition solutions. There is also an indication to promote urine flow in patients with oliguric acute renal failure. TPN solutions containing 50% dextrose are extremely hypertonic and can cause an irritation to the blood vessel if given in a small peripheral vein, such as cephalic or saphenous. Hypertonic solutions are typically given in larger veins such as the jugular vein in which blood flow is faster to dilute the hypertonicity of the infused solution and reduce irritation to the lining of the blood vessel.

DHI Records Generic term used to refer to records computed by the Dairy Record Processing Centers.

DHI supervisor An officially trained and DHIA-certified employee qualified to collect milk samples and record milk weights for all official types of testing plans.

Diabetes A chronic health condition where the body is unable to produce insulin and properly breakdown sugar (glucose) in the blood. Symptoms include hunger, thirst, excessive urination, dehydration and weight loss. The treatment of diabetes requires daily insulin injections, proper nutrition and regular exercise. Complications can include heart disease, stroke, neuropathy, poor circulation leading to loss of limbs, hearing impairment, vision problems and death.

Diabetes insipidus Inadequate secretion of, or resistance to the effects of, antidiuretic hormone (ADH or Vasopressin). This hormone stimulates the kidney retain water in the body. Consequently, the dog passes a large volume of urine with a low specific gravity, and also exhibits great thirst. It may be acquired, inherited, or idiopathic. mellitus due to a failure of the pancreas to produce sufficient insulin, or the cells resistance to the effects of insulin the body is unable to properly process glucose. May require insulin injections, or may be controlled with diet. May be acquired or possibly inherited.

Diabetes mellitus Also known as sugar diabetes. An insufficient amount of insulin is produced by the pancreas resulting in a high blood sugar level.

Diagnostic plans Diagnostic plans are made in order to determine if a certain disease is present. For example you may plan to perform bile acid analyses to determine if liver failure is present.

Diagnostic tests These are tests performed to find the cause of a pet's problem. Diagnostic tests may include analysis of blood, urine, and other body fluids; x-rays (the correct term is radiographs); biopsies, etc.

Diagonal A pair of legs at the trot, such as the right front and the left hind. When posting, the rider sits as the inside hind hits the ground or "rise and fall with the (front) leg on the wall." Riding across the diagonal is a maneuver from one corner of an arena to another through the center.

Dialysis A process which involves removing waste products from the body.

Diamond eyes A combination of severe entropion and ectropion involving both upper and lower eyelids. Most commonly seen in Saint Bernard dogs.

Diaphragm The diaphragm is a large transverse muscle at the base of the thorax, used in respiration to draw air into the lungs.

Diarrhea A condition in which the movement of food through the digestive system is faster than normal; often results in the frequent passing of abnormally loose or watery stool.

Dicoumarol A chemical compound found in spoiled sweet clover and lespedeza hays. It is an anticoagulant and can cause internal hemorrhages when ingested by cattle.

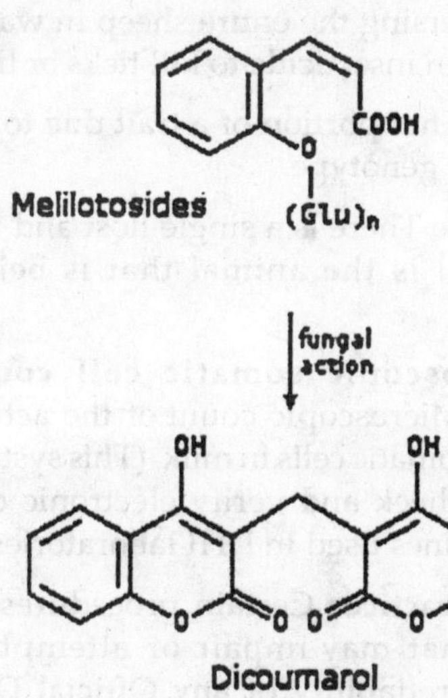

Fig. Dicoumarol

Diestrus The stage of the estrous cycle which follows estrus. In the bitch diestrus lasts 62-63 days from the LH peak.

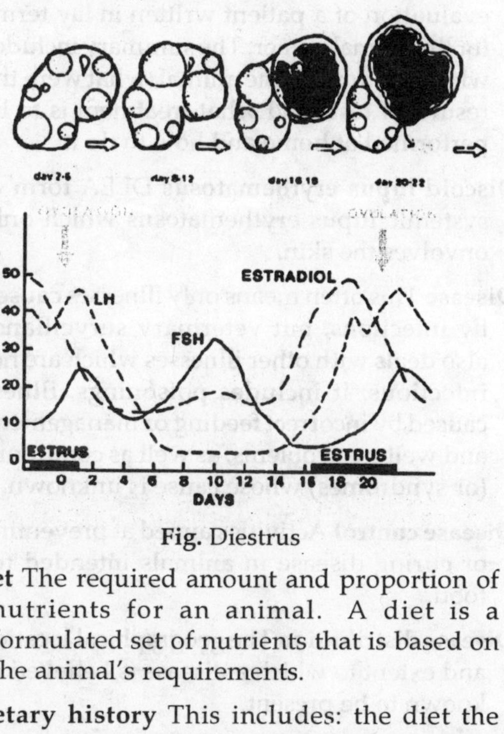

Fig. Diestrus

Diet The required amount and proportion of nutrients for an animal. A diet is a formulated set of nutrients that is based on the animal's requirements.

Dietary history This includes: the diet the animal is currently receiving and for how long? Have they ever home cooked a hypoallergenic diet (potato and pinto beans, lamb and rice)?

Dietary indiscretion Eating what one should not. Dogs with dietary indiscretion eat garbage, dead fish on shore, etc.

Dietary scours When the calf is getting so much nutrient intake they can not absorb it all and it is fermenting in the colon producing gassy, large volume, smelly diarrhea.

Differential diagnosis Differential diagnoses are also known as rule-outs and are possible causes for the problems displayed by a patient. For example, kidney failure is one possible cause for polyuria in a dog or cat.

Differentiated A cell that has developed into a particular cell type, e.g. a neuron or heart muscle cell.

Diff Quik stain A 3-step staining process to stain cytology samples.

Digestibility Expressed as a percent, is a measure of the content of food that is retained in the body after food is eaten. The difference between the weight of food eaten and the weight of stool produced, divided by the weight of the food.

Digestible energy Energy that is available to the animal by digestion; measured as the difference between gross energy content of a feed and the energy contained in the animal's feces (gross energy minus fecal energy.)

Digestible protein (DP) The amount of protein of feed that is absorbed by the digestive tract; it may be computed using the formula: Percent DP = percent crude protein of feed x digestion coefficient for protein in the feed.

Digestion The changes in a feed that must take place before the nutrients can be absorbed and used by the animal.

Digestion coefficient The digestion coefficient of feed ingredients (DCFI) may be calculated using the formula: Wt. of ingredient consumed − Wt. of undigested ingredient in feces.

Digestive system An organ system that absorbs and digests food. The digestive system includes the esophagus, stomach, intestine, liver and pancreas.

Digital examination Using gloved fingers to examine. Usually refers to rectal or vaginal exams.

Digital manipulation Manually stimulating the penis in order to obtain a semen sample for analysis.

Digitalis glycosides Class of drugs including digitoxin and digoxin, which are drugs derived from the Digitalis purpurea plant, and used in the treatment of congestive heart failure.

Dihydrotestosterone DTHThe form of testosterone utilized by the prostate gland.

Dilated cardiomyopathy A heart condition in which the heart enlarges, but the heart muscle becomes thinner.

Dimensions of pain There are 3 dimensions of pain: sensory-discriminative, motivational-affective and cognitive-evaluative, which influence how an individual interprets and responds to a painful stimulus.

Dimethyl sulfoxide DMSO An organic solvent used to deliver other substances that themselves are less soluble.

Dinoflagellate Single-celled algae, mainly marine and often with a cellulose shell; some species may be luminescent, and some cause the red tides that are extremely toxic to marine life.

DIP Degradable intake protein. That protein or nitrogen degraded in the rumen by micoorganisms into microbial protein or freed as ammonia.

Diphenhydramine HCL Benadryl. An antihistamine.

Diploe Diploe is the anatomical term for the spongy substance between flat bones.

Dipping Immersing the entire sheep in water containing an insecticide to kill ticks or lice.

Direct Effect That portion of a trait due to an individual's genotype.

Direct lifecycle There is a single host and the host animal is the animal that is being infected.

Direct microscopic somatic cell count (DMSCC) Microscopic count of the actual number of somatic cells in milk. (This system is used to check and verify electronic cell count machines used in DHI laboratories.)

Disallowed practices Certain procedures or practices that may impair or attempt to impair the reliability of any Official DHI record.

Disbudding The practice of removing the horns on a goat.

Discharge summary A written overview of the evaluation of a patient written in lay terms for the animal owner. The summary includes what was done to the animal, what were the results of tests and what treatment is to be performed at home and how to do it.

Discoid lupus erythematosus DLEA form of systemic lupus erythematosus which only onvolves the skin.

Disease This often means only illnesses caused by infections, but veterinary surveillance also deals with other illnesses which are not infectious. It includes poisonings, illness caused by incorrect feeding or management, and welfare problems, as well as conditions (or syndromes) whose cause is unknown.

Disease control Activities aimed at preventing or curing disease in animals intended for food.

Disease distribution The geographical location and extent to which a disease is believed or known to be present.

Disease triangle Interactions between the host, the pathogen, and the environment.

Disinfectant A germicidal chemical that destroys microorganisms and the potential infectivity of a material.

Diskospondylitis Infection of the intervertebral disk with concurrent osteomyelitis of contiguous vertebrae.

Disposable syringe An all-plastic syringe designed for a single use, with a separate steel needle. Because there is no mechanism to prevent re-use, this type of syringe may be used more than once.

Disposal The collection, storage, and subsequent destruction of all syringes and needles to avoid any accidents.

Disposition The temperament of an animal.

Disqualification A quality that makes a cat ineligible for show. Disqualifications are often mentioned in the breed standard. For example, a Maine Coon with an incorrect number of toes is disqualified from show.

Disseminated intravascular coagulation DIC Concurrent stimulation of the cloting and fibrinolytic systems by a disease leading to either thrombosis or abnormal bleeding.

Disseminated intravascular coagulation DICConcurrent stimulation of the cloting and fibrinolytic systems bu disease.

Distemper Canine distemper is a viral disease that causes a severe and often fatal systemic illness in dogs and their close relatives. Distemper is also fatal in animals such as raccoons, and mustelids including skunks, mink, and ferrets.

Distichiasis An extra row of cilia or eyelashes grow from the meibomian gland openings on the eyelid margin.

Disunited Cantering or loping on different leads front and hind.

Diuresis Increased urine production. This can occur naturally in the animal, or can be induced using special drugs or fluid administration.

Diuretic Agent which increases the secretion of urine, ridding the body of excess fluid.

Diurnal Active during the day, opposite of nocturnal, which means active during the night.

Diverticulum Blind pouch (a pocket or closed branch).

Divisional Veterinary Manager The veterinary surgeon in charge of an Animal Health Divisional Office of the State Veterinary Service. The equivalent in Northern Ireland is called a DVO – Divisional Veterinary Officer.

DMI Dry matter intake.

DNA (deoxyribonucleic acid) The molecule that encodes the genes responsible for the structure and function of living organisms and that transmits genetic information from one generation to the next. DNA molecules, localized mainly in cell nuclei, are constructed of a double helix held together by hydrogen bonds between purine and pyramidine bases which project inward from two chains containing alternate links of deoxyribose (a sugar) and phosphate.

DNA vaccine (nucleic acid vaccine) Direct injection of a gene(s) coding for a specific antigenic protein(s), resulting in direct production of such antigen(s) within the vaccine recipient in order to trigger an appropriate immune response.

Dock To remove a cow's tail. This practice may keep cows udders cleaner, but may also result in cows being less content, especially in fly season.

Docking Removing the tail for sanitation purposes.

Doe A sexually mature female goat.

Doeling A female goat from one to two years old, or from one year old until first parturition.

Dog and cat travel and risk information A voluntary scheme for vets to report exotic diseases of dogs and cats.

Dog Walk Slang term that is used to describe a walk that is so slow that there is movement front to rear when sitting on the horse. This gait is used to get the horse to work on the fundamentals of the rhythms and build reach on both ends or break up a pace.

Domboro's solution Aluminum acetate solution. A topical drying agent (astringent).

Domestic animal An animal that has been housed and fed by man for generations and has little fear of man as a result. Some domestic animals learn to depend on human provision so completely that they have little ability to survive if returned to a natural habitat.

Domestic long hair (DLH) A longhair of unknown or mixed parentage.

Domestic medium hair (DMH) A semi-longhair of unknown or mixed parentage.

Domestic short hair (DSH) A shorthair of unknown or mixed parentage.

Dominance A dominant gene affects the appearance of the sheep (phenotype). A dominant gene from only one parent will change the phenotype, even if the corresponding gene from the other parent is different.

Dominant Describes a gene that covers up the physical expression of its paired allele or recessive gene. For example, black-and-white, Holsteins (B) is dominant over red-and-white (b). Thus, BB and Bb Holsteins are black-and-white, whereas bb individuals are red-and-white.

Dominant follicle The largest follicle on the ovary that secretes hormones that will suppress the other follicles so that the female will have only one egg and will prevent twinning.

Dominant gene A gene that is expressed when present either in its heterozygous or homozygous form.

Dong quai A Chinese herbal remedy made from the root of Angelica sinensis, a large plant in the carrot family. It is often called "female ginseng" because it is a general tonic for women and the female reproductive system in much the same way that ginseng acts as a tonic for men and the male reproductive system. Mixed with astragalus, it may provide a tonic for treating fatigue and other symptoms associated with blood loss.

Donor dams Genetically superior cows from which embryos are collected and transferred to recipients to allow these cows to produce a greater number of offspring than possible in a normal reproduction scheme.

Dorsal roots Nerve fibers that come into the spinal cord from the body and send sensory information to the brain.

Double To bend the horse sharply.

Double bridle. Bridle consisting of two separate headstalls and bits. The snaffle bit (bradoon) is very small.

Double dressed weight A method of selling lambs in which the shrunk dressed weight is doubled. This is the live pay weight regardless of the actual live weight.

Double standardization This refers to standardization of milk for both fat and nonfat solids (or protein).

Double tree Device that connects two single wiffletrees.

Down The soft, fur-like fluff covering a newly hatched chick; also, the fluffy part near the bottom of any feather.

Downer Cow Animal which cannot stand or walk due to sickness or injury.

Doxapram A respiratory stimulant. No longer recommended for use in CPR.

Draft Large muscular animals with adult weighing 2000 to 2600 lbs used for farm tillage and field work.

Draft horse A horse of one of the breeds of "heavy horses" developed for farm or freight work, such as Percheron, Belgian, and Clydesdale. Draft horses weigh 1,500–2,200 pounds and can be as tall as 17 hands.

Drag To hang back. Also, at the end of a column of riders, to "ride drag" or be a "drag rider."

Drenching Treating sheep for internal parasites with an oral dose of deworming medicine.

Dressage French for "training" or "schooling." The systematic art of training a horse to perform prescribed movements in a balanced, supple, obedient, and willing manner.

Dressed weight Hanging Weight

Dressing precentage The carcass weight divided by the live weight.

Dried milks Dried milk is made from whole milk; nonfat dry milk is manufactured from skim milk. In drying milks, about 95 to 98 percent of the water is removed by concentrating the solids in vacuum pans and then drying by spraying milk into a chamber of hot air or onto a slowly revolving heated drum under vacuum.

Driving Description of a horse or pony used to pull a wagon or cart.

Drop band or bunch These are smaller groups of animals separated from a larger herd or flock.

Drop the shoulder To shift weight on the forehand and lean too much to the inside during a turn.

Dropped noseband Piece of tack worn lower than a caves-son and used in conjunction with a snaffle bridle. Worn over and below the bit, it enhances sensitivity to the snaffle by positioning it on the bars and encouraging salivation.

Droppings Chicken manure or "poop".

Drove Group of swine.

Drove/droving To move sheep.

Drug resistance Drug resistance is the result of microbes changing in ways that reduce or eliminate the effectiveness of drugs, chemicals, or other agents to cure or prevent infections.

Dry Describes a nonlactating female. The dry period of cows is the time between lactations (when a female is not secreting milk).

Dry Cow A cow that is not lactating or secreting milk after it has completed a lactation period following calving.

Dry cow therapy Antibiotic therapy given at the onset of the nonlactating period of the cow. It is intended to cure and protect against intramammary infection.

Dry date First calendar day the cow is not milked (See dry period).

Dry ewe/doe A female that is not producing milk.

Dry Eye Keratoconjunctivitis sicca (KCS) is the technical term for a condition also known as 'dry eye.' It occurs because of inadequate tear production. Symptoms include a thick, yellowish discharge from the eye.

Dry Lot An open lot that may be covered with concrete, but that has no vegetative cover. Generally used as exercise areas in most of US, but may be used as primary cow housing in the more arid climates.

Dry Matter (DM) The portion of feed that is not water.

Dry matter basis An expression of feed nutrient content after the moisture has been removed by drying. Used to compare nutrient composition or animal intake of feeds differing in moisture content.

Dry off To change a lactating animal to a nonlactating one. Usually done 6 to 8 weeks prior to freshening. See involution.

Dry period A period of 45-60 days when lactation is halted before the next lactation begins. The dry period is required for rejuvenation of secretory parenchyma.

Drying off End of lactation when milking is stopped and udder is allowed time to regenerate milk-producing tissue.

Drylot A relatively small area in which cattle are confined indefinitely as opposed to being allowed to have free access to pasture.

DTH response Delayed T helper cell responses.

Dual purpose Sheep that have been bred and selected for the economic production of both wool and mutton.

Dub To trim the comb.

Duck Any of a diverse species of wild and domestic waterfowl. Ranging from tiny Call Ducks to large Muscovie and Rouen Ducks they are omnivorous. In the wild, they are found form the near arctic through the tropics near both fresh and salt water. Ducks have been domesticated for a long time.

Duckling A baby duck.

Dun A yellow or gold body and leg color, often with a black or brown mane and tail, and usually with a dorsal stripe and stripes on the legs and withers.

Duodenum The first portion of the small intestine extending from the stomach to the jejunum; most chemical digestion and absorption of nutrients occurs here.

Dura Mater The dura mater is the membrane which covers the brain.

Duration of immunity Length of time an animal is protected from a disease. Vaccines for some diseases provide long durations of immunity (years), while vaccines for some other diseases only provide immunity that lasts for 6 months.

Dusting The act of thrashing around in the dirt to clean their feathers and discourage body parasites.

Dutch collar Similar to breast collar.

Dysecdysis Abnormal shedding of the skin in reptiles.

Dysfibrinogenemia, factor I deficiency Fibrinogen, or Factor I, is an important component of the "clotting cascade" which allows your body to stop bleeding. This disease is due to either an abnormally low amount of fibrinogen, or its complete absence, or the presence of a normal amount of an abnormal and less effective fibrinogen. Symptoms include easy or excessive bleeding or no symptoms at all.

Dysmature cria A cria that has developed too slow inside the uterus. They are born weak and lacking vigor.

Dysphagia Difficulty eating and swallowing.

Dysplasia An abnormal tissue development, common in the bones of the canine.

Dyspnea Difficult or labored respiration.

Dystocia Abnormal or difficult labor, causing difficulty in delivering the fetus.

Dystrophic Disorder caused by incorrect nutrition.

Dysuria Difficult or painful urination.

E

E. coli Bacterium causing mastitis in cows and diarrhea in calves.

E. Coli scours disease that effects lambs in first 5-7 days of life causing watery, yellow diarrhea, dehydration and rapid death.

E.E.E. Eastern Equine Encephalomyelitis, viral disease of horses affecting the brain.

E.I.A. Equine Infectious Anemia, known as swamp fever. Equine infectious anemia is a disease which is caused by a virus. It can be spread by 3 principle means. Through blood sucking flys or insects. In-utero or Colostral infection, or careless use of needles or other equipment in contact with open wounds.

E.V.A. Equine viral arteritis.

Ear canal The tube that connects the external ear with the ear drum.

Ear The ear is the organ used for hearing. It converts sound into electrical impulses that are fed to the brain.

Egg tooth A horny cap on a chick's upper beak that helps the chick pip through the shell.

Ear drum The membrane that divides the outer ear from the inner ear, where the mechanism of hearing takes place. The membrane prevents infection from reaching the inner ear, as well as vibrating to amplify sounds.

Ear mites Small parasitic insects that live in the ear canal of an animal, and that are able to survive outside the ear for only very short periods of time.

Early maturing Reaches high proportion of mature size quickly: opposite of late maturing.

Earmark A distinctive mark clipped out of the ear of an animal.

Eartag A tag that generally is attached to the ear of a dairy cow for easy and accurate identification.

Earthdog Events Non competitive tests that gauge the trained and natural abilities of Dachshunds and small terriers to follow game to ground.

Earthen storage basin An earthen pond or basin for storing animal waste. Difers from an anaerobic treatment lagoon in that wastes are not stored for and extended period and microbial breakdown or treatment does not occur.

East West Front Incorrect positioning that causes the feet to turn outwards.

Easyboot A brand name for a vinyl boot that encloses the horse's hoof.

Ecdysis Shedding of the external layers of the skin in reptiles.

ECG A printout of an analysis of the electrical activity in the heart.

Echinacea An herb frequently used by Native Americans of the southwest plains and is now often seen as a garden perennial. Herbalists value the dried root for its actions against many types of viral and bacterial illnesses. It has antibiotic properties and also appears to enhance the immune system. Echinacea products come in a variety of forms: tinctures, capsules, tablets, extracts of fresh or dried roots.

Echocardiogram The image produced by performing an ultrasound examination of the heart.

Echocardiography An ultrasound exam of the heart. Passing sound waves through the heart to see the internal structure of the heart. A plain radiograph (x-ray) only shows the shape of the heart but not its internal structure.

Eclampsia Low blood calcium occuring in female dogs and cats at the end of gestation, or more commonly during early lactation. Small breed dogs are more commonly affected. Low calcium causes signs of muscle tetany.

ECP A type of estrogen sometimes used to mismate.

Ectoparasites They live outside of the body. Many of the arthropod parasites are ectoparasites; they land on your skin and cause an infestation.

Ectopic Non-malignant tissue growing in an unusual location (e.g., an ectopic pregnancy is conception of a normal embryo outside the normal location, which is the uterus).

Ectopic cilia Abnormal eyelashes originating from the upper lid on the conjunctival side, usually just a few millimeters in from the eyelid margin, about mid way along the upper lid.

Ectropion Eyelid turns outward. Allows for the accumulation of foreign matter causing eye irritation.

Edema The presence of abnormally large amounts of fluid in the intercellular tissue spaces of the body, as in a swelling of mammary glands commonly accompanying the initiation of the birthing process in many farm animals.

Effector arm The part of the immune system that recognizes and responds to infection.

Efficacy In vaccine research, the ability of a vaccine to produce a desired clinical effect, such as protection against a specific infection or disease, at the optimal dosage and schedule in a given population. A vaccine may be tested for efficacy in Phase 3 trials if it appears to be safe and shows some promise in smaller Phase 1 and 2 trials.

Efficacy Effectiveness Usually refers to the effectiveness of an AED in controlling seizures.

Efficacy rate A measure used to describe how good a vaccine is at preventing disease.

Effluent The liquid outflow or discharge of a waste treatment process.

Egg The reproductive element of birds Millions of chicken eggs are produced each year in the United States for human consumption. Duck eggs are popular fare in many parts of the world and Goose eggs are valued for their uses in baking. Hatching eggs refer to fertile eggs that will be set by a hen or hatched in an incubator. A chicken egg must be incubated for 21 days while geese require 30-31 days to hatch.

Ejaculate The movement of semen through the urethra to outside the penis.

Ejaculation Emission of semen from the stallion's urethra.

EKG A printout of an analysis of the electrical activity in the heart.

Elastrator Instrument used to apply heavy rubber bands (elastrator rings/bands) to tail and scrotum for docking and castration. Some breeders also used this method for disbudding.

Elbow Joint between the humerus and the radius and ulna, located on the foreleg between the shoulder joint (scaputahumeral) and the knee (carpal joint).

Elbow dysplasia, ED Asynchronous growth of the bones of the foreleg causing the joint to meet improperly.

Elbows Out Turning out or off from the body; not held close.

Electrocardiogram A printout of an analysis of the electrical activity in the heart.

Electrocardiography ECGA test that measures the electrical activity of the heart. ECG or EKG.

Electrocautery An instrument with a very hot tip, heated by electricity, is applied to a tissue. Electrocautery may be used to make an incision, remove a mass, or to stop bleeding.

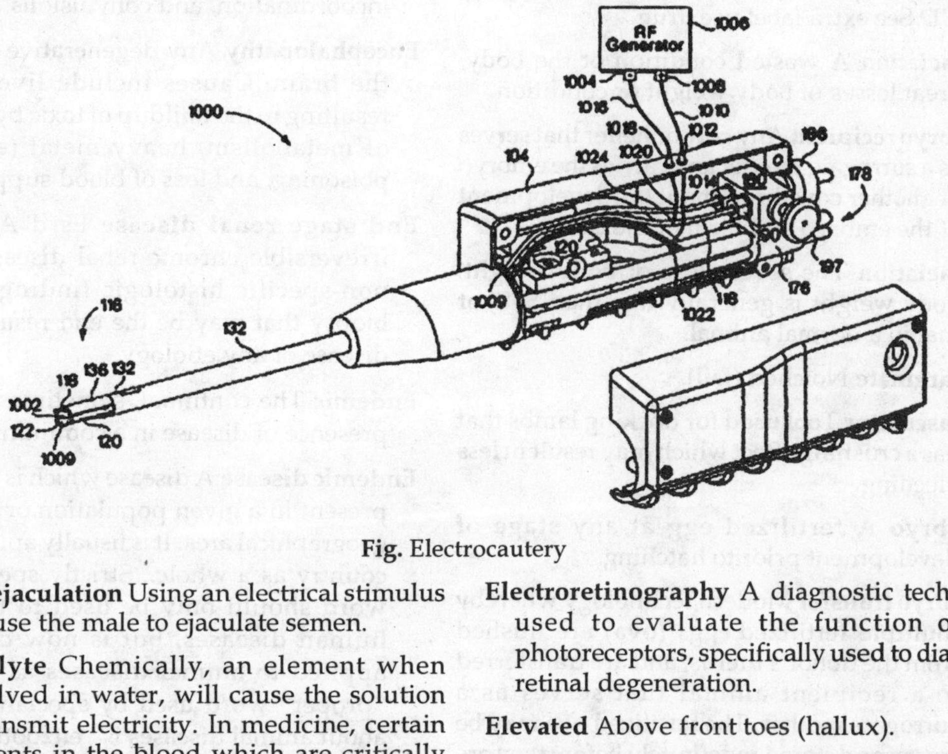

Fig. Electrocautery

Electroejaculation Using an electrical stimulus to cause the male to ejaculate semen.

Electrolyte Chemically, an element when dissolved in water, will cause the solution to transmit electricity. In medicine, certain elements in the blood which are critically important to life, including sodium, potassium, chloride, calcium, and phosphorous.

Electronic Collar A collar that provides a warning sound and/or an electric stimulation to the dog upon receipt of an electronic signal given by the user. Used as a training device.

Electronic Feeders Stations in which cows are fed specified amounts of feed by a computer that recognizes their unique electronic identification transponders.

Electroretinography A diagnostic technique used to evaluate the function of the photoreceptors, specifically used to diagnose retinal degeneration.

Elevated Above front toes (hallux).

Elimination Disqualification from placings because of an infraction of a specifically stated rule, such as a fall, going off pattern, etc.; a process of selecting semifinalists from a very large number of riders.

ELISA (Abbreviation for enzyme linked immunosorbent assay) A serological assay in which bound antigen or antibody is detected by a linked enzyme that converts a colorless substrate to a colored product.

ELISPOT assay An adaptation of ELISA in which cells are placed over antibodies or antigens attached to a plastic surface. The antigen or antibody traps the cells secreted products, which can then be detected by using an enzyme-coupled antibody that cleaves a colorless substrate to make a localized colored spot.

Elizabethan collar A large, plastic, cone-shaped collar used on cats, dogs, and birds to prevent them from licking or biting at skin, wound dressings, or casts.

ELUD See extra label use drug.

Emaciation A wasted condition of the body; great losses of body weight or condition.

Embryo recipient Any cow or heifer that serves as a surrogate mother and carries the embryo of another cow throughout the development of the embryo and birth of the calf.

Emaciation The severe loss of body weight; body weight is generally less than 50% of that in a normal animal.

Emarginate Notched (tail).

Emasculator Tool used for docking lambs that has a crushing effect which may result in less bleeding.

Embryo A fertilized egg at any stage of development prior to hatching.

Embryo transfer Modern technology whereby multiple fertilized eggs (ova) are flushed from the donor's uterus, and are transferred to a recipient animal that serves as a surrogate mother. The fertilized ova may be frozen and stored indefinitely before they are thawed and transferred to recipients.

Embryonic stem cells Stem cells derived from blastocysts (early embryos).

Embryonic vesicle The sac containing the embryo which later in pregnancy develops into a fetus.

Emerging disease A disease which has only recently been discovered, or which was previously rare but now appears to be getting more common, or which is changing in the way it affects animals.

Emesis A synonym for vomiting.

Emollient A softening agent.

Empirical therapy Therapy that is initiated based on observation of clinical symptoms and patient history only, without previous confirmation of diagnosis by laboratory or other methods.

Encephalitis Inflammation of the brain usually with severe signs such as fever, incoordination, and convulsions.

Encephalopathy Any degenerative disease of the brain. Causes include liver disease resulting in the buildup of toxic by-products of metabolism, heavy metal (e.g., lead) poisoning, and loss of blood supply.

End stage renal disease Esrd Advanced, irreversible chronic renal disease. Also a non-specific histologic finding on renal biopsy that may be the end result of renal disease of any etiology.

Endemic The continual, sometimes low-level presence of disease in a community.

Endemic disease A disease which is constantly present in a given population or in a given geographical area. It is usually applied to the country as a whole.. Strictly speaking, the word should only be used to talk about human diseases, but is now commonly applied to animal diseases as well. The "proper" word used by specialists to talk about animal diseases is "enzootic".

Endocarditis When the endocardium or inner surface of the heart becomes inflamed or irritated.

Endochondral Relating to bone formation that take place on a cartilage scaffold.

Endocrine The body system that produces hormones. Endocrine organs include the pancreas, thyroid gland, parathyroid glands, and adrenal glands. Diseases of the endocrine system may lead to the production of too much or too little hormone.

Endocrine gland An endocrine gland is one which secretes hormones into the body.

Endocytosis Incorporation of substances into a cell by a process where the cell membrane invaginates to form vesicles.

Endogenous Originating within the organism, here meaning the regeneration that would happen without intervention

Endometritis Uterine inflammation or infection due to bacteria or fungi.

Endoparasites They live within the animal.

Endorphin A morphine-like peptide that is produced in the brain and which binds to certain receptors to reduce the sensation of pain.

Endoscope A long flexible instrument which can be passed into the body to view various structures through the use of fiber optics.

Endoscopy Passing an instrument into a cavity to see the insides.

Endosome A cellular structure that is involved in the transport of proteins from the outside to the inside of the cell.

Endothelial cells Polygonal, elongated cells that form the entire lining of the vascular system (the endothelium). Their structure and functional integrity is fundamental to the integrity of vessel wall and the circulation.

Endothelial dystrophy An inherited condition seen mainly in older dogs characterized by death of endothelial cells allowing water to enter the stroma resulting in permanent edema.

Endothelium The epithelial cells lining the inside of a blood vessel.

Endotoxemia A type of shock caused by absorbing endotoxin which is released from some types of bacteria in the intestine when those bacteria die.

Endotoxin A substance released from some types of bacteria in the intestine that when absorbed into the blood causes fever and shock called endotoxic shock.

Endotracheal tube This tube is placed into the animal's trachea (windpipe) to allow the oxygen and gases to be breathed into the lungs.

End tidal CO_2 Monitoring CO_2 of exhaled gases provides information about the patient's approximate CO_2 levels and is an indirect indicator of cardiac output and blood flow.

Energy A nutrient essential for maintenance, growth, production and reproduction. Energy is required in larger amounts than any other nutrient except water, and is often the limiting factor in livestock production.

Energy medicine Therapies which use an energy field (electrical, magnetic, sonic, acoustic, microwave, infrared) to detect or treat illness. A practitioner would identify imbalances in the energy fields of the patient's body and then correct them.

Energy terminology Gross Energy (GE) The total combustible energy in a feed, determined by measuring the amount of heat produced when a feed sample is completely burnt in a bomb calorimeter.

Engage To shift weight to the hindquarters, to work off the hindquarters and stride forward with the hind legs.

Engagement Use of the horse's back and hindquarters to create energy and impulsion to forward movement. An engaged horse has a rounded top line, dropped croup, flexed abdominals, and elevated head and neck.

English Referring to riding with English tack and attire.

Enophthalmos Retraction of globe into the orbit resulting in a sunken eye.

Ensilage A green chop (forage) preserved by fermentation in a silo, pit, or stack, usually in chopped form. Also called silage.

Enteral Delivery of drugs or nutrients to the intestianl tract by deposition in the mouth, stomach or jejunum.

Enteral feeding A method to feed an animal in which a tube is placed through the body wall into the intestine, and a nutritious liquid is forced through the tube into the intestine.

Enteric A pathogen that is related to E. coli.

Enteritis An inflammation of the intestinal tract.

Enteropatogenic E. coli Specific strains of E. coli that attach very tightly to gut wall and secrete various toxins, causing both excess secretion and malabsorption as well as general systemic effects on the calf.

Enterotoxemia Actually misnamed "overeaters", it is a toxin in all healthy goats, that multiplies with a stressor to cause stomach cramps and death.

Enterotoxemia Type C Disease that affects goats in the first two weeks of life causing bloody infection of the small intestine and rapid death.

Enterotoxemia type D disease that affects unvaccinated lambs that have been placed on high energy diets.

Enterotoxigenic E. coli A specific strain K99 that attaches to intestinal cells and causes a hypersecretory diarrhea.

Entropin A heritable trait in which the lower eyelid is inverted, causing the eyelashes of the lower lid to brush against the eye.

Entropion Eyelids turn inward causing hair to irritate the surface of the eye. Normally requires surgical correction, and sometimes requires multiple surgeries.

Enucleation Removing the eye from the orbit: leaves most of the orbital contents behind.

Envenomation The act of injecting a poisonous material (venom).

Environment The total of circumstances surrounding an organism or a group of organisms, including the physical, social, and cultural conditions affecting the nature of the organism.

Environmental Derived from the animal's environment, bedding, housing, etc.

Environmental history This includes a travel history of the animal, a description of the home environment, the percentage of time the patient spends indoors vs outdoors, and the presence of other pets in the household.

Environmental mastitis Mastitis caused by coliforms and environmental Streptococci.

Environmental medicine An approach to medicine which focuses on the role of dietary and environmental allergens on health and disease. Skilled use of environmental medicine may help improve many chronic illnesses.

Enzootic disease An animal disease which is constantly present in a given population or in a given geographical area - usually applied to a country as a whole.

Enzyme A complex protein compound produced in living cells which speeds up chemical reactions without itself being changed or destroyed. It is added to animal feeds to supplement low enzyme production by some young animals or to improve utilization of feeds.

Enzyme linked immunosorbent assay ELISA An immunological technique for measuring the amount of a substance such as antibody or antigen in blood.

Eosinophil A type of white blood cell that commonly increases in numbers as a response to parasites and allergies.

Eosinophilia A condition in which there are more than the usual number of eosinophils in the circulating blood.

Epidemic An outbreak of disease. As commonly used, the word implies a large outbreak which spreads rapidly. However, epidemiologists use it to mean any number of cases of a disease which is more than expected in a population in a given period of time. So if the disease is normally absent, then just a few cases can be called an epidemic. Strictly speaking, the word should only be used to talk about human diseases, but is now commonly applied to animal diseases as well. The "proper" word used by specialists to talk about outbreaks of animal diseases is "epizootic".

Epidemiologist Someone who studies the way diseases occur in defined populations of animals or people. The study involves questions like "which animals are affected? How many are affected? When are they affected? Where are the affected animals?"

Epidemiology The study of the frequency and distribution of disease in human population. Epidemiologists are thought to be important chiefly in defense against parasitic infections; they are activated by the lymphocytes of the adaptive immune response.

Epidermal membrane Also called the fourth membrane. A membrane that covers the cria entirely at birth.

Epidermis The outer most layer of skin which is made of sequential layers called the stratum corneum, stratum granulosa, stratum spinosum, stratum basalie, and basal lamina.

Epididymitis Inflammation of the epidiymis often resulting in infertility in rams.

Epidural On the surface of the spinal cord

Epidural anesthesia Injection of an anesthetic agent into the space outside the dura mater of the spinal cord.

Epiglottis The epiglottis is a fibro-cartilaginous lid shaped like a leaf which covers the upper opening of the larynx.

Epilate Removing hair.

Epilepsy Abnormal electrical function of the brain causing disturbances of the nervous system.

Epinephrine A vasopressor drug which via alpha stimulation increases systemic vascular resistance and improves coronary and brain blood flow.

Epiphora An overflow of tears upon the cheeks due to a blockage or narrowing of the tear ducts.

Epistaxis Bleeding from the nose.

Epithelial cells Cells that line the surface of an organ such as the epithelial cells lining the vagina.

Epithelium Epithelium is an anatomical term a basic type of bodily tissue. It comprises the external surface of the skin, the internal surfaces of the digestive, respiratory and urogenital systems and others. The constituent cells of an epithelium are always closely packed together and the intercellular substance is reduced to a minimum.

Epitope A site on an antigen recognized by antibody; epitopes are also called antigenic determinants. A T-cell epitope is a short peptide derived from a protein antigen. It binds to an MHC molecule and is recognized by a particular cell.

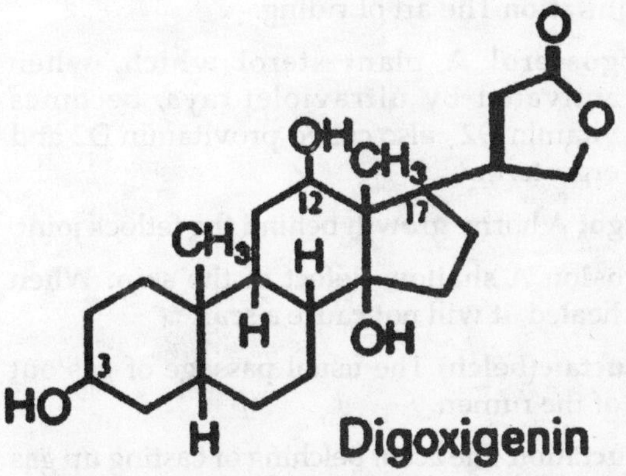

Fig. Epitope these for antibody binding

Epitope spreading Describes the fact that responses to autoantigens tend to become more diverse as the response persists.

Epizootic Designating a widely diffused disease of animals spreading rapidly and affecting many individuals of a kind concurrently in any region, thus corresponding to an epidemic in man.

Equestrian Of or pertaining to horseman or horsemanship; a rider.

Equestrienne Female rider or performer.

Equine The family of Equidae, horses, asses, and zebras.

Equine encephalomyelitis A viral disease causing inflammation of the brain and spinal cord.

Equine influenza A viral disease affecting the respiratory tract of the horse.

Equine viral arteritis A viral disease of the horse, usually mild but often causing abortion in the mare.

Equipment Sanitization The removal of microorganisms and fat, protein, and mineral residues in milking equipment through use of water, heat, and chemicals.

Equitainer A container originally designed for shipping horse semen; also used to maintain temperature control of semen from other species.

Equitation The art of riding.

Ergosterol A plant sterol which, when activated by ultraviolet rays, becomes vitamin D2 , also called provitamin D2 and ergosterin.

Ergot A horny growth behind the fetlock joint.

Erosion A shallow defect in the skin. When healed, it will not cause a scar.

Eructate(belch) The usual passage of gas out of the rumen.

Eructation The act of belching or casting up gas from the stomach.

Erysipelas A specific acute cutaneous inflammatory disease caused by b-hemolytic Streptococci and characterized by hot, red, edematous, brawny and sharply defined eruption; usually accompanied by severe constitutional symptoms.

Erythema Multiforme A medical condition characterized by inflammation of the skin or mucous membranes (including the mouth, throat and eyes). Erythema Multiforme has been reported following infection. Symptoms persist anywhere from 2 days to 4 weeks and include skin lesions, blisters, itching, fatigue, joint pain and fever.

Erythema Redness of the skin caused by blood clogging in small blood vessels.

Erythrocyte Red blood cell; contains hemoglobin, which carries oxygen to the tissues.

Escape rhythm When the SA node is firing at an abnormally slow rate, another location in the heart takes over pacing the heart. This may be the AV node or a ventricular focus.

Escutcheon The part of a cow that extends upward just above and back of the udder where the hair turns upward in contrast to the normal downward direction of hair. Also called milk mirror.

Esophageal feeder Tube placed down the esophagus of a lamb to administer milk or other liquid.

Esophageal reflux A condition in which stomach contents move backward into the esophagus, i.e., heartburn.

Esophagus The muscular tube for the passage of food from the mouth to the stomach.

Essential amino acids Amino acids that must be supplied in the diet, as the animal either cannot synthesize them or cannot synthesize them in sufficient quantities to meet requirements.

Essential host Humans are an essential element of the organisms life cycle. Example: Taeniasis - cysticercosis.

Estimated Breeding Value (EBV) An estimate of an animal's genetic merit for a particular trait based on the individual's performance and the performance of relatives. This value is expressed as a difference from the breed average.

Estimated crude protein from non-protein source ECP from NPS Non-protein nitrogen sources such as urea or ammonia; used in ruminant diets in limited amounts to enhance dietary protein levels.

Estrogen A female hormone produced by the ovaries, which results in the onset of estrus.

Estrous cycle Describes all parts of the heat cycle whereas estrus is just the stage of the heat cycle during which the female is receptive to the male.

The recurrent, restricted sexual receptivity (heat) in female mammals, commonly marked by intense sexual urge. Estrous pertains to the entire cycle of reproductive changes in the nonpregnant female animal.

Ether extract (EE) Fatty substances or lipids of foods and feeds that are soluble in ether.

European breeds Those native to Great Britain or continental Europe such as Charolais, Simmental, Limousin, Jersey, Holstein, and Guernsey.

Ether extract laboratory test A test to measure the total fat content of a feed.

Ethyl lactate A topical agent that alters follicular environment to reduce bacterial flora.

Etiology Origin or cause of.

Evaporated milk The liquid food obtained by partial removal of water from milk. The MF and TMS contents are not less than 7.5 and 25.5 percent, respectively. It contains 25 IU vitamin D per ounce and is homogenized. The food is sealed in a container and is so processed by heat, either before or after sealing, as to prevent spoilage.

Evasion Avoidance of an aid; for example, a horse that overflexes or gets "behind the bit" to keep from accepting contact with the bit.

Evening Primrose Oil The oil from the seeds of the evening primrose plant is used for a variety of ailments. Supplements may benefit arthritis and brittle hair and fingernails, and Native Americans used the oil to treat asthma, gastrointestinal ills, and bruises. The oil contains gamma linolenic acid which is a fatty acid often lacking in Western diets.

Eventing Combined training including dressage, cross country, and stadium jumping.

Eversion Turned inside out.

Ewes Female sheep which are part of the breeding herd for raising lambs.

Excoriation Superficial loss of the epidermis caused by physical damage such as scratching.

Exenteration Removal of the entire orbital contents, the globe and everything within the orbit.

Exhibition breeds Chickens kept and shown for their beauty rather than their ability to lay eggs or produce meat.

Exhibitor Someone who shows cats.

Exocrine Secreting outwardly, into, or through a duct.

Exocrine gland An exocrine gland is one which secretes onto a surface. Such as a sweat gland.

Exon A genetic sequence that codes information for the formation of a protein and that is copied and spliced together with other such sequences to form messenger RNA.

Exophthalmos Bulging of the eye. May be due to a space-occupying lesion that pushes the eye forward or may be a specific breed attribute (e.g. Pekingnese dogs).

Exophthalmos The abnormal outward protrusion (bulging) of the eye.

Exostoses/osteochondromas A specific type of benign bony outgrowth from a bone that occurs near the growth plates by an endochondral process.

Exotic An animal not native to the geographical area where it is living.

Exotic disease A disease which is not usually present in the UK but which does occur in other countries. The most important ones are notifiable diseases.

Expected Progeny Difference (EPD) The expected difference between the progeny performance of a breed average animal and the performance of an individual's progeny for any given trait(s).

Exposure Exposure does not equal poisoning, it is the dose. If you smell ammonia you have been exposed but you have not been poisoned with ammonia gas.

Expression system In genetic engineering, the cells into which a gene has been inserted to manufacture desired proteins.

Extended Longer and taller.

Extensor Muscle responsible for opening the angle of a joint.

Extensor rigidity A condition in which muscles contract and tend to straighten the limb, prevent it from relaxing.

Extensor tendons Tendons located at the front of a limb.

Extention Faster, longer strides in any gait while maintaining the original rhythm.. The outline of the horse should appear to lengthen. with the head and neck stretching forward. The stride should have more impulsion.

External Parasite Parasites that may be found on the hair, skin and in the nasal and ear passages.

Extra label use drug An antibiotic or other chemical used on the advice of a veterinarian in a dosage, route of administration, for a disease, or in some other manner not included on the approved printed package label.

Extracelluar fluid ECF Includes fluid around cells and in the plasma. Comprises 1/3 of total body water.

Extracranial Originating external to the cranial (brain) cavity.

Extrahepatic Outside of the liver.

Extra-Label Drug Use An antibiotic or other chemical used on the advice of a veterinarian in a dosage, route of administration, for a different disease or in some other manner not included on the approved printed package label.

Extroversion The process of exposure of tissues inside the streak canal of cows' teats. It is usually caused by prolonged milking and excessive milking vacuum or inadequate pulsation.

Exudate A thick fluid that is produced in response to a disease or infection.

Eye The eye is the organ of vision.

Eyelid agenesis Born without part of the upper eyelids.

F

Feather legged Having feathers growing down the shanks, i.e., Cochins and Brahmas.

F1 Progeny resulting from the mating of a purebred ram and a purebred ewe of different breeds.

Face The horse's head. Also, to turn toward a cow.

Facial fold trichiasis Seen in brachycephalic breeds that have a large facial fold and the hair from the facial fold touches the medial aspect of the cornea.

Facing correcting wool blindness by removing wool from the face.

Fading puppy syndrome An apparently normal puppy gradually weakens and dies within a week or two of birth. Not a specific disorder, but generally applied to infectious causes.

Fall For a horse, shoulder and hindquarter on the same side touch the ground; for a rider, separation between the rider and horse necessitating remounting.

Fallopian tubes The Fallopian tubes are two tubes in mammals which carry eggs from the ovary to the uterus. Eggs are fertilised in the Fallopian tubes by sperm, and then moved to the ovary by way of cilia.

Fallow Pale cream to light fawn color; pale yellow; yellow-red. Color definitions may vary by breed. Always check the breed standard for the definitive color description.

False heat The display of estrus by a female animal when she is pregnant.

Fancier A person especially interested and usually active in some phase of the sport of purebred dogs.

Fang See Canines Teeth

Far side The horse's right side.

Farm A farm includes stock, dairy, poultry, fish, fruit, and truck farms, plantations, ranches, ranges, orchards and plant nursery. This includes growing, feeding, protecting, tending, etc., the product of the farm, not just the harvesting.

Farm cat Helps keep the barns free of mice and rats.

Farrier A skilled horse shoer.

Farrow When a sow gives birth to pigs.

Farrowing area Where the sow furrows.

Fat A term used in a general sense to refer to both fats and oils. Fat supplied 2.25 times as much energy as carbohydrates. Both fats and oils share the same general structure and chemical properties, but have different physical properties, i.e., oils are liquid at room temperature.

Fat corrected milk The estimated quantity of milk calculated on an equivalent energy basis. It is a means of evaluating milk production records of different dairy animals and breeds on a common energy basis.

Fat differential The amount added to or subtracted from the blend price for each 0.1 percent that the milk fat is above or below 3.5 percent. For example, if the blend price is $9.00/cwt and the fat differential is 10›, a dairyman with milk of 4.0 percent milk fat would receive $9.50/cwt.

Fat soluble vitamins Includes vitamins A, D, E and K. Vitamins A, D and E are supplemented in many livestock rations. Fat soluble vitamins are stored in body fat reserves.

Fault Scoring unit to keep track of knockdowns, refusals, or other offenses.

Favor To limp slightly.

Fawn A brown, red-yellow with hue of medium brilliance. Color definitions may vary by breed. Always check the breed standard for the definitive color description.

Feathering Longer fringe of hair on ears, legs, tail, or body.

Febrile Relating to fever; feverish.

Fecal coliform bacteria See coliform bacteria.

Fecal flotation A procedure, performed by a veterinarian, used to identify various parasite eggs in a fecal (manure) sample.

Fecal Pertaining to feces.

Fecal oral transmission cycle A cycle of disease spread where the pathogen is shed in the sick animal's feces and infects other animals when they ingest something contaminated by the infected feces.

Feces The manure or excrement produced by an animal.

Fecundity Efficiency of an individual in production of young. Animals that bring forth young frequently, regularly, and, in case of those that bear more than one offspring at a birth, in large numbers, are said to be fecund.

Federation of cooperatives An organization of cooperatives that provides for joint activities but allows each cooperative to manage its own affairs.

Feed Food for animals. Amount will be determined by number of animals, age, etc.

Feed additives Products added to basic feed mixes to improve the rate and/or efficiency of gain, prevent certain diseases, or preserve feeds.

Feed bag A sack usually of canvas and leather held on the horse's nose by a strap behind its ears allowing it to eat grain without a manger or other container.

Feed efficiency (feed conversion) The units of feed consumed per unit of weight increase or unit of production (milk, meat, eggs).

Feed grade Term to describe the quality of feedstuffs suitable for animal, but no human, consumption.

Feed processing Physical or chemical changes in feedstuffs which influence their nutritional value.

Feeder lamb A lamb lacking in weight and/or finish that is usually placed in a feedlot for finishing to slaughter weight and grade.

Feeder pig Young pig that is ready to feed and get ready for the market. Feeder pigs weigh from 40 to 120 pounds.

Feeder/finisher pigs Pigs from weaning age (25 40 pounds) to market size (220+ pounds)

Feedlot Type of farm where a large number of young cattle can be fed gain type feeds, such as corn, oats, or barley.

Feedstuff An edible material that contributes nutrients to animals' diets.

Feline Immunodeficiency Virus A virus that chronically suppresses the immune system of cats resulting in secondary infections.

Feline Pertaining to cats.

Fell The thin parchment like membrane (tissue or skin) covering lamb. It should be removed on all cuts.

Felting The property of wool fibers to interlock with each other if they are rubbed together under pressure and in moist condition while heated.

Femininity Possession of well-developed secondary female sex characteristics.

Feminization A male showing signs of being under the influence of the female hormone, estrogen.

Femur The femur is the thigh bone in the human leg.

Fender Part of the Western saddle that protects a rider's leg from the rigging. The wide leather strap, on the western saddle, between the saddle seat and the stirrup on which the riders leg rests.

Fenoxycarb An insect growth regularor recently withdrawn from the market.

Fentanyl patches A sticky patch impregnated with the narcotic fentanyl which is applied topically for sustained release and absorption of the drug.

Fenthion A "pour-on" organophosphate preparation.

Fermented feed Fodder preserved by storing in piles or air-tight structures causing it to ferment and heat; also any feed that has become damp accidentally, causing it to ferment.

Fertile Capable of producing a chick.

Fertility Capable of conceiving and bearing offspring.

Fertilization The process of sperm combining with eggs.

Fertilization rate The percentage of females bred that get pregnant. A 90% fertilization rate means that 9 out of 10 females bred get pregnant.

Fertilized Containing sperm.

Fetal Refers to a puppy or kitten before birth.

Fetch 1. The retrieving of game by the dog.

2. The command to retrieve game.

Fetlock The tuft of hair on the back side of the fetlock joint.

Fetlock joint Between the cannon (metacarpus or metatarsus) and the pastern (first phalanx) including the sesamoid bones; sometimes referred to as ankle.

Fetotomy Dissection of a dead fetus into smaller pieces to allow for easier removal from the mother

Fetus The unborn young of a viviparous vertebrate having a basic structural resemblance to the adult animal.

Fever In dogs, a body temperature reading over 103Æ'.

Feverfew A perennial with small blossoms and leaves that are medicinal. The leaves are helpful in the treatment of migraine headaches. This may be due to its ability to block release of inflammatory substances from the blood. Although recommended for routine use, it may help dogs with pain from arthritis.

Fiador Knotted rope throatlatch, used in conjunction with a basal, browband headstall, and horsehair reins. The knots of the fiador are the hackamore, the fiador, and the sheet bend.

Fiber The portion of a feed that is indigestible or slowly digested by ruminants. May be expressed as crude fiber, non-detergent fiber, acid detergent fiber, or effective fiber.

Fiberoptic Bundles of glass fibers that transmit light and permit one to see around corners.

Fibroblast growth factors (FGF) A family of protein growth factors involved in new blood vessel formation, wound repair, lung maturation, and the development of skeletal muscle, specific lineages of blood cells and bone marrow stroma. FGFs are recognized by a family of cell surface receptors that have the ability to catalyze reactions inside the cell after they are activated by the FGFs.

Fibroproliferative Of or relating to the growth and proliferation of fibroblasts, the most basic connective tissue cell.

Fibrosarcoma A malignant tumor arising from collagen-producing fibroblasts (an immature fiber-producing cell of connective tissue).

Fibrous a. Containing, consisting of, or resembling fibers.

b.Characterized by fibrosis.

c. capable of being separated into fibers.

Fibrous Joints In anatomy, fibrous joints are articulations in which the surfaces of the bones are fastened together by intervening fibrous tissue, and in which there is no appreciable motion. For example between the bones of the cranium.

Fibula The fibula is the lateral bone of the leg. It is slender, compared to the tibia. It's purpose is to give attachment to the muscles.

Figure eight nose band. Noseband popular with eventers; straps cross in an 'X' on the bridge of the horse's nose for better leverage and control.

Figure of 8 suture pattern A suture pattern used on wedge resections of the lower eyelid. It gives good apposition and the eyelid eyelid margin remains continuous.

Filamentous Very long and slender.

Fill A term designating the fullness of the digestive tract of an animal. Also used to identify a phase of packaging milk and/or milk products in which containers are filled with product.

Filled milk Milk from which milk fat has been removed and replaced with other fats or oils.

Filly Female horse 4 years and under that has never produced a foal.

Filoplumes Hairlike feathers.

Filter DNA A mastitis screening test useful in determining somatic cells present in milk by filtering and measuring the amount of deoxyribonucleic acid (DNA) produced.

Finasteride A 5 alpha-reductase inhibitor that prevents the conversion of testosterone to dihydrotestosterone.

Fine needle aspirate Suction is applied to a hollow needle which has been inserted into tissue and a core of the tissue is withdrawn to culture and/or examine microscopically.

Finish The amount of fat beneath the skin of a meat bird.

Finishing The act of feeding an animal to produce a desirable carcass for market.

Fipronil Trade name is Frontline. A phenylpyrazole insecticide which acts as a neurotoxin.

First calf A term commonly used to indicate the first calf born to bovine females.

First generation First generation: A description of medications developed from an earlier form of the medication. First generation medications were developed from the original form of the drug; second generation medications are adaptations of first generation drugs; third generation drugs are adaptations of second generation, etc.

Fissure Splitting of the skin surface.

Fistula An artificial opening into an animal, e.g. the rumen.

Flag Rhythmic motion of stallion's tail when he ejaculates.

Flagellum Flagellum are a small hair-like organ on the surface of certain cells. They are the motile organs of the sperm cells of higher animals.

Flank (1). In roping, to hold a calf by its flank and leg and place it on its side.

Flank (2). The area of a horse's barrel between the rib cage and the hindquarters.

Flash noseband Cross between a cavesson and a figure-eight noseband.

Flat Class without jumping.

Flat Barn An area for milking cattle where the person milking is on the same level as the cow. May be used with a pipeline or bucket milking system. Generally the same area is used for cow housing.

Flat barn milking area An area for milking cattle where the person milking cattle is on the same level or floor as the cattle. May be used with pipeline or bucket milking systems.

Flat bone In human anatomy, flat bones occur where the principal requirement of the skeleton is to protect delicate structures or provide broad surfaces for muscular attachment. The bones are comprised of two thin layers of compact bone separated by a variable quantity of spongy substance.

Flat foot walk A true flat foot walk is a four-beat gait in which each foot is picked up and set down in an even cadence. The rear end movement should be smooth and close to the ground without any snap or pop. Each stride should reach forward and slide in as it is set down, over striding the track of the front foot. The head shake is in time with the rear feet and should be smooth. The tail should set still and flow.

Flatulence Passing gas from the intestinal tract. May be a sign of disease of the small intestine.

Flaxen A golden mane or tail on a darker-bodied horse.

Flea dip A solution made to kill fleas, applied to an animal and not rinsed off, to allow it to have residual action.

Fleece The wool from one sheep. The coat of the sheep usually removed as one unit. The term "fleece" correctly applies only to wool fabrics, although there are so-called fleeces of other fibers.

Flehmen A reaction to odd smells or tastes; horse curls upper lip upward.

Flex To bend the horse to the inside. Also, to give in the poll and yield to rein contact.

Flexion Characteristic of a supple and collected horse, there are two types of flexion 1. vertical or longitudinal, which is often mistakenly associated with "headset," when in reality it is an engagement of the entire body abdomen, hindquarters, back, neck, and head

2. lateral, which is side-to-side arcing or bending characteristic of circular work.

Flexor Muscle responsible for closing the angle of a joint.

Flexor tendons Tendons located at the rear of a limb.

Flight Zone Maximum zone of comfort or security of animals.

Float To file a horse's teeth to remove sharp points; (n.) a file like instrument used to float teeth.

Floating The process of filing off sharp edges of a horse's teeth.

Flock A group of sheep that are managed together. Sheep have inborn ability or desire to flock, or gather, together. This is also known as gregariousness.

Flow sheets Flow sheets are records of patient data over time. These may include a tabular summary of laboratory test results, vital signs or drugs administered.

Fluid milk Milk commonly marketed as fresh liquid milks and creams. It is the most perishable form of milk and commands the highest price per unit volume. Also called market milk.

Fluid milk products Milk, flavored milk, concentrated milk, filled milk, skim milk, fortified skim milk, lowfat milk, buttermilk, milk drinks, and cream products.

Fluid therapy Fluid therapy is broadly defined to include the administration of many types of fluids including crystalloids and colloids. Fluid therapy may be given to prevent or correct fluid deficits or electrolyte abnormalities. Correct water imbalance from excessive fluid loss or inadequate intake Hemorrhage Vomiting Diarrhea Polyuria Expand blood volume - shock Correct electrolyte imbalance(s) Correct acid-base imbalance Supply blood components Supply calories and nutrients Renal disease - promote renal blood flow

Fluorescein stain A stain applied to the cornea to assess for corneal and conjunctival epithelial defects or to assess the patency of the nasolacrimal ducts.

Fluoroscopy An x-ray procedure in which x-rays are transmitted through the body onto a fluorescent screen; beneficial in that movement of joints or organ systems can be observed (e.g., the movement of material through the esophagus, stomach, and intestines).

Flush season Time during the year, usually spring and early summer, of maximum milk production.

Flush System A manure removal system in which an area is cleaned by high volumes of fresh water, or gray water that is recycled from a manure pit or lagoon.

Flushing The practice of conditioning ewes before breeding by turning them to better pasture or feeding small amounts of grain. Flushing is done to increase the number of twin and triplet lambs that will be born.

Flutd Feline lower urinary tract disease; a condition in cats characterized by blood in the urine, urination outside of the litter box, and straining to urinate. The name for this condition was previously called feline urological syndrome (FUS).

Fly back A bad habit in which a horse will suddenly pull back, often resulting in a broken halter or tie.

Fly snapping Repeated snapping at non-existent flying object has been associated in BMDs with partial seizures, in some cases with ear infections, and in a few cases with food allergies. Some forms may be alleviated by seizure medications. A few have been alleviated with behavioral modification techniques, which may indicate that some forms are simply behavioral problems often caused by boredom.

Fly strike Cutaneous myiasis. A result of cutaneous parasitism by larvae of flesh flies, blow flies and/or the screwworm fly.

Flying change A change of lead at the lope, without slowing to the trot.

Flying lead change Change from one lead to another without changing gait.

Foal A young, nursing horse of either sex. (v.) the act of foaling, when a mare delivers her young.

Foal colic Abdominal pain in a mare, following foaling. due to the rapid contracting of the uterus.

Foal heat Estrus that occurs in most mares 9 days after foaling.

Foaling The process of a mare giving birth.

Focal Seizures Also called partial seizures. These seizures affect a part of the brain and thus just a part of the body – like the flicking of an ear. Focal seizures are more likely from secondary epilepsy than primary.

Fodder Coarse food for cattle or horses, such as corn stalks or straw.

Foetus A foetus is an unborn offspring of an animal.

Folic acid One of the vitamins in the B complex. It is involved in the synthesis of amino acids and DNA.

Follicle A follicle is a small group of cells that surrounds and nourishes a structure such as a hair (hair follicle) or a cell such as an egg (Graafian follicle).

Follicle stimulating hormone FSHFSH has the primary responsibility for promoting growth of follicles on the ovaries.

Follicular cycle The series of events that occur when the ovary produces a follicle (an egg) and the follicle goes through a series of changes.

Folliculitis Superficial bacterial dermatitis associated with the hair follicle.

Fomite A vector of disease transmission that has no part in the pathogen's life cycle. A contaminated milking towel that spreads disease from cow to cow with each subsequent use is a fomite.

Fontanelle The fontanelle is a membrane covered vault in the skull. It normally closes during infancy.

Food chain The path along which food energy is transformed between two or more species.

Food hypersensitivity An allergy. An adverse reaction to food with a proven immunologic basis.

Food intolerance An adverse reaction to food that does not have a proven immunologic basis.

Food poisoning An adverse reaction to a food caused by a direct effect of a toxin.

Food producing animal Animals raised for the purpose of providing food for humans. Most commonly this refers to poultry, swine, cattle and sheep, but does not exclude other domestically managed animals.

Foot bath A long shallow tub or depression in the concrete where cows walk through a mild solution (usually including copper sulfate or formalin) to promote foot health. Usually located along an alley where cows return from the milking parlor.

Foot rot An inflammation occurring between the toes and in the hooves of sheep and cattle. It is caused by a combination of fungus and bacteria.

Forage Roughage of high feeding value. Grasses and legumes cut at the proper stage of maturity and stored to preserve quality are forage. A crop that is high in fiber and grown especially to feed ruminant animals.

Forced air incubator A mechanical device for hatching fertile eggs that has a fan to circulate warm air.

Forcing Pen Pen used to confine animals prior to moving them into treatment chutes.

Forehand That portion of the horse from the heart girth forward.

Foreign body Any abnormal substance within the body. Examples include wood slivers, ingested cloth or balls, glass in the feet, etc.

Forelock The hair growing between a horse's ears that falls on the forehead; a horse's "bangs."

Forequarters The two front quarters of a cow. Also called the fore udder.

Foresaddle Unsplit from half of lamb or mutton.

Forestripping Expressing streams of milk from the teat prior to machine milking to determine visual quality and to stimulate "letdown."

Fork Part of the swells of a saddle that makes up the gullet.

Foster mother A mother that is rearing a lamb or kid other than her own.

Founder Another word for laminitis, a serious disease affecting a horse's hooves and often caused by a horse's eating too much grain or green pasture.

Four beat lope An incorrect lope, where the horse strikes the ground in a broken rhythm.

Fovea The fovea is a small depression in the retina where vision is most acute.

Fowl 1. Domesticated birds raised for food.

2. A stewing hen.

Fox Trot The fox trot is a broken diagonal gait with a distinctive rhythm that is created by a horse moving its front foot a split second before its opposite rear foot. The fox trot is a smooth gait because the horse is in contact with the ground at all times. A horse that is foxtrotting correctly will never have more than two feet off the ground at any given time. On both the front and back ends the horse will sit one foot down as it picks the other foot up and for a moment both feet will be touching the ground.

Fracture A break in the bone; generally caused by trauma, twisting, or weakened bone structure due to disease.

Fragmented coronoid process, FCP The coronoid process fragments forming a loose body in the elbow joint, called a joint mouse.

Free choice(ad libitum) Feed made available to an animal at all times (same as self-fed).

Free mating free mating Also called paddock mating. A single male is introduced with a band of females.

Free radical Atom which carries an unpaired electron; free radicals can potentially injure cells and may be responsible for numerous age-related diseases.

Free range To allow chickens to roam a yard or pasture at will.

Free stalls Resting cubicles or "beds" in which dairy animals are free to enter and leave, as opposed to being confined in stanchions.

Free stall barn Housing for cattle where cows can freely enter unoccupied stalls. Most common housing barn in the Northwest.

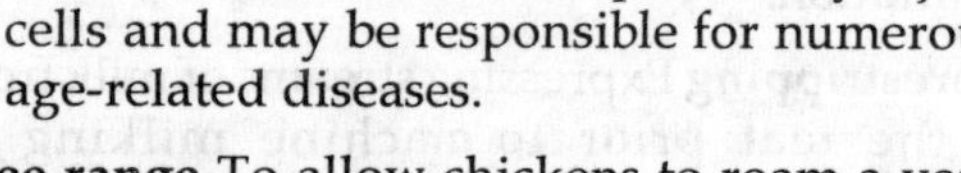

Fig. Free stall barn

Free walk Walk on a loose rein to allow the horse to stretch its neck and lower its head.

Freemartin Female born twin to a bull calf (about 9 out of 10 of these will not conceive). A sterile heifer born twin with a bull.

Freeze branding A method of identification with a cold iron to aid in easily identifying dairy cattle

Freeze drying The evaporation of water from a frozen product with the aid of high vacuum. Also called lyophilization.

Freight Expense of hauling milk, grain, or livestock. Watch for netted sales with freight also deducted separately.

Frenching Removing one-and-a half inches of meat from the end opposite the loin eye of roast or rib chop.

Frenulum A piece of tissue that maintains adhesion between the penis and prepuce.

Fresh A cow that has recently given birth to a calf. Also refers to dairy products having original qualities unimpaired and those recently produced or processed.

Fresh Cow A cow that has recently given birth to a calf.

Fresh frozen plasma Plasma that has been separated from the RBC shortly after blood collection and then frozen. Coagulation factors are preserved in this blood product.

Fresh Milk Dairy products having original qualities unimpaired and those recently produced or processed.

Freshen Commonly used to designate the act of calving (parturition); to give birth to a calf and concurrently initiate lactation.

Freshening Parturition, calving.

Frizzle 1. Feathers that curl rather than laying flat.

2. A breed of chicken.

Frog Wedge-shaped pad in the sole of the hoof which acts as a shock absorber for the hoof. It contacts the ground first at each step and aides in pumping blood.

Frontal bone The frontal bone is the plate at the front of the top of the human skull. It forms the forehead.

Frontline spray Generic name is Fipronil.

Frozen plasma Plasma that has been separated from RBC after blood collection but not with the intent of preserving the labile coagulation factors. Used primarily to provide plasma protein in hypoproteiemic patients.

Fryers Chicken raised from 90 120 days, then sold for meat.

Full sibs Animals having the same sire and dam, such as full brothers, full sisters, and/ or a full brother-sister pair.

Functional antibody An antibody that binds to an antigen and has an effect that can be demonstrated in laboratory tests.

Fungi Single-celled or multicellular organisms. Fungi can be either opportunistic pathogens (such as aspergillosis, candidiasis, and cryptococcosis) that cause infections in healthy persons. Fungi are also used for the development of antibiotics, antitoxins, and other drugs used to control various human diseases.

Fungicide A substance that kills fungi.

Furuncle A painful, nodular adcess in the skin.

FUS (Feline urologic syndrome) A collection of signs in cats resulting in blood in the urine, straining to urinate, and urinating in abnormal locations. The more current term is feline lower urinary tract disease (FLUTD).

Futurity A show class or event for young horses that requires entering long (often years) before the actual event.

G

Gizzard An organ that contains grit for grinding up the grain and plant fiber a chicken eats.

Gait Any forward movement of a horse, the rhythmic movement of the feet and legs, natural or acquired by training. The three natural gaits are walk, trot, canter and or gallop.

Gaited horse An animated horse such as the American Saddlebred, Morgan, or Tennessee Walking Horse with flashy gaits.

Galactopoietic Stimulating or increasing secretion of milk.

Gall Bladder The gall bladder is a small muscular sac attached to the liver.

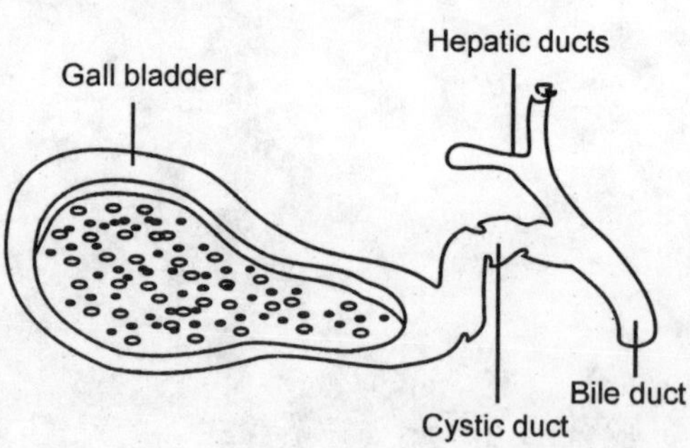

Fig. Gall Bladder

Gallop Fastest of dog gaits; has a four-beat rhythm and often an extra period of suspension during which the body is propelled through the air with all four feet off the ground.

Galls Sores and/or swelling.

Galvayne's groove V-shaped groove that appears at the gum line of the corner incisor at age of 10.

Gambrel Restrainer Restraining device that is a gambrel-shaped piece of plastic that is placed over the top of the animal's neck, with slots on either side to hold both front legs of the animal.

Game Hunted wild birds or animals.

Gamebirds Any of several species including Pheasant, Quail and Partridge/Grouse that have traditionally been hunted for food and sport. Gamebirds may be raised in captivity but are not domestic in the senses that chickens are. The term can also be used for Wild turkey and some species of wild waterfowl.

Gametocytes Precursors of the sexual forms of the malaria parasite, which release either male or female gametes within the stomach of the mosquito.

Gammalinolenic acid A fatty acid which found in evening primrose oil or black currant oil. Gammalinolenic acid is an effective anti-inflammatory agent. It also promotes healthy growth of skin, hair, and nails. It may be good for skin conditions, arthritis, and autoimmune disorders; however, it takes six to eight weeks to see changes after the addition of gammalinolenic acid to the diet.

Gander A male goose.

Ganglion A ganglion is an enlargment occuring somewhere in the course of a nerve, and containing nerve cells in addition to nerve filaments.

Garget A common term for an inflammation of the udder of the cow or the resulting abnormal milk. More accurately referred to as mastitis.

Garlic This herb is valued as a pungent culinary spice, but it has also gained recognition as a medicinal remedy. Raw garlic is antibacterial and anti-fungal, but this action is lost when garlic is cooked or dried. Raw garlic can also have an anti-inflammatory action. It is also thought to strengthen the cardiovascular system by reducing cholesterol and lowering blood pressure.

Gas colic Colic caused by excessive amounts of gas in the stomach and/or intestines.

Gaskin The heavy muscular area between the hock and the stifle.

Gastric Another term for stomach.

Gastric dilatation Gastric dilatation means stomach distention or enlargement, caused by expanding gas. This may or may not be accompanied by volvulus, or torsion, or twisting of the stomach on its long axis.

Gastric Juice Gastric Juice is a clear, colourless fluid secreted by the mucous membrane of the stomach, and is the chief agent in digestion.

Gastric lavage To flush out the stomach.

Gastric System The Gastric System refers to all parts of the body which contribute to digestion.

Gastritis Inflammation of the stomach.

Gastrocnemius The Gastrocnemius is a muscle forming most of the human calf.

Gastroenteritis Chemical, bacterial, or viral inflammation of the mucosa of the stomach and intestines.

Gastrointestinal Also known as GI. Pertaining to the stomach and intestines. The term 'digestive system' includes the mouth, gastrointestinal tract, anus, pancreas, and liver.

Gay Tail A tail carried above the horizontal level of the back.

Geld To castrate a male horse.

Gelding A castrated or neutered male horse. This is done to make the horse safer to work or ride.

Gene A specific sequence of DNA or RNA that is located on a chromosome. A gene is the functional unit of inheritance controlling transmission and expression of one or more traits by specifying the structure of a particular protein.

Gene pool The collective genetic information contained within a population of sexually reproducing organisms.

Gene therapy The insertion of normal or genetically altered genes into cells, usually to replace defective genes especially in the treatment of genetic disorders.

Genealogy Recorded family descent. Pedigree.

Generalized Seizure Also called Tonic-Clonic seizures. If the whole brain is involved in the seizure, it is a generalized seizure. Can be Grand Mal or Mild, but are usually associated with primary epilepsy.

Generation Interval Average age of parents when the animals that will replace them in the flock are born. This represents the average turnover rate of a flock.

Genes A hereditary unit consisting of a sequence of DNA that occupies a specific location on a chromosome and determines a particular characteristic in an organism. Genes undergo mutation when their DNA sequence changes.

Genetic appraisal Cows and sires are evaluated by researchers at the Animal Improvement Programs Laboratory, ARS-USDA, to determine their genetic values.

Genetic base The average genetic merit of a population (usually a breed) at a specific period, which is used as a reference point to express a genetic difference from a base population (genetic merit of cows and bulls).

Genetic Correlation Relationships between traits that arise because some of the same genes affect both traits.

Genetic Merit The genetic worth of an animal for a particular trait can be expressed as an EPD, EBV or ABC.

Genetic Progress An increase in the average genetic merit of a population for a particular trait as a result of selective breeding.

Genetic trend Genetic change per year for a trait in the population.

Genetically Linked Defects Problems with health or temperament that are passed to offspring by their ancestors.

Genetics The branch of science concerned with the means and consequences of transmission and generation of the components of biological inheritance.

Genic Producing, formic; produced by.

Genome The complete set of genes present in a cell, parasite, or virus.

Genome Wide Linkage Analysis The study of the relationship between genetic markers of affected vs. unaffected individuals in a family with a genetic disease in order to localize chromosomal region of the gene responsible for the disease.

Genotype Environment Interaction Changes in the ranking of performance of genotypes in different environments. For example, one genotype may perform the best in one environment and only average in another environment.

Genotype The actual genetic constitution (makeup) of an individual as determined by its germ plasm. For example, there are two genotypes for black-and-white Holsteins—BB and Bb. See dominant.

Geographical information system A computer system capable of assembling, storing, manipulating, and displaying geographically referenced information (i.e. spatial data).

Geographical location A place or site that is spatially referenced to the earth's surface.

Germicidal A substance that has the ability to kill germs.

Germs Any microscopic organism that can potentially cause disease; includes viruses, bacteria, and fungi.

Gestation Period of pregnancy beginning at conception and ending with birth (142-152 days).

Gestation Pregnancy (gravidity) The period from conception to birth. The period of fetal development betweenfertilization of the ovum and birth of the offspring.

Get The offspring of a male A get-of-sire refers to given number (commonly four) of progeny from a sire.

Ghee Concentrated milk fat prepared by melting butter, decanting the fat after gravity separation from the serum, and driving off most of the remaining moisture by heating. About 1 percent moisture remains. It is used mostly in Asia and Africa.

Gills Gills are a respiratory organ found in animals which obtain oxygen from water, such as crustaceans, molluscs, fish and amphibians.

Gilt Female pig less than 1 year old that has never had a litter of pigs.

Ginger An herb valued as a culinary seasoning and also considered a remedy for a variety of illnesses. Dry ginger is a good anti-inflammatory, and together with garlic it can replace the need for aspirin-like (NSAID) drugs. Fresh or pickled ginger is good as an anti-emetic compound and calms an upset stomach. It relieves motion sickness and dizziness and improves digestion.

Gingiva The gums.

Gingival Relating to the gums.

Gingivitis Inflammation and swelling of the gums surrounding the teeth. The gingiva are normally pink and become red when inflamed.

Ginkgo Extracts of leaves from the ginkgo tree (Ginkgo bilboa) are able to increase the blood flow to the brain. It is able to increase vasodilation and thus improve the blood flow in peripheral areas such as the lower legs and feet.

Ginseng There are two species of ginseng: Oriental ginseng (Panax ginseng) and American ginseng (Panax quinquefolium). Both contain compounds that work on the pituitary-adrenal axis to increase resistance to stress and to affect metabolism, skin and muscle tone, and hormonal balance. Oriental ginseng is more of a stimulant and can raise blood pressure in some humans. The oriental ginseng strengthens the immune system and increases the body's ability to deal with fatigue and stress.

Girth Belly band – strap around horse's body (heart girth) just behind front legs, which holds saddle or harness in place.

Giving milk Lactating, or the act of yielding milk by a mammal.

Gizzard An organ located between the stomach and the intestines inside the chicken's body. The gizzard grinds the food of the chicken and serves as the "chicken's teeth."

Glabrous Hairless areas of skin.

Gland A gland is a bodily organ that manufactures and secretes enzymes, hormones or other chemicals.

Glans penis The end of the penis.

Glaucoma Increased pressure within the eye caused by an accumulation of fluids; can lead to blindness if left untreated.

Glia Nervous system support cells; make up approximately 90% of nervous system cells

Glipizide An oral medication that can be used to control blood glucose levels in some diabetic cats who still have some insulin production.

Glomerular filtration rate GFR The rate at which the glomeruli form filtrate from blood in glomerular capillaries. GFR correlates with renal function and to renal blood flow. Kidney disease and dehydration both result in a decrease in GFR.

Glomerulonephritis Inflammatory disease of the glomerulus, part of the kidney, which filters toxic waste from the blood. Tests of the urine can show a variety of abnormalities. Complete loss of kidney function can occur.

Glomerulus This literally means a small cluster; commonly used to refer to the renal glomerulus, the area of blood filtering in the kidney.

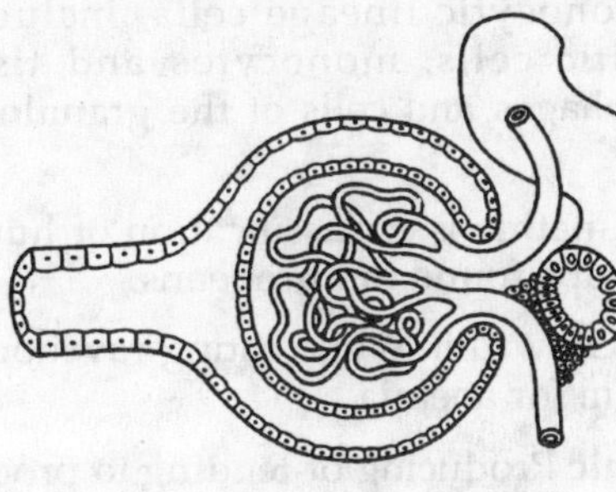

Fig. Glomerulus

Glucocorticoid Hormones produced by the adrenal gland which regulate protein, carbohydrate and fat metabolism, and are important to almost every function of cells and organs. They also stabilize cell membranes which is an important part of their function in treating allergic reactions. Also called glucocorticosteroids.

Glucocorticosteroid Hormones produced by the adrenal gland which regulate protein, carbohydrate and fat metabolism, and are important to almost every function of cells and organs. They also stabilize cell membranes which is an important part of their function in treating allergic reactions. Also called glucocorticoids.

Glucosamine One of the building blocks the body uses to make new cartilage.

Glucosuria Glucose in the urine. (Also called glycosuria.)

Gluteus maximus The Gluteus maximus is a large muscle in the human back-side.

Glycogen A storage form of glucose in the body.

Glycoprotein A protein-conjugate with a carbohydrate (sugar) component.

Glycosaminoglycans Compounds which serve as the building blocks of cartilage, which covers the ends of bones within a joint. Glucosamine and chondroitin are necessary for the body to make glycosaminoglycans.

GM CSF Granulocyte macrophage colony stimulating factor is a cytokine involved in the growth and differentiation of myeloid and monocytic lineage cells, including dendritic cells, monocytes and tissue macrophages and cells of the granulocyte lineage.

Gnathic Gnathic is a classification of human skull shape found in Europeans.

Go light Grow thin while eating ravenously; synonym for anemia.

Goitrogenic Producing or tending to produce goiter (enlargement of the thyroid gland).

Goldenseal A small perennial with white flowers and red berries. The dried roots and rhizomes are used to treat respiratory and skin infections. It acts as a stimulant, dries up secretions of mucous membranes, reduces inflammation, and fights infection . Goldenseal also promotes the production of saliva, bile and digestive enzymes.

Gonadotropin releasing hormone GnRH A hormone released from the hypothalamus that stimulates the release of follicle stimulating hormone (FSH) and luteinizing hormone (LH).

Gonioscopy A technique used to evaluate the iridocorneal angle to help judge the risk for glaucoma in an eye.

Gonys Lower edge of mandible.

Good management/farming practices Routine practices that minimize risk from harmful antimicrobial resistant bacteria or resistance genes through good farm management and hygiene practices (e.g. optimal housing conditions and feeding strategies) and other non-antimicrobial disease preventive strategies, whilst maximizing the productivity of food animal production.

Goose The singular of geese or a female goose.

Go round A preliminary or elimination round (or heat) in a class with a large number of entries. Some events have two or three go-rounds, and scores are averaged.

Gosling A baby goose.

Gossypol A toxic yellow pigment found in cottonseed. Heat and pressure tend to bind it with protein and thereby render it safe for animal consumption.

Gourth membrane Also called epidermal membrane. A membrane that covers the cria entirely at birth.

GPD (gaseous products of digestion) These include the combustible gases produced in the digestive tract during fermentation of the ration. Methane constitutes the major proportion of the combustible gases produced by ruminants; however, nonruminants also produce methane. Trace amounts of hydrogen, carbon monoxide, acetone, ethane, and hydrogen sulfide are also produced.

Graafian Vesicles The Graafian Vesicles are numerous small globular transparent follicles found in the ovaries of mammals. Each follicle contains one ovum whic is expelled when it reaches maturity.

Grade Animals showing the predominant characteristics of a given breed. They usually have at least one purebred parent, ordinarily the bull.

Grade A milk Milk produced and processed under rigid sanitary regulations. Milking and processing facilities are approved and inspected by public health officials. Fluid milk products must meet this inspection standard.

Grade cattle An animal possessing the distinct characteristic of a particular breed but not registered with a breed association. Sometimes called commercial cattle.

Grade cow A cow that is not registered.

Gradient Change in the concentration of a substance with distance from the cell that makes the substance.

Grading up The continued use of purebred sires on grade dams.

Graduated Feathers successively shorter from center to outside (tail).

Graft A procedure in which a mother raises a newborn that is not her own.

Grafting Fostering a kid onto a doe that is not its natural mother.

Grain 64.798918 mg. Sometimes referred to as 60 mg, 62 mg, 64 mg or 65 mg. The term comes from the weight of a grain of wheat.

Gram A measure of weight. 28 grams = 1 oz.; 454 grams = 1 lb.

Gram negative A classification of bacteria based upon their lack of retention of a certain stain in the laboratory. The staining quality is based on the structure of the cell wall surrounding the bacteria. This structure of the cell wall influences which antibiotics will kill the bacteria. This laboratory staining method was developed by Hans Gram in 1884.

Gram positive A classification of bacteria based upon their uptake of a certain stain in the laboratory. The staining quality is based on the structure of the cell wall surrounding the bacteria. This structure of the cell wall influences which antibiotics will kill the bacteria. This laboratory staining method was developed by Hans Gram in 1884.

Grand Mal Seizure Also called Tonic-Clonic. This is a generalized seizure, associated with primary (idiopathic) epilepsy.

Grand Prix Top caliber classes in dressage and show jumping, often offering large cash prizes.

Granny ewe When a pregnant ewe close to lambing tries to claim another ewe's newborn lamb.

Granuloma An excessive amount of non-healing tissue in a wound.

Grape The plant is cultivated in temperate regions around the world. The medicinal parts are the leaves, fruit and juice. Extract from grape seeds can reduce free radicals and decrease the chances of developing chronic diseases. Flavonoids in the leaves have an anti-inflammatory effect.

Grass tetany A magnesium-deficiency disease of cattle characterized by hyperirritability, muscular spasms of legs, and convulsions.

Gravel An abscess of the hoof wall extending from the white line to the coronet.

Gray A color in which the skin is black, and the hair is a mixture of black and white.

Gray matter Inner part of the spinal cord, looks grey because of the cell bodies located in that area

Gray Water Water that is considered waste and not to be used for cleaning milking systems. Usually including recycled water from a lagoon or milk house waste. Even water only used to cool milk in a plate cooler is considered gray water, though it is often fed to cows to reduce total usage.

Graze To consume standing vegetation, as by livestock or wild animals.

Greasy wool The wool as it comes off the sheep. It contains yolk (wool grease lanolin) suint (sweat) and dirt and vegetable fiber.

Green cheese A term applied to the fresh uncured product. It refers to flavor, odor, body, and texture, not color.

Green chop (fresh forage) Forages harvested (cut and chopped) in the field and hauled to livestock. This minimizes the loss of moisture, color, nutrients, and wastage. Also called zero grazing or soilage.

Green or green broke An inexperienced horse or rider, relatively speaking. In hunter classes, the horse can be any age and is rated according to awards won in past performances.

Green Tea A tea which subjected to a heating process without previous special withering and fermenting. The plant Camellia Sinesis was orignially cultivated in China and is now grown as a tea plant in many countries. Green tea has some cholesterol lowering effects, and it also contains theophylline which can help boost energy.

Greenhouse Barn Commonly referring to any of a group of hoop type barns with translucent or plastic covers over a tubular steel frame.

Gremlin The name of a specific secreted BMP antagonist (inhibitor).

Grey A horse with a truly grey coat.

Grey roan A horse with a coat of mixed grey and white hairs.

Griseofulvin Oral treatment for dermatophytes.

Grit Sand and small pebbles eaten by a chicken and used by its gizzard to grind up grain and plant fiber.

Grooved Concrete Floor surfaces with grooved patterns cut or depressed into concrete to provide better traction for cattle.

Gross energy (GE) The amount of heat, measured in calories, released when a substance is completely oxidized in a bomb calorimeter.

Ground tie To stand in one place, with reins dropped on the ground.

Ground training When the trainer works the horse from the ground, rather than being mounted. Includes in-hand work, barn manners, longeing, and ground driving.

Group Fed Feeding system where all animals in a group are fed at one time.

Growth cone Tip of a regenerating axon

Growth factor Proteins involved in cell differentiation and growth.

Growthy Describes an animal that is large and well-developed for its age.

Grullo A type of dun with a smoky or mouse-colored body, and usually having a black mane, tail, lower legs, and dorsal stripe.

Guaranteed yield Selling lamb on the basis of a guaranteed dressing percentage (yield). Adjustments in price are made for lambs exceeding or not meeting the guaranteed yield.

Guard Dog A dog that stays with the goats without harming them and aggressively repels predators.

Guillain Barre Syndrome (GBS) A rare neurological disease characterized by loss of reflexes and temporary paralysis. Symptoms include weakness, numbness, tingling and increased sensitivity that spreads over the body. Muscle paralysis starts in the feet and legs and moves upwards to the arms and hands. Sometimes paralysis can result in the respiratory muscles causing breathing difficulties. Symptoms usually appear over the course of one day and may continue to progress for 3 or 4 days up to 3 or 4 weeks. Recovery begins within 2-4 weeks after the progression stops. While most patients recover, approximately 15%-20% experience persistent symptoms. GBS is fatal in 5% of cases.

Guinea Fowl A pheasant like bird from Africa raised for ornamental qualities, meat, feathers for crafts and fly tying, or vermin control. They are gregarious, and very interesting. They are watchful and territorial making them good natural alarms. They can be noisy, tend to be only partially domesticated and if allowed to roam will cover a fairly wide range.

Gular sac Bare skin on throat and base of mandible.

Gullet Area under the fork, swells, or pommel of the saddle.

Gulps Exaggerated swallowing movements. In BMDs, it often is accompanied by a desperate need to eat anything, especially grass.

Gutter A shallow to deep channel located behind cows in tiestall barns capture manure and urine.

Gymkhana A program of competitive games on horseback, usually timed events.

H

Hackles A rooster's cape feathers.

H2 antagonist A compound which binds (attaches) to the area on a cell at which histamine also binds. By binding at the same site, the antagonist blocks histamine from binding and prevents histamine from producing its effects, which include the production of stomach acid.

Habitat The place where an organism lives.

HACCP (Hazard Analysis Critical Control Point) An internationally recognized and recommended approach to food safety that anticipates and prevents hazards associated with ingredients.

Hack Class A flat class.

Hackamore A device to guide a horse without a bit, in effect a bitless bridle. A bridle featuring a nosepiece, instead of a bit to control the horse.Americanization of jaquima, which is Spanish for the composite of a bosal, fiador, headstall, and mecate.

Hackles Hairs on neck and back raised involuntarily in fright or anger.

Hackney Action A high lifting of the front feet accompanied by flexing of the wrist like that of a Hackney horse.

Haemoglobin Haemoglobin is the protein that carries oxygen in the blood.

Haemophilus influenza type b (Hib) A bacterial infection that may result in severe respiratory infections, including pneumonia, and other diseases such as meningitis.

Half hitch A knot, also called a "hooey."

Half Life The time that it takes for one half of the original concentration of a given drug to dissipate through the body. The shorter the half-life of a drug, the more frequently you have to administer the drug.

Half pass Variation of travers, executed on the diagonal instead of along the wall. The horse should be nearly parallel to the long sides of the arena, with the forehand slightly in advance of the haunches.

Half prick Ear Also known as the semi-prick ear, ears carried erect with just the tips leaning forward.

Half sib In genetics, a half brother or half sister.

Half sibs Individuals who have the same sire or dam (i.e. half brothers and half sisters).

Hallmark A distinguishing characteristic.

Hallux The hallux is the innermost of the five digits which normally compose the hind foot of a vertebrate. In humans the big toe, in a bird the hind toe.

Halter Harness that fits over the horse's head by which it may be tied or handled.

Halter class Conformation class.

Halter pulling A bad habit in which a horse pulls violently backward on the halter rope when tied.

Hamate bone The hamate bone is one of the bones in the human wrist.

Hame Metal or wooden curved piece to fit the collar on a draft harness.

Hame strap A short strap which connects the right and left hames together on top and bottom.

Hand Four inches of height on a horse. Horses are measured from the highest point of the withers to the ground in units called hands. 14.2 means (14 hands x 4 inches) + 2 inches, which is 56 inches + 2 inches = 58 inches.

Hand breeding Also called hand mating. The females are completely supervised during the mating process and the male is led to the female and controlled during the breeding process.

Hand Milking The manual milking of an animal as opposed to the use of mechanical milking devices.

Hand twitch Using your hand to hold the horse's nose (as a twitch).

Handle The degree to which all the attributes which comprise quality, such as softness, fineness, length and elasticity, are noticeable when wool is judged by feel.

Handlers Processors or dealers of milk who commonly purchase raw milk and sell pasteurized milk and milk products.

Handy Prompt and athletic in response to the rider.

Hanging weight The weight of the carcass before any fat and bone have been trimmed.

Hapten A substance that becomes antigenic when it complexes with proteins.

Hard keeper An animal that requires more than the usual amount of food to stay in good condition.

Hard trot Slang term referring to all of the mutations of the fox trot or another gait that result in a rough ride for the rider i.e., long trot, cow trot, and square trot.

Hard Mouthed A dog that crushes or renders game unfit for consumption.

Hard-pad disease Crusty, dry footpads that may occur as a consequence of canine distemper infection.

Hardware disease Commonly, an inflammation of the body cavity by an animal eating metal objects and perforation of the digestive tract.

Hare Foot Foot on which the two center digits are appreciably longer than the outside and inside toes of the foot, and the arching of the toes is less marked, making the foot appear longer overall.

Harlequin Patched or pied coloration, usually black or gray on white. Color definitions may vary by breed. Always check the breed standard for the definitive color description.

Harness A leather, nylon or cloth strap shaped around the shoulders and chest, with a ring at its top for the lead.

Harvester Machines that have blades to cut plants.

Harvestore Silo A brand of oxygen limiting (air tight) upright silos with bottom unloading.

Hatch 1. The process by which a chick comes out of the egg.

2. A group of chicks that come out of their shells at roughly the same time.

Hatchability Percentage of fertilized eggs that hatch under incubation.

Hatchery A company that hatches baby chicks and sells them to farmers.

Haunch Bones The hip bones.

Haunches Hindquarters.

Havanese A small breed of dog with a soft coat originating in Cuba.

Haversian Canals The Haversian Canals are a network of minute canals, which traverse the solid substance of bones and proceed from the central cavity. They convey nutrient vessels to all parts.

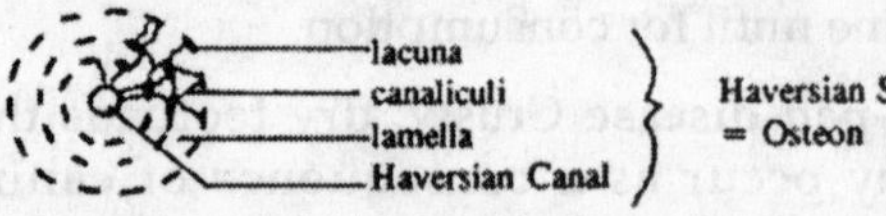

Fig. Haversian Canals

Haw A third eyelid or membrane on the inside corner of the eye.

Hawthorn A European shrub with thorny branches of the Crataegus species. The herb may be prescribed as a mild heart tonic.

Hay Dried feed consisting of the entire plant. Alfalfa, clover, grass, and oat hay are used in dairy rations.

Hay additives Organic acids or acid-forming compounds designed to allow hay to be harvested at higher than normal moisture contents by preventing the microbial activity responsible for spoilage.

Hay Dried forage (grasses, alfalfa, clovers) Used for feeding farm animals.

Haylage Low-moisture silage (35 to 55 percent moisture). Grass and legume crops are cut and wilted in the field to a lower moisture level than normal for grass silage, but the crop is not sufficiently dry for baling. It is commonly stored in a sealed, or airtight, storage system.

Hazard The likelihood or the probability that a substance, i.e., the poison, will induce a disease state under conditions of use.

Head mange Common name for notoedric mange.

Head pressing Pressing the head against a wall or other hard object.

Head shy Description of a horse who shies away from having his head touched.

Header In team roping, this rider ropes the steer's horns.

Headlocks Self-locking stanchions along a feed alley in which cows voluntarily enter the head slot when going to eat. All cows may be held until herd health work is completed, and then all cows may be simultaneously released. Headlocks may be adjusted to remain open, allowing cows to come an go at will, when restraining the cows is not necessary.

Headstalls Another name for bridles.

Health Protection Agency A new, independent organisation which brings together experts on infectious diseases, poisons, chemicals, and biological and radiation hazards. It provides laboratory services, research, and advice on all aspects of human health and disease control, as well as planning for health emergencies.

Heart block A condition in which the electrical impulses of the heart are not properly conducted from the atria (chambers which receive the blood) to the ventricles (chambers which pump the blood).

Heart girth The circumference of the body just back of the shoulders of an animal. It is used to estimate body weight.

Heat A queen's estrus period, during which time she is fertile and receptive to the advances of a tom. Queens in heat usually call, and some may spray.

Heartworm A species of parasitic worm (Dirofilaria immitis) that lives and reproduces in the chambers of the heart of an animal. Microscopic, immature worms (microfilariae) circulate in the blood and are taken in by mosquitoes that bite the animal. Microfilariae mature in the mouthparts of the mosquito and infect another susceptible animal bitten by the same mosquito.

Heat detection Identification of females in heat for artificial insemination.

Heat increment (HI) The increase in heat produced following consumption of food. It consists of calories released in fermentation and nutrient metabolism. When environmental temperature is below critical temperature, this heat may be used to keep the body warm; therefore, it is not wasted. Also called work of digestion.

Heat period That period of time when a female will accept a male in the act of mating. Also called in heat or estrus.

Heating Temperature rises as hay or fodder ferments, dries, or cures.

Heaves Damage to the lungs, resulting in labored breathing.

Hectare A metric unit of land measurement (2.47 acres).

Hedging Entering into the purchase of commodity futures contracts to reduce the risk of an unfavorable price fluctuation.

Heeler In team roping, this rider ropes the steer's heels.

Heifer A bovine female less than three years of age who has not borne a calf. Young cows with their first calves are sometimes called first-calf heifers.

Heinz body A condition in which the red blood cells are destroyed and this results in anemia. The specific type of anemia is called 'Heinz body anemia' because the red cells develop an abnormality called a 'Heinz body' which can be seen under the microscope. This anemia can occur as a reaction to certain medications and also in cats who eat onions.

Helminth A category of parasitic worms.

Helminthiasis Parasitic worm infestation.

Helper T cells Also known as CD4 T-cells or helper CD4 T-cells. These are cells that can help B cells make antibody in response to challenge. The most efficient helper cells are also known as Th2, cells that make the cytokines IL-4 and IL-5. Some experts refer to all CD4 cells as helper cells, regardless of function. Function determination requires cellular assays that show that some CD4 T cells kill the cells they interact with, and therefore not all CD4 cells are helper cells.

Hemangiosarcoma A malignant tumor of endothelial cells (the layer of cells that lines the cavities of the heart and of the blood and lymph vessels). (Epithelial cells cover all body surfaces, inside and out.)

Hematocrit PCV (Packed Cell Volume), hematocrit: A laboratory test to monitor relative number of red blood cells present in the blood. A blood sample is placed in a tiny glass tube and spun in a centrifuge. The cells are heavier than the plasma and are compacted at one end of the tube. After the tube is spun, it is examined and the packed cell volume is determined as the percentage of the red cellular portion relative to the total amount of blood in the tube (i.e. remainder being the plasma). The normal for dogs is 40-59 and cats is 29-50.

Hematology The study of blood, its physiology and pathology.

Hematoma Localized collection of blood, a lump. Dogs can get them in their ear flaps from violent and repeated shaking of the head, from such things as ear infections or insect stings.

Hematuria Blood in the urine. The blood may or may not be seen with the naked eye.

Hemocytometer A piece of equipment that is used to count white blood cells and can also be used to count sperm.

Hemodialysis A process used to remove waste products from the blood.

Hemoglobin A protein inside of red blood cells, responsible for the binding and transport of oxygen to the body tissues (Hb).

Hemolysin 1.a substance liberated by a living agent and capable of causing lysis of red blood cells and liberation of their hemoglobin

2. a sensitizing antibody that combines with red blood cells of the antigenic type that

stimulated formation of the h., affecting the cells in such a manner that complement fixes with the antibody-cell union and causes dissolution of the cells, with liberation of their hemoglobin.

Hemolysis Breaking or destruction of red blood cells.

Hemolytic Causing the red blood cells to break open.

Hemophilia The blood lacks coagulating factors, causing a strong tendency to bleed, and difficulty in getting the bleeding to stop. hepatitis inflammation of the liver. This can result from a variety of causes including infections (particularly viral), drugs, autoimmunity and genetics. The liver stores and filters blood, secretes bile, converts sugars, processes fat, produces proteins which help to control blood volume, and produces some of the clotting factors.

Hemorrhage To bleed excessively; may be the result of injury or blood clotting abnormalities.

Hemorrhagic follicle Also called a corpus hemorrhagicum. A follicle that has been present on the ovary and has not been given the chance to ovulate so it will continue growing and becomes large and cyst-like and bleeds inside.

HemostatA surgical instrument used to pinch small blood vessels to stop bleeding (hemostasis is to stop bleeding). Hemastats may be used in non-surgical procedures, for example to pluck hair from the ear canals.

Hen A female chicken (sometimes applied to other species) over 1 year of age.

Hen feathered The characteristic of a rooster having rounded rather than pointed sex feathers.

Heparin Sulfate Proteoglycans (HSPGs) Ubiquitous macromolecules associated with the cell surface and extracellular matrix of a wide range of cells of vertebrate and invertebrate tissues. They are essential cofactors in cell-cell recognition systems, in receptor-growth factor interactions, and in internalization of receptors.

Heparin Type of long chain sugar that is found especially in liver, that prolongs the clotting time of blood, and that is used medically.

Hepatic fibrosis Scarring of the liver

Hepatic Pertaining to the liver.

Hepatitis An inflammation or infection of the liver.

Hepatitis B Hepatitis caused by a virus and transmitted by exposure to blood or blood products or during sexual intercourse. It causes acute and chronic hepatitis. Chronic hepatitis B can cause liver disease, cirrhosis, and liver cancer.

Hepatitis Inflammation of the liver.

Hepatocerebellar degeneration Death of liver cells causing poisoning of the white matter of the brain.

Hepatocyte Liver cell.

Hepatomegaly Enlargement of the liver.

Herbal medicine It involves the use of natural plants or plant-based substances to treat illness and to enhance the body's function. Medicines are prepared from plant materials including leaves, stems, roots, and bark. These treatments usually contain many biologically active ingredients. The herbs can be prepared in many ways and may be found in many forms including pills, capsules, powders, and extracts. The strengths of herbal remedies can vary depending on the species of herbs used, how and when they were gathered, and how they were prepared. Herbal remedies should be used under the guidance of a practitioner familiar with herbal medicine.

Herbivore Animal that eats primarily plants and vegetation.

Herd A group of animals (especially cattle), collectively considered as a unit.

Herd average Average milk and component production per cow for all cows in the herd unit for 12 months.

Herd bound When a horse is too dependent on being with other horses and doesn't want to be separated from them.

Herd code An exclusive reference number that identifies every DHI herd. The first two numbers identify the state, the next two, the association, and the final numerical series identifies the herd within an association.

Herd owner The declared owner of a herd of dairy cattle as recorded on a legal document, registration papers or other official documents.

Herd summary Summary statistics for herd production, reproduction, health, and demographic factors.

Herdmate comparison Method of estimating the genetic transmitting ability in which a cow's yield is compared to that of other cows in the same breed from different sires that calved in the same herd during the same season.

Heredity The transmission of characteristics from parents to their offspring through genes.

Heritability The proportion (fraction) of difference among animals for a trait, such as milk production, due to genetic difference rather than environmental factors. The fraction of variation in a trait that is genetically transmissible from parent to offspring.

Hermaphrodism A condition where reproductive structures of both the male and the female are in one body.

Hernia Abnormal protrusion of organs through a weak spot or abnormal opening, usually in the abdominal or groin areas.

Herpes Zoster A disease characterized by painful skin lesions that occur mainly on the trunk (back and stomach) of the body but which can also develop on the face and in the mouth. Complications include headache, vomiting, fever and meningitis. Recovery may take up to 5 weeks. Herpes Zoster is caused by the same virus that is responsible for chickenpox. Most people are exposed to this virus during childhood. After the primary infection (chickenpox), the virus becomes dormant, or inactivated. In some people the virus reactivates years, or even decades, later and causes herpes zoster. Also known as the shingles.

Herringbone milking parlor A raised, zigzag-designed milking stall which allows the group milking of several cows at one time in a pipeline milking system.

Hetastarch A colloid solution of hydrolyzed amylopectin containing a range of particle sizes, from 10,000 daltons to over 3 million daltons.

Heterogenous Consisting of dissimilar or diverse ingredients or constituents.

Heterosis (Hybrid Vigour) The increase in performance observed for a specific crossbred above the average performance of the parental lines.

Heterotopic Ossification Bone formation that occurs in an abnormal place. Synonymous with ectopic.

Heterozygote An animal is said to be heterozygous for a certain gene if both sites at which the gene might be expected are occupied by different genes.

Heterozygous Having two different alleles at corresponding loci on homologous chromosomes in a cell.

High lope A gallop.

High moisture silage Silage usually containing 70 percent or more moisture.

High titer vaccine A modified live vaccine that contains a higher number of virus particles than the 'average' vaccine. High titer vaccines can generally elicit an immune system response in young animals who have a maternal antibody level that would prevent them from responding to an 'average' vaccine.

High/low string High/low producing cows are split into feeding groups to optimize ration inputs for milk output.

Hindsaddle The area of the lamb or carcass from the last rib back, includes loin, leg and rump.

Hinny Cross between a stallion and a female donkey.

Hip dysplasia, CHD, HD Improper development of the hip joint, typically, the acetabulum (socket) is not deep enough for the femoral head (ball) to fit fully into place.

Hippocampus Part of the brain critical for learning and memory

Hippomanes Normal formations in the cavity of the placenta where the fetus was located.

Histamine H2 receptor antagonist A compound which binds (attaches) to the area on a cell at which histamine also binds. By binding at the same site, the antagonist blocks histamine from binding and prevents histamine from producing its effects, which include the production of stomach acid.

Histiocytomas A small wart-like skin growth that will eventually disappear. (Note: NO growths or lumps on a BMD should ever be ignored!)

Histiocytosis Abnormal appearance of histiocytes in the blood. (Histiocytes are produced by the bone marrow and are normally immobile until stimulated by inflammation. They are a type of antigen presenting cell.)cutaneous benign proliferation of nodules in or under the skin.malignant a rapidly invasive proliferation of neoplastic (new growth) histiocytes. No known treatment, always fatal.systemic proliferation of histiocytes invading the skin and lymph nodes. Can go into remission for years, or progress to the malignant form. Can be treated, but not cured.

Histocompatibility Literally means the ability of cells to get along with each other. Used to determine whether a transplanted tissue or organ will be acceptable by the recipient. Histocompatibility is determined by the major histocompatibility complex molecules.

Histology/Histopathology A branch of anatomy that deals with the minute structure of animal and plant tissues as discernable with the microscope.

HIV Abbreviation for human immunodeficiency virus, the causative agent of acquired immunodeficiency syndrome. A retrovirus of the lentivirus family that selectively infects CD4 T cells leading to their depletion, which eventually results in immunodeficiency.

HIV gag A structural component of the HIV genome coding for various structures on the surface of the virus functionally necessary for attachment of the virus to a susceptible cell, such as p24, p17. Other examples of the genome include env (envelope genes) and pol (polymerase enzymes).

HLA The acronym for Human Leukocyte Antigen is the genetic designation for the human MHC. Individual loci are designated by upper case letters, as in HLA-A and alleles are designated in numbers, as in HLA-A 201.

Hob A male ferret.

Hobbles. Rope, cloth, or leather loops that fasten the forelegs together.

Hock Tarsal joint between the tibia and cannon, corresponding to human heel.

Hodgkins disease A malignant disease on which antigen presenting cells resembling dendritic cells seem to be the transformed cell type.

Hodgkins lymphoma A form of Hodgkins disease in which lymphocytes predominate, and it has a much better prognosis than the nodular sclerosis form of this disease in which the predominant cell type is non-lymphoid.

Hogback Three-rail jump with the center element the highest.

Hogget Sheep 12 to 24 months of age.

Hogtie To tie three legs with a narrow rope.

Holding area An area to hold cows prior to entry into the milking parlor. Sometimes called a holding pen. May also include a wash pen.

Holding Pen An area in which cows congregate prior to entering a milking parlor to be milked.

Holistic The approach of taking into consideration the whole body and environment when offering treatment. Sometimes called the Eastern approach.

Holistic medicine A healing philosophy which views the patient as a whole body rather than as a disease or a collection of symptoms. A patient's emotional and spiritual state can affect the patient's condition. Also, nutrition, environment, and lifestyle may contribute to an illness. Holistic practitioners may combine traditional forms of treatment (medicication and sugery) with alternative forms of treatment including homeopathy, acupuncture, chiropractic, massage, and herbal medicine.

Hollow back A back which is unduly dipped.

Homeopathy A system of therapeutics founded by a German physician named Samuel Hahnemann (1755-1843). It is a philosophy of "like heals like". In this system, the treatments are composed of substances which, in their undiluted state, actually produce the symptoms of the disease in a healthy individual. The substances are diluted to infinitesimal amounts in solutions and vigorously shaken (successed) before they are given to the patient. Many homeopaths also believe that an individual's mental, physical, and emotional constitution may also need to be treated. The potency is based on the dilution ratio and it is believed that the more diluted the dose, the more potent the effect. A dilution ratio written as 1x is 1 part substance to 9 parts dilution medium, 1c is 1 part substance to 99 parts medium, and 1m is 1 part substance to 999 parts medium. A remedy labeled 20c has first been mixed as 1 part substance to 99 parts dilution base. Then, 1 part of this mixture is then mixed with 99 parts of the base and this dilution process is continued for a total of 20 times.

Homogenization Breaking up the fat in the milk into tiny globs. This is done so that the cream in the milk will not rise to the top when milk is put in the refrigerator.

Homogenized milk Milk that has been treated to ensure breakup of fat globules to such an extent that, after 48 hours of quiescent storage at 7øC, no visible cream separation occurs on the milk. The reduced size of fat particles results in formation of a softer curd in the stomach.

Homozygous Each gene of a specific gene pair is the same in an individual (i.e. AA).

Homozygote An animal is said to be homozygous for a certain gene if both sites at which the gene might be expected are occupied by that gene.

Hondo The eye on the end of a rope that forms the loop. Also called "honda."

Honest A quality in a horse which makes him dependable and predictable.

Hooey A half-hitch knot.

Hoof The hard horny covering of the horse's foot.

Hoof dressing A preparation designed to be applied to the hoof either for conditioning or for appearance.

Hoof packing Material, usually claylike, to be applied to the bottom of the horse's hoof.

Hoof pick A metal one-tined "rake" to clean debris from a horse's hoof.

Horizontal Transmission Ways infections are spread between animals i.e. direct, indirect, or airborne horizontal transmission.

Hormone A chemical formed in one part of the body that is carried in the blood to other parts of the body where it has its effect.

Horn The highest part of the pommel, of the western saddle, around which the rider can dally a rope.

Horner's Syndrome Loss of sympathetic innervation resulting in miosis, ptosis and enopthalmos.

Horses 1 For registration purposes, all Thoroughbreds, Arabians, Tennessee Walking Horses, etc. are one year old on January 1 regardless of when born during the prior year.

2. Many times the stallions may be syndicated for breeding purposes. Generally, up to 40 shares of a stallion are sold. Each share, breeding, entitles the holder of the right to 3 "tries" at impregnating the same mare per year. A breeding right is an intangible, depreciable asset. The purchase of a breeding right many times guarantees a live foal. This means the foal has to stand and nurse the mare.

3. Mares are eligible to be bred at age two, but are generally bred at age three. The mare usually gives birth to one offspring each year.

4. Teaser ponies are used by the breeder to prepare the mare forservice by the stallion. A teaser pony is a depreciable asset.

5. A gelding is a male horse that has been castrated. It cannotbe depreciated for breeding purposes. It can be depreciated if it is used as a show, work or race horse.

Horsemanship Exhibition of a rider's skill, usually referring to the Western style of riding.

Host The organism in or on which a parasite lives. For example, dogs and cats are hosts for fleas and roundworms.

Hot horse A horse sweaty, warm, and puffing from a recent workout; also a slang term for a horse who may be hard to handle or temperamental.

Hot nursery A nursery where piglets are raised until they are 4 weeks old and the ambient temperature is very warm.

Hot Quarter A quarter of the udder that is infected and may actually feel hard or hot to the touch due to elevated temperatures.

Hot spots Inflammation of the skin, dermatitis. Frequently caused by flea bites, or a hypersensitivity to an allergen. Can also be caused by bacteria building up in an area that the dog bites or scratches. Some BMD owners have linked it to the dog having wet fur for prolonged periods of time.

Hot blooded Refers to horses having ancestors that trace to Thoroughbreds or **Arabians.** Characteristics might include fineness of bone, thin skin, fine hair coat, absence of long fetlock hairs, and blood that makes it well-suited for speed and distance work.

Hothouse lamb A lamb born and raised out of the normal season and marketed at six to ten weeks of age.

Hotweight basis The weight of a dressed carcass immediately after slaughter prior to cooler shrinkage.

Hotz Celsus technique A surgical procedure for correction of lower lid entropion.

Hotz Celsus A surgical technique used to repair entropion.

Household pet (HHP) The household pet class at a North American show is open to all cats, purebred or not, that are not eligible to compete in any other class. The term "household pet" is also used to refer to mixed-breed cats.

HPV Human papilloma virus the causative agent of genital warts (condylomata acuminata) a sexually transmitted infection.

HPV-16 Serotypes 16 and 18 commonly associated with progression to cancer of the cervix in women.

HTST (high-temperature short-time) The temperature and time combination for pasteurization of milk and milk products. The minimum for milk is 71.7øC (161øF) for at least 15 seconds. Higher temperatures are used in pasteurizing products of high solids because of the protection afforded bacteria by solids.

Human albumin A colloidal solution prepared from pooled human plasma and heated to kill many types of blood borne diseases.

Human Chorionic Gonadotropin stimulation test HCG stimulationA stimulation test which measures testosterone in response to HCG administration. Used to detect retained testicles.

Humane twitch A clamp-type twitch.

Humerus The humerus is the long bone in the upper region of the human arm. It joins with the shoulder at the glenoid cavity.

Humoral immunity Is the antibody-mediated immunity made in a humoral immune response. Humoral immunity can be transferred to unimmunized recipients by using immune serum containing specific antibody.

Hundredweight Generally refers to milk sold off the farm in 100 pound units.

Hunter A type of horse, not a breed, which is suitable for field hunting or show hunting.

Hutch An individual housing unit for young calves. Often made of white fiberglass or polyvinyl.

Hybrid A cross breed - typically used for a purposeful crossing of two species to produce offspring with a unique set of characteristics. Mating two hybrid birds will not produce offspring with the same characteristics of the parents. (See Breed)

Hybrid vigor (heterosis) The increased growth or production exhibited by the first generation over the average of its two parent breeds. It is usually expressed as a percentage.

Hybridomas Myeloma cells cultured in the lab survive indefinitely. Myeloma cells can be fused with a normal B cell. The resulting hybridoma produces large quantities of monoclonal antibody.

Hydatitosis cysts found in the body cavity of sheep.

Hydrocephalous The accumulation of fluid in the ventricles of the brain. The head may appear to be large and dome shaped. Many small breeds of dogs have a degree of hydrocephalous that is normal for the breed. Severe hydrocephalous damages brain tissue.

Hydrolyzed Breaking a compound into smaller and simpler compounds by a chemical reaction with water.

Hydrops An abnormality during pregnancy where the uterus retains large amounts of water. This can be caused by defects in the fetus and/or in the mother.

Hydroxyzine HCl An antihistamine.

Hymen A thin membrane partially occluding the opening to the vagina in a virgin.

Hyper This prefix is used in conjunction with many terms and means an increase, for example, hyperthermia means an increase in temperature.

Hyperalgesia Unexpected increased pain intensity from a stimulus. Excessive sensitivity to pain.

Hypercalcemia Elevated blood calcium. The most common cause is the production of a biochemical substance by tumors, resulting in the retention of calcium. This is called pseudohyperparathyroidism, most commonly occurring in patients with lymphoma or tumors of the apocrine anal sac. Pseudohyperparathyroidism has been reported associated with other tumor types. Primary hyperparathyroidism occurs uncommonly.

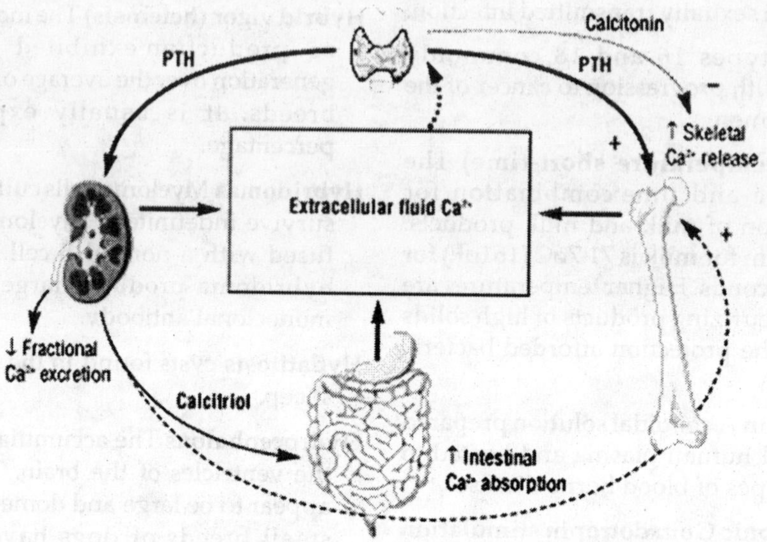

Fig. Hypercalcemia

Hyperesthesia Increased sensitivity to stimulation. Is most commonly seen with peripheral nerve diseases, such as, tumors and polyradiculoneuritis.

Hyperglycemia Elevation of blood glucose. There are numerous causes of hyperglycemia including diabetes mellitus, hyperadrenocorticism, excitement and the administration of glucose or glucocorticoids.

Hyperkalemia Increased level of potassium in the blood.

Hyperkeratosis Increased thickness of the horny layer of the epidermis.

Hypermagnesemia Elevated blood magnesium.

Hypermotile Something that is overactive.

Hypernatremia Elevated blood sodium. Hypernatremia is uncommon in dogs and cats and most often is iatrogenic from the repetitive administration of high sodium containing solutions. Animals who have severe hypernatremia in excess of 170 meq/L show nervous system signs of depression progressing to coma.

Hyperosmolarity An increase in the osmotic concentration of the blood. Hyperosmolarity of the blood can draw water from RBC's causing lysis or from neurons causing neurologic signs such as coma.

Hyperosmotic agents Drugs such as mannitol and glycerine which draw water to themselves. Used to control edema and swelling.

Hyperphosphatemia Elevated phosphorus.

Hyperpigmentation An increased dark color in the skin caused by the pigment 'melanin.'

Hyperplasia Proliferation of cellular elements usually accompanied by increased size of the organ.

Hyperplastic Abnormal increase in the amount of tissue, e.g., a hyperplastic ear would have increased numbers of cells in the ear canal, sometimes to the point of closing off the ear canal. In prostatic hyperplasia, the prostate enlarges due to an increased number of normal, not cancerous, cells.

Hypersensitive A type of allergic condition in which the body overreacts to a certain agent such as a bee sting or medication.

Hypersensitivity A condition in which the body has an exaggerated response to a substance (e.g. food or drug). Also known as an allergy.

Hypersensitivity type IV An exagerated reaction of the cellular components of the immune system.

Hypertension Elevated blood pressure.

Hypertensive Elevation in blood pressure.

Hypertensive retinopathy Retinal damage caused by edema or hemorrhages beneath the retina causing it to detach. Systemic hypertension is the cause of the detachment.

Hyperthermia An increase in body temperature above normal.

Hyperthyroidism Increased production of thyroid hormone. Hyperthyroidism occurs commonly in geriatric cats but is rare in dogs.

Hypertonic A fluid that contains a ratio of electrolytes to water that is greater than extracelluar fluid. A fluid that contains a concentration of electrolytes greater than extracellular fluid.

Hypertonic dehydration Dehydration that develops after a hypotonic fluid is lost from the body. The fluid lost from the body contains a ratio of electrolytes to water that is less than extracelluar fluid. The osmolality of ECF is hypertonic after the electrolyte-poor fluid is lost. This is a rare form of dehydration in dogs and cats.

Hypertonic Hypertonic solutions have higher osmolalities than extracellular fluid/plasma.

Hypertonic saline Hypertonic saline has a concentration of sodium and chloride greater 0.9% and is used in states of hypovolemic shock. A very small volume of hypertonic saline administered IV to a hypovolemic patient will result in the mobilization of fluid from the cells into the extracellular fluid compartments, causing an expansion of blood volume and maintenance of blood flow to vital organs. Hypertonic saline solutions must subsequently be followed by the administration of isotonic solutions to reestablish fluid balance in intracellular and extracellular fluid locations.

Hypertrophic A thickening or an enlargement of an organ.

Hypertrophic osteodystrophy, HOD Inflammation of the growth plates, and can be accompanied by depression, weight loss, and fever. The joints may be swollen and feel hot. Mild cases usually resolve with no lasting ill effects. However, in the rare case of severe HOD, permanent damage to the bone joints can result in limb deformities.

Hypertrophy An increase in the size of a tissue or organ due to the enlargement of existing cells.

Hyperventilate An increase in the rate and/or depth of respiration such that the body loses too much carbon dioxide.

Hyperventilation Fast breathing. Also called hyperpnea.

Hyphema Blood in the anterior chamber.

Hypnozoite A form of the malaria parasite that remains inactive within the liver and can produce relapses.

Hypo This prefix is used in conjunction with many terms and means a decrease, for example, hypothermia means a decrease in temperature.

Hypoalbuminemia Low concentration of blood albumin.

Hypocalcemia Low blood calcium. Hypocalcemia causes tetany (rigidity of muscles) in dogs and cats but flaccid muscle weakness in cattle.

Hypodermoclysis A synonym for subcutaneous.

Hypoglycemia Abnormally low blood glucose.

Hypokalemia Low blood potassium. A hallmark sign of hypokalemia is weakness.

Hypomagnesemia Low blood magnesium.

Hypomotile Something that is not as active as it normally should be.

Hypomyelination, tremblers Reduction in the amount of myelin (cover or sheath) on the nerves. The disease has an early onset, in BMDs is considered to be an autosomal recessive trait.

Hyponatremia Low blood sodium. The most common cause is Addison's disease or iatrogenic from the administration of electrolyte free solution, such as 5% dextrose.

Hypoplasia Inadequate or defective development of tissue.

Hypopyon Pus in the anterior chamber of the eye.

Hyposensitivity A condition in which the body has a weakened or delayed reaction to a substance.

Hyposensitization The administration of increasing doses of antigen to reduce sensitization to the antigen.

Hypothalamus The hypothalamus is the region of the human brain below the cerebrum which regulates rhythmic activity and physiological stability within the body, including water balance and temperature.

Hypothermia Inability to keep warm often caused by cold or wet weather.

Hypothyroid Low function of the thyroid gland.

Hypothyroidism A condition, more common in dogs, in which the thyroid gland does not produce enough thyroid hormone.

Hypotonic A fluid that contains a ratio of electrolytes to water that is less than extracellular fluid. A fluid that contains a concentration of electrolytes less than extracellular fluid.

Hypotonic dehydration Dehydration that develops after a hypertonic fluid is lost from the body. The fluid lost from the body contains a ratio of electrolytes to water that is greater than extracellular fluid. The osmolality of ECF is hypotonic after the electrolyte-rich fluid is lost. The best example of this type of dehydration is hypoadrenocorticism (Addison's Disease).

Hypotonic Hypotonic solutions have lower osmolalities than extracellular fluid/plasma.

Hypotony Decreased intraocular pressure.

Hypovitaminosis A A condition in which the body suffers from a deficiency in Vitamin A.

Hypovolemia Reduced circulating blood volume either due to blood or fluid loss or to redistribution of blood flow as occurs during shock.

Hypoxia Low oxygen level in blood and tissues.

Hysteropexy A surgical procedure during which the uterus is "tacked" to prevent prolapse.

I

I.D. Abbreviation for intradermal, a mode of delivery of therapy.

I.M. Abbreviation for intramuscular. Intramuscular, within the substance of muscles a mode of delivery for therapeutic agents.

I.P. Abbreviation for intraperitoneal within the peritoneal cavity.

I.V. Abbreviation for intravenous, within the venous system.

IAAAM International Association of Aquatic Animal Medicine.

Iatrogenic A condition resulting from the action of the doctor; e g., an allergic reaction resulting from administration of an injection by a veterinarian.

Iatrogenic infection Infections that are acquired through human intervention. Also referred to as nosocomial infections.

ICAM Abbreviation for intercellular adhesion molecule. ICAM-1, ICAM-2, and ICAM-3 are cell surface ligands for the leukocyte integrins and are crucial in the binding of lymphocytes and other leukocytes to certain cells, including antigen-presenting cells and endothelial cells. They are members of the immunoglobulin superfamily.

Ice milk A frozen product resembling ice cream, except that it contains less fat.

2. to 5 percent versus 10 percent) and more SNF (12 percent versus 10 percent) than ice cream. Both ice milk and ice cream contain stabilizers and emulsifiers and about 15 percent sugar.

Icterus A yellow discoloration of the gums and white of the eye that is often associated with liver problems and some types of anemia.

IDDM Insulin dependent diabetes mellitus (IDDM): A form of diabetes in which so little insulin is produced that supplemental insulin must be given for the animal to live. Also called Type I diabetes mellitus.

Idiopathic Epilepsy Seizures for which there is no known cause. Also called primary, inherited, genetic or true epilepsy.

Idiopathic When the exact cause of the problem or disease is not known.

Idiosyncrasy to food A qualitatively abnormal response to a food or food additive that resembles a hypersensitivity.

IFN Abbreviation for Interferon. Interferons are cytokines that can induce cells to resist viral replication. Interferon-a and -b are produced by leukocytes and fibroblasts respectively as well as by other cells.

Ig Standard abbreviation for immunoglobulin.

Iiritis Inflammation of the iris

IL Interleukin, a type of cytokine produced by leukocytes that influences a variety of cells.

Ileus A condition in which there is an absence of muscular contractions of the intestine which normally move the food through the system; can result in an intestinal obstruction.

Iliacus The Iliacus is a muscle in the human thigh.

IM Intramuscularly, in the muscle shot.

Imidocloprid Advantage, Bayer) is a neurotoxin available as a topical "pour-on" for use in dogs and cats over 4 months of age.

Imitation milks Mixtures of nondairy ingredients (other than milk, milk fat, and nonfat milk solids) which are combined forming a product similar to milk, lowfat milk, or skim milk. Sodium caseinate, though derived from milk, is commonly termed a nondairy ingredient and is often used as a source of protein in imitation milks. Vegetable oils are commonly used as the source of fat.

Immune complex The result of the malaria parasite that remains inactive within the liver and can produce relapses.

Immune globulin A protein found in the blood that fights infection. Also known as gamma globulin.

Immune mediated The immune system is supposed to protect against disease by destroying foreign objects such as bacteria. If the immune system attacks normal parts of the body such as red blood cells, the disease is immune-mediated.

Immune mediated disease Immune mediated indicates that the immune system is involved in the genesis of disease. Immune mediated diseases can be due to a foreign antigens (viruses, drugs) acting as haptens, adhering to or altering the surface of cells so that antibodies form against the hapten - cell complex or against cell antigens that become exposed. True autoimmunity indicates that the immune system is damaging unaltered "self". Often it is not possible to differentiate between true autoimmunity and immune mediated diseases.

Immune response The reaction of the immune system to foreign substances.

Immune system The complex system in the body responsible for fighting disease. Its primary function is to identify foreign substances in the body (bacteria, viruses, fungi or parasites) and develop a defense against them. This defense is known as the immune response. It involves production of protein molecules called antibodies to eliminate foreign organisms that invade the body.

Immune mediated Immune-mediated reaction or disease: A condition or disease caused by abnormal activity of the immune system in which the body's immune system either over-reacts (e.g., immune-mediated contact dermatitis) or starts attacking the body itself (e.g., autoimmune hemolytic anemia). See also autoimmune.

Immunity A condition in which the animal's immune system has been primed and is able to protect the body from a disease-causing agent such as a certain virus or bacteria. An animal could have immunity to one agent, such as parvovirus, but not have immunity to another agent, such as rabies.

Immunization The process of rendering an animal protected (immune) against a certain disease. Vaccination is a way to produce immunization. However, just because an animal has been vaccinated (received a vaccine) does not necessarily mean the animal is immune. If the body did not correctly react to the vaccine or if the vaccine was defective, immunity would not occur. No vaccine produces immunity in 100% of the population to which it was given. 'Vaccination' is not the same as 'immunization.'

Immunodeficiency Reduced function of the immune system of an animal, making it more susceptible to infectious disease. Can be an inherited defect or caused by drugs, radiation, or viruses.

Immunogen A substance capable of provoking an immune response. Also called an antigen.

Immunogenicity The ability of an antigen or vaccine to stimulate immune responses.

Immunoglobulins There are several kinds that contribute to immunity overall: IgG most abundant in serum and colostrum. IgM "early" antibody; the first one to appear when there is an infection. IgA secreted on mucosal surfaces of respiratory, intestinal and genital tracts. IgE allergic antibody to allergens.

Immunology A science that deals with the immune system.

Immunoprophylaxis Administration of vaccines to confer protection against infectious agents.

Immunostimulant A compound which stimulates the immune system to work more effectively to kill bacteria, viruses, or cancer cells.

Immunosuppression Any failure of the immune response usually becomes apparent through increased susceptibility to infection and disease.

Immunosuppressive Something, for instance a drug, hormone, or virus, that reduces the function of the immune system of an animal. An animal with reduced function of its immune system is called 'immunosuppressed.'

Immunotherapy Cancer treatment that produces antitumor effects primarily through the action of natural host defense mechanisms or by the administration of natural mammalian substances.

Impaction Blockage of a body passage or cavity, such as the crop or cloaca. Also see "pasting".

Impaction Constipation See compaction.

Imperforate Separated by a septum (nostrils).

Impetigo Superficial pustular pyoderma seen in dogs less than 9 months of age.

Imported Semen Frozen semen that is imported from another country.

Impulsion The energy and thrust forward characterized by a forward reaching rather than a backward pushing motion.

In In, within, inside.

In the hole Third in line to enter the pen; after "on deck."

In vitro In an artificial environment, referring to a process or reaction occurring therein, as in a test tube or culture medium. Cf. in vivo. [L. in glass].

In vivo Within the living body.

In Whelp Pregnant.

Inactive problems Inactive problems are unresolved problems that are not being addressed diagnostically or therapeutically. Usually they are problems of a minor nature.

Inactive vaccine A vaccine made from viruses and bacteria that have been killed through physical or chemical processes. These killed organisms cannot cause disease.

In and Out Combination fence.

Inapparent infection The presence of infection without symptoms. Also known as subclinical or asymptomatic infection.

Inbreed To mate together closely related cats, for example brother and sister, or father and daughter.

Inbreeding Production of progeny from closely related parents. Inbreeding increases the number of homozygous gene pairs and decreases the number of heterozygous gene pairs. Inbreeding increases prepotency and the expression of undesirable recessive genes.

Incidence The proportion of sampled animals that develop a condition of interest over a defined period of time. It is the measure of the occurrence of disease over time in a defined group of suscept·ble animals. Incidence can also be applied to measuring the occurrence of new cases of disease in an ever-changing population over time.

Incisions A wound made by something sharp like glass fragments or a scalpel blade, that penetrates all layers of the skin.

Incomplete record A cow's production in a lactation that is terminated early for some reason. (Lactations not yet completed may be referred to as a "record in progress.")

Incontinence The inability to control the excretion of wastes; generally used to describe the inability to control urination.

Incubate To maintain favorable conditions for hatching fertile eggs.

Incubation period The time between the exposure to a disease, causing agent, and the onset of signs of the disease.

Incubator Machine used to keep eggs warm so that baby chicks will hatch from them.

Incumbent At level of other toes (hallux).

IND (investigational new drug) The pre-approval status of an experimental drug or biologic (e.g. vaccine) after the U.S. Food and Drug Administration (FDA) agrees that it can be tested in people (generally done in order to collect sufficiently data for licensure.) "IND" often refers to the application to obtain this pre-approval status.

Indications for use The situations when and how a specific product can be used.

Indirect lifecycle There are multiple hosts and so the parasite is actually required to pass from one host to another host, and sometimes to another host, before it comes back to the original host in this lifecycle.

Indirect transmission A mode of disease transmission where the environment is somehow part of the transmission cycle; i.e. contaminated water in a water trough spreads the disease.

Indolent ulcer Ulcerative lesions found most frequently on the upper lips, but also seen in the skin elsewhere or in the oral cavity.

Induced lactation A lactation that is artificially initiated by the use of hormones, not by birth.

In milk Designating a lactating female.

Induced ovulator An animal such as the queen that requires vaginal stimulation in order to ovulate.

Inducible NO synthase or iNOS Macrophages and other cells have an iNOS, which is induced by many different stimuli to activate NO synthesis. This is a major mechanism of host resistance to intracellular infection in mice, and probably in humans as well.

Infection An invasion of an organism by a pathogen such as bacteria or viruses. Some infections lead to disease.

Infection Control The activities aiming at the prevention and the spread of pathogens between patients, from healthcare workers to patients, and from patients to healthcare workers in the healthcare setting.

Infectious agents The organisms that cause infection; can be viruses, bacteria, fungi, or parasites.

Infectious Capable of invading living tissue and multiplying therein, causing disease.

Infectivity/Infectiousness Capacity of parasite to become established in the animal's tissues – e.g. rotavirus and coronavirus in calf scours, are carried in the gastrointestinal tract of calves (> 4 weeks of age) and older cattle without clinical signs of disease.

Infertility Inability to conceive and bear offspring.

Inflammation A condition in which tissue reacts to injury and undergoes changes during the healing process. As an example, a toe with a sliver of wood in it would be inflamed and show the signs of inflammation which include redness, increased temperature, pain, swelling, and a loss of or disordered function. The toe is swollen, red, hot, painful, and the animal is reluctant to walk on that toe.

Inflammatory Bowel Disease (IBD) A general term for any disease characterized by inflammation of the bowel. Examples include colitis and Crohn's disease. Symptoms include abdominal pain, diarrhea, fever, loss of appetite and weight loss.

Informed consent An agreement signed by prospective volunteers for a clinical research trial that indicates their understanding of 1. Why the research is being done,

2. What researchers want to accomplish,

3. What will be done during the trial and for how long,

4. What risks are involved,

5. what, if any, benefits can be expected from the trial,

6. What other interventions are available, and

7. The participant's right to leave the trial at any time.

Infusoria Microscopic organisms which are cultured as a food for the fry of freshwater fish.

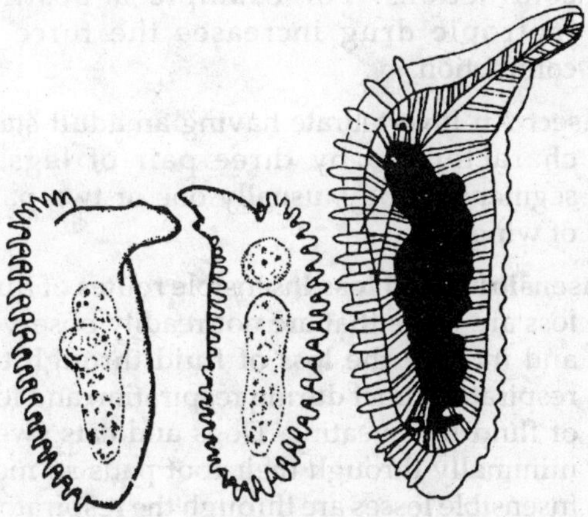

Fig. Infusoria

In hand class A class in which the horse is led by the exhibitor.

Inherited A trait passed from one generation to the next in the genes from each parent.

Initial database The initial information collected on a patient when the patient is first seen. The minimum amout of information that will be collected should be defined in advance and may differ for different types of patients.

Initial problem list A listing of problems identified from history and physical examination. This list becomes more specific as the results of diagnostic tests become available.

Initiation A stage in the development of acute renal failure defined as the time from renal insult to recognition of decreased GFR, decreased urine output and increased BUN and creatinine. This phase lasts 1-2 days.

Injection The administration of a substance into the skin, subcutaneous tissue, muscle tissue, or veins.

Innate A permanent characteristic that is present because of the genetic make-up of the animal.

Innate immunity Components of the immune system that everyone is born with.

Inotropic Affecting the force of muscle contractions. For example a positive inotropic drug increases the force of contraction.

Insect An invertebrate having an adult stage characterized by three pair of legs, a segmented body, usually one or two pairs of wings.

Insensible fluid loss Insensible routes of fluid loss are those that are not readily observed and include the loss of fluid through the respiratory tract during respiration and loss of fluid by sweating. Dogs and cats sweat minimally through their foot pads so most insensible losses are through the respiratory tract. The fluid lost during breathing is close to pure water and does not contain many solutes (a hypotonic loss). The basal loss of water through breathing is about: 10-15 ml/lb/day. High environmental temperatures, fever and activity result in increased insensible losses.

Insoluble carbohydrate Also, insoluble fiber. Fiber that resists enzymatic digestion in the small intestine.

Institute of Animal Health This is the largest research institute in the United Kingdom dedicated to the study of infectious diseases of farm animals. It has three laboratory sites at Compton, Pirbright, and Edinburgh.

Insulin A hormone produced by the pancreas which is necessary for glucose to be able to enter the cells of the body and be used for energy.

Insulin resistance A condition in which the blood glucose level remains higher than it should at an insulin dosage of 2 units/pound of body weight per day in cats.

Insulinoma Insulin-producing tumor of the pancreas; the increased production and blood level of insulin resulting from these tumors can cause low blood sugar (hypoglycemia).

Intake protein (IP) Total protein or nitrogen consumed without regard to quality.

Integrins Cellular sensors that act as signalling molecules.

Intensity of lay The number of eggs a hen lays during a given time.

Inter estrus interval The duration between consecutive estrous cycles, usually about 4 months in the bitch.

Inter trochanteric fossa A depression located between the greater and third trochanters of the femur. This is the site at which a needle penetrates into the femur for intraosseous administration or for collection of bone marrow.

Interbreeding The breeding of dogs of different breeds.

Interceptor Generic name is Milbemycin oxime.

Interdental space The space on the horse's jawbone between the incisors and pre-molars where there are no teeth, making room for the bit.

Interdigital pyoderma Bacterial infections between the toes.

Interferon (abbreviation IFN) A class of small glycoproteins that exert antiviral activity at least in homologous cells through cellular metabolic processes involving synthesis of double stranded RNA, which is an intermediate in replication of RNA viruses. IFN's are classified in three groups alpha, beta, and gamma based on their reactivities with antibodies as well as their physico-chemical properties and their cells of origin and method of induction.

Interferon A glycoprotein produced by macrophages, lymphocytes and epithelial cells in response to viral infection.

Inter-ictal The time period between seizures.

Interleukins They are also referred to as cytokines. These are regulatory proteins that are secreted primarily by lymphocytes to help the interaction between the lymphocyte and a macrophage.

Intermediate Host In the life cycle of some parasites, the immature form of the parasite must pass through a different type of host (animal, insect, snail, etc.), called the intermediate host, before it can re-enter and infect the type of animal it came from. An example would be heartworms. The adult worm lives in the dog or cat. The immature form, laid by the adult heartworm, is taken up by the mosquito. The immature form develops within the mosquito, and is then reintroduced into another dog or cat where it develops into the mature adult and the cycle repeats itself. The intermediate host for heartworms, then, is the mosquito.

Internal cooking temperature Lamb can be served rare (140 degrees), medium (150 degrees), or medium well (160 degrees) - never well done.

Internal Parasites One celled protozoan, larvae and worms that survive by living off the host animal's meals or blood.

Internal parasites Parasites located in the stomach and intestines of sheep.

International unit IUA standard unit of potency of a biological agent. Example: vitamin, hormone, antibiotic, antitoxin. Also called a USP unit.

Interossei Interossei are muscles in the human hand and foot.

Interposed abdominal compression CPR In CPR, interposed abdominal compressions with chest compressions with an alternating rhythm between the abdomen and the chest.

Interstitial Between parts or within the spaces of tissue.

Interstitial cell tumor A type of cancer of the testes.

Interstitial cystitis ICa condition of the bladder resulting in hematuria and pollakiuria that resembles the condition in humans with the same name.

Interstitial fluid Interstitial fluids are a subset of extracelluar fluids that surrounding cells and includes fluid in: dense connective tissue, bone, cartilage, cerebrospinal fluid, the gastrointestinal tract, and bile.

Interstitial space A subset of extracellualr fluid including fluid surrounding cells, in connective tissue, in bone, in cartilage, cerebrospinal fluid, fluid in the gastrointestinal tract and bile.

Intertriginous pyoderma Skin fold pyoderma occurring in lip folds (spaniels), facial folds (brachycephalic breeds), vulvar folds (obese, spayed females) and corkscrew tails (brachycephalic breeds).

Intervertebral disk disease, IVDD Pain and often paralysis resulting from displacement of the center of a vertebral disk.

Intestinal flora The normal bacteria found in the intestine.

Intestine The intestine is the convoluted membranous tube which extends from the stomach to the anus and which receives the ingested food from the stomach, mixes it with bile, pancreatic juice and intestinal secretions, gives origin to the chyle and delivers the indigestible products from the system.

Intra Inside within, opposite of extra.

Intra mammary antibiotics Antibiotics instilled directly into the mammary gland.

Intracardiac route The administration of drugs directly into the heart through the chest wall.

Intracellular An action taking place within a cell.

Intracellular fluid ICFF luid located inside cells. Comprises 2/3 of total body water.

Intracellular parasites Parasites that reside with in the hosts cells.

Intracellular vaccines Vaccines within a cell or cells.

Intracranial Originating within the cranial (brain) cavity.

Intradermal skin testing IDST Injection of known amounts of allergens intradermally and comparing the reaction to a positive (histamine) and negative control (saline).

Intralipid™ A solution of lipids available in 10 or 20% solution that can be administered IV.

Intramedullary A route of drug or fluid administration into the bone marrow cavity which is considered to be confluent with the vascular space. Fluids or drugs administered via this route, enter the blood stream very rapidly.

Intramuscle (im) injections The route of administration of an injection This is accomplished by inserting the needle straight into the skin and deep into the muscle.

Intramuscular (IM) In the muscle.

Intramuscular injection An injection made into the body of a muscle.

Intraocular pressure IOP The pressure within the globe. IOP is increased in glaucoma.

Intraosseous A route of drug or fluid administration into the bone marrow cavity which is considered to be confluent with the vascular space. Fluids or drugs administered via this route, enter the blood stream very rapidly.

Intratracheal route The administration of drugs into the trachea usually using a catheter placed near the tracheal bifurcation.

Intravascular IV Given directly into the blood stream.

Intravascular space The vascular space. Space located in the blood vessels.

Intravenous (iv) injections Are sometimes used. Some medications are labeled for intravenous injection only, because they are strong irritants to muscle and tissue and can cause damage. The IV route of administration provides a rapid means of getting the medication into the system of a sick animal as well as eliminating the chance of tissue damage. IV injections are given directly into the bloodstream.

Intravenous IV. Giving a drug or other substance into a vein for a rapid effect.

Intromission The act of placing the penis in the vagina.

Intron A segment of a gene that is transcribed to RNA but then is removed from the primary RNA transcript by splicing together the sequences (exons) on either side of the intron.

Intussusception A condition in which one part of the intestine 'telescopes' into another.

Inversion A dangerous condition where a horse's respiration rate is higher than its pulse rate.

Investigational vaccine A vaccine that has been approved by the Food and Drug Administration (FDA) for use in clinical trials on humans. However, investigational vaccines are still in the testing and evaluation phase and are not licensed for use in the general public.

Involution A decline in size or activity of tissues and/or organs. For example, the mammary gland tissues normally involute with advancing lactation. It is part of the process of lactating cows wherein they dry off.

Iodinated casein Milk protein (casein) to which iodine is bound. It is commonly referred to a thyroprotein and can be used to stimulate dairy cows to secrete more milk.

Iodine Disinfectant used on navels of newborn goats that helps dry up the navel, thus closing the passageway into the body of the goat. Also applied to hooves of newborns by some breeders. Veterinary iodine contains 7% iodine while common iodine for humans contains 2% iodine.

Ionofores One of the most common feed additives that we give cows to increase production, to increase efficiency, and increase rate of gain.

Ionophore A carboxylic polyether antibiotic that affects the transport of ions across cellular membranes and inhibits the growth of some gram positive bacteria. It is used in growing cattle to enhance feed efficiency and stimulate growth. Examples: Bovatec, Rumensin.

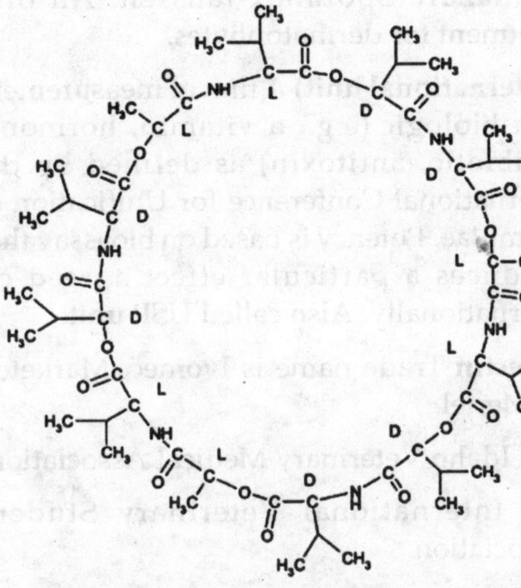

Fig. Ionophore

IR genes Immune response genes are genetic polymorphisms that control the intensity of the immune response to a particular antigen. Virtually all Ir phenotypes are due to the differential binding of peptide fragments of antigen to MHC molecules, especially MHC class II molecules. The term is little used now. An immune response gene defect is usually, but not always due to failure to bind an immunogenic peptide, so that no T cell response is observed.

IRB (Institutional Review Board) A committee of physicians, statisticians, community advocates and other that reviews clinical trial protocols before they can be initiated and is responsible for monitoring the safety of clinical trials at that institution. IRBs ensure that the trial is ethical and that the rights of participants are adequately protected.

Iridencleisis Treatment for glaucoma in which a window is made in the sclera and the iris pulled through and sutured under the conjunctiva.

Iris bombe Posterior synechiae that occur all the way around the pupil and aqueous cannot flow through.

Iris hypoplasia In blue-eyed animals: may see iris hypoplasia where the iris fails to develop properly and the irises of these young animals are almost transparent.

Iris prolapse Prolapse of the iris through a defect (ulcer) in the cornea.

Iris The colored portion of the eye is called the iris. As with humans, dogs' iris colors vary. In the center of the iris is the black opening called the pupil. This opening can be made larger or smaller by muscles called ciliary bodies, that attach to the colored iris, causing it to expand or contract.

Irish Setter Any of a breed of setters having a silky reddish-brown or red and white coat.

Irons Stirrups on an English saddle.

Irregular bones In anatomy, irregular bones are bones which do not fit into any of the other bone types. They are comprised of a spongy substance enclosed within a thin layer of compact bone.

Irritable bowel syndrome Soft or watery feces, often with mucus. Associated with stress. Also called colitis.

Isabella Usually used to describe Doberman Pinschers, this color is similar to fawn or light bay, but has more saturation and brilliance (similar to a bay-colored horse). Color definitions may vary by breed. Always check the breed standard for the definitive color description.

Iso ionic Iso-ionic refers to a similar concentration of a particular electrolyte in a solution compared to extracellular fluid; therefore solutions which are iso-ionic with regard to sodium will have sodium concentrations comparable to the sodium concentration of extracellular fluid and plasma, which is approximately 145 mEq/l in the dog and cat.

Isoerythrolysis A condition in which antibodies in the mare's colostrum destroy the foal's red blood cells.

Isoflavone An estrogen-like substance produced by pasture plants; a type of phytoestrogen.

Isomer Different spacial configurations of a drug or chemical compound.

Isosthenuria Urine with the same specific gravity as glomerular filtrate indicating that the renal tubules have performed no work to either concentrate or dilute glomerular filtrate. There are also non-renal causes of isosthenuria.

Isothermalizer Part of the Equitainer semen container system.

Isotonic Isotonic or iso-osmotic fluids have the same tonicity or osmolality as does extracellular fluid, which in the dog and cat is approximately 280-310 mOsm/l.

Isotonic dehydration Dehydration characterized by the loss of water and electrolytes in a ratio similar to extracellualar water. Dogs and cats most often have isotonic dehydration as water and electrolytes are lost.

Isotretinoin (Accutane-Roache. A retinoids which is a synthetic derivatives of vitamin A.

Itraconazole Sporanox-Janssen. An oral treatment for dermatophytes.

IU (international unit) A unit of measurement of a biologic (e.g., a vitamin, hormone, antibiotic, antitoxin) as defined by the International Conference for Unification of Formulae. Potency is based on bioassay that produces a particular effect agreed on internationally. Also called USP unit.

Ivermectin Trade name is Ivomec. Marketed by Meriel.

IVMA Idaho Veterinary Medical Association.

IVSA International Veterinary Student Association.

J

Jabot The apron of the Schipperke; the part situated between the front legs.

Jack A male donkey.

Jack Russell Terrier A terrier originating in England, having a small sturdy body, straight legs, and a smooth, mostly white coat that has brown or black markings.

Jacobsens Organ A sense organ located in the roof of the dog's mouth that functions somewhere between smell and taste.

Jaundice The condition in which there is a buildup of waste products in the body called bilirubin. Bilirubin is yellow in color, therefore, an animal with jaundice will have yellow gums, skin (often seen on the inside flap of the ear), and a yellowish cast to the 'whites' of the eyes. It can occur if a large number of red blood cells are destroyed, the liver is not functioning normally, or the bile ducts are blocked.

Jejunum The jejunum is the second part of the human small intestine. It is about 9 feet long.

Jen Chung An acupunture technique also referred to as governing vessel 26 which causes sympathetic stimulation.

Jenny A female donkey.

Jerk To pull or yank a rope or rein.

Jet injector Needleless device that allows the injection of a substance under pressure through the skin without a needle.

Jill A female ferret.

Jog A slow Western trot.

Jog cart Two-wheeled cart used to exercise Standardbred horses, heavier than a race sulky.

Johne's disease (Mycobacterium paratuberculosis) A bacterial disease causing severe weight loss and sometimes diarrhea.

Johnes A wasting disease of ruminants, contagious in their fecal matter (poop).

Joining Putting the rams and ewes together for mating. Tupping is the same thing.

Joint A joint is a structure where two bones meet.

Joule J A unit adopted by Systeme International (SI) for expressing energy. The Joule is more commonly used in Europe than in North America (4.184J = 1 calorie).

Jowls Flesh of the lips and jaws.

Jug A small pen used to confine a ewe and her newborn lamb(s).

Jugular A large vein on the bottom surface of the neck that may be used to collect blood samples or to place catheters.

Jugular vein The jugular vein returns blood from the head to the heart in vertebrates.

Jumper Horse judged on jumping performance based only on faults and time. Touch faults are sometimes also used. Preliminary jumpers are those horses having won up to $1,000; Intermediate up to $3,000; Open over $3,000.

Jump off In the event of a tie, a course may be altered and the two tied horses asked to jump again.

Junior Rider under eighteen years of age as of January 1. Horse four years of age and under.

Juvenile cellulitis Moist juvenile Pyoderma or Puppy strangles. Lesions of erythema, draining tracts, alopecia, and edema of the chin, lips, ears and eyelids seen in puppies less than 6 months old. Lesions are located on the muzzle and head, although abdominal, axillary and inguinal regions can be affected.

Juveniles An immature weaned llama.

K

Keel The breastbone, which resembles the keel of a boat.

Kava A beverage brewed from the dried roots and rhizomes of the plant Piper methysticum has been consumed in some areas of the South Pacific for many centuries. It can act as an antidepressant and may be used to treat anxiety and tension. Kava may have sedative properties.

KBr Potassium Bromide. An AED.

KCS Keratoconjunctivitis sicca is the technical term for a condition also known as 'dry eye.' It occurs because of inadequate tear production. Symptoms include a thick, yellowish discharge from the eye.

Keds Bloodsucking ticks that pierce the skin causing serious damage to the pelts.

Keel The rounded outline of the lower chest.

Keepers Fixed loops, used to keep the ends of the straps of a bridle (or saddle) in place.

Keet a Guinea Fowl chick.

Kelp A form of iodine-rich seaweed. Extracts of kelp have been used as a goiter remedy.

Kemp An opaque and structureless fiber present in badly bred wools which appear not to absorb dye and consequently is prominent in the finished fabric unless further treated in some way.

Kennel Building or enclosure where dogs are kept.

Kennel Cough Tracheobronchitis of dogs or cats.

Keratic precipitates Clusters of inflammatory cells on the back (endothelial surface) of the cornea.

Keratin A cystine rich protein produced by the epithelial cells.

Keratinization disorders Cutaneous disorders characterized by scaling.

Keratitis Inflammation of the cornea of the eye; may be caused by infection, trauma, or an allergic reaction.

Keratoconjunctivitis sicca KCS Dry eye which may be a consequence of prior exposure and infection with canine distemper virus.

Keratoconjunctivitis sicca Keratoconjunctivitis sicca (KCS) is the technical term for a condition also known as 'dry eye'. It occurs because of inadequate tear production. Symptoms include a thick, yellowish discharge from the eye.

Keratolytic Softens and loosens crusts and scales on the skin.

Keratotomy Removal of part of the thickness of the cornea.

Kerry Blue Terrier A breed of terrier of Irish origin, having a dense, wavy bluish-gray coat.

Ketoacidosis A life-threatening condition in which ketones, which result from the breakdown of fat for energy, accumulate in the bloodstream and the pH of the blood decreases.

Ketoconazole Nizoral-Janssen. An oral treatment for dermatophytes.

Ketones Compounds found in the blood of pregnant sheep suffering from pregnancy toxemia

Ketonuria The presence of ketone bodies in the urine, as with ketosis in high-producing cows.

Kid A goat up to one year old.

Kid(s) Baby goats, either sex.

Kidding Having babies.

Kidding Parturition in the goat; the act of giving birth to young.

Kidney The kidney is a gland used for filtering urine from the blood.

Killed vaccine A vaccine that contains antigen of the infectious agent that has been killed by chemical or physical means and does not replicate in the host.

Killed Virus Vaccine (KV) A vaccine containing dead viruses which cannot multiply when administered in an animal, but can stimulate an immune response to prevent future infection by the virus.

Killer T cell Another term used for cytotoxic T cells.

Kilocalorie (kcal) Equivalent to 1000 calories.

Kinase An enzyme that is important in regulating cell functions, specifically can transfer a phosphate from a high energy phosphate such as ATP

Kindling A process where having repetitive seizures lowers the threshold for having more seizures. This is one reason for getting early control of the seizures.

Kinesiology An investigation of the muscle-gland-organ link for an indication of the cause of illnesses. Practicioners of applied kinesiology believe muscles reflect the flow of ch'i and that by measuring muscle resistance one can determine the health of bodily organs. Once a problem has been identified, various treatment techniques are used to strengthen the muscles involved and restore health.

Kinetic skull Having mobile joints between various parts of the skull, e.g., being able to unhinge the jaws. This allows the mouth of the animal, e.g., snake, to open wider so that it can eat large prey.

Kink Tail A deformity of the caudal vertebrae producing a bent tail.

Kiss A smacking noise made with the lips, to cue the horse to move forward also known as "clucking."

Kiss Marks Tan spots on the cheeks and over the eyes. Color definitions may vary by breed. Always check the breed standard for the definitive color description.

Kit A baby ferret.

Kitten A young, immature cat. The kitten class at a North American show is open to purebred and registered kittens that are between the ages of four and seven months (inclusive) and meet the standard for their breed. Adult cats compete in the championship or premiership (alter) classes.

Knee boot Leather or plastic device used to protect knees from bruising each other as horse jogs or races.

Knee The carpal joint, between the radius and the cannon of the foreleg.

Knee cap The stifle, with the bone known as the patella.

Knee Joint See Stifle

Knock in Transgenic animal in which a gene has been added, or the process of adding a gene

Knock out Transgenic animal in which a gene has been removed, or the process of deleting a gene

Known Carrier An animal that has produced offspring with a genetic defect.

Knuckling Over Faulty structure of wrist joint allowing it to flex forward under the weight of the standing dog.

Koch's postulates Used in infectious diseases to determine if the parasite will cause disease. The traditional criteria used are as follows:The organism must be regularly isolated from cases of the disease. The organism must be grown in pure culture or free of the animal host. Such a pure culture should cause disease upon inoculation into susceptible animal. The same organisms must be re-isolated from the experimentally induced disease.

Kur Musical freestyle in dressage.

Kuvasz A long-established Hungarian breed of tall, light-footed but sturdy white dog; used also as a hunting dog.

Ky1 adjuvant A form of adjuvant.

L

Labrador Retriever A breed of dog originating in Newfoundland, having a short, yellow, black, or brown coat and a tapering tail and used in hunting to retrieve felled game.

Labrum The labrum is the ventral lobe in the front of an insect's head which covers the mouth parts.

Laceration Cut.

Lachrymal gland The lachrymal gland is a gland beneath the upper eye lid which secretes tears which drain from the inner corner of the eye through the Lachrymal duct to the nose.

Lachrymation The act of tearing; secreting and conveying tears.

Lacrimal system Consists of 2 glands that produce the aqueous tear film component, one in the dorsolateral orbit and one on the bulbar surface of the nictitans. Tears flow through the nasolacrimal duct to the nose

Lactate To secrete or produce milk; also, salt of beta-hydroxy propionic acid.

Lactated ringer's solution Lactated ringer's solution is one of the most common crystalloid solutions used in a small animal practice. It has an osmolality comparable to extracellular fluid, so it is considered an isotonic solution. Most lactated Ringer's solution that are commercially available are marketed for people, therefore the actual osmolality of lactated Ringer's solution is slightly less than the osmolality of canine and feline extracellular fluid/plasma. The sodium, potassium, and chloride concentrations of lactated Ringer's solution are comparable to extracellular fluid, although the sodium concentration is iso ionic to human extracellular fluid/plasma and is slightly lower than the sodium concentration of canine and feline extracellular fluid/plasma. Lactated Ringer's solution contains lactate, which is converted by the liver to bicarbonate.

Lactated Ringers Solution Used for adding body fluids to a dehydrated goat (known as LRS).

Lactating Producing milk.

Lactation The period of time when the doe is producing milk. Normally from birth of kid to weaning.

Lactation average Actual 305-day average milk and component production for all cows in the herd that was completed during a 12-month period. (Since dry days are not included, lactation averages usually are 8 to 15 percent higher than rolling herd averages).

Lactation curve A graphic plot of days in milk vs. pounds of milk produced.

Lactation period The number of days an animal secretes milk following each parturition. Usually 11 to 12 months.

Lactation record The total milk and components produced by a cow beginning on the day of calving and ending on the day the cow goes dry. For purposes of genetic comparison, 10-month (305-day) lactation records are the standard of the industry. A 306 to 365-day lactation record may be used for promotion. Lactation records greater than 365 days will not be published.

Lactation totals to date The production totals for milk and components through the current test date.

Lacteals Lacteals are small lymphatic vessels which arise from the mucous membrane lining of the small bowel.

Lactogenic immunity A form of local immunity in milk (post colostrum) that bathes the intestinal tract and prevents colonization by virulent bacteria and neutralized viruses passing through the gut.

Lactogenic Stimulating the secretion of milk.

Lactose intolerance A condition in which lactose is not adequately hydrolyzed in the intestine because of insufficient lactase enzyme.

Lactose The 12-carbon sugar unique to milk; a disaccharide composed of glucose and galactose. Average milk contains about 5 percent lactose which varies little by breed.

Lagophthalmos Inability to fully close the eyelids over the eyeball.

Lamb Any sheep less than a year old. Produced on the farm or purchased at about 20 pounds and raised until 8 9 months old. Normal selling weight is 90 100 pounds. Usually purchased in early summer and sold in late fall of same year.

Lamb bed Uterus.

Lamb marking The act of earmarking, docking, and castrating lambs.

Lambdoidal suture The lambdoidal suture is a fissure which divides the parietal bone from the occipital bone in the human skull.

Lambing Ewes giving birth to young.

Lamellate Coarse or fine parallel ridges or plates (at cutting edge of bill).

Lameness Unevenness in the horses stride when moving.

Laminitis Founder, inflammation of the sensitive laminae, or plates of vascular tissue, of the wall of the horse's hoof.

Landseer Newfoundlands that are white dogs with black markings, named in honor of Sir Edward Landseer, the 19th Century artist who used these dogs as models

Langerhans cells Phagocytic dendritic cells found in the epidermis. They can migrate from the epidermis to regional lymph nodes via the lymphatics. In the lymph node they differentiate into dendritite cells.

Lanolin Grease that is on the fleece of sheep. Lanolin is used in make up and lotions and also to "waterproof" shoes.

Laparascopy Examination of the contents of the peritoneum with a laparoscope passed through the abdominal wall. A laparoscpe is a type of endoscope, a tube down which light is reflected. Fitted with grasping and cutting tools, the laparascope can perform minor surgery, take tissue samples for biopsy and remove eggs from the ovary.

Laparotomy A surgical procedure to open the abdominal (belly) cavity.

Large Fowl The original sized chicken (as opposed to Bantams) Large fowl typically range in size from four pounds to 13 pounds. They encompass most of the varieties of chickens people are familiar with but are often larger than many people realize. Light breeds of large fowl are primarily egg layers and lay white shelled eggs. Heavier breeds include the utility and meat breeds and typically lay brown eggs.

Large intestine The lower part of the intestinal tract, usually made up of the colon, cecum, and rectum. Bacteria that live harmlessly in the large intestine help to digest complex carbohydrates.

Larva The worm-like offspring of an insect (plural larvae).

Larvae Insects or parasites that have hatched from eggs but are not yet mature. For example, maggots.

Larynx The larynx is a muscular tube in the neck that allows air to pass from the throat to the trachea (windpipe). The larynx contains the vocal cords, which allow people and animals to make sounds. The larynx has cartilage that opens to allow air into the trachea.

Latency A virus which remains hidden and does not cause disease but which may reactivate and cause clinical signs of disease at a later time.

Latent A dormant stage of disease; the patient is infected with an organism, but is not yet ill.

Lateral Movements Work in which the horse moves with the forehand and haunches on different tracks. Shoulder-in, haunches-in (travers), haunches-out (renvers), and half-passes are the lateral movements.

Lateral Pertaining to the side.

Lateral recumbent Laying down on the side.

Lateral torsion Twisted or rotated out.

Latigo Cinch strap on a Western saddle.

Layback The angle of the shoulder blade as compared with the vertical plane viewed from the side.

Layer A bird kept for egg production - most commonly chickens and ducks. Common layer breeds such as leghorn chickens and Khaki Campbell ducks have been developed to lay many eggs and generally do not set a nest well.

Layon The angle of the shoulder blade as compared with the vertical plane viewed from the front.

Leaching The process of removal of soluble materials by the passage of water through soil.

Lead A specific footfall pattern at the canter or lope in which the inside legs of the circle reach farther forward than the outside legs. When working to the right on the right lead, the horse's right foreleg and right hind leg reach farther forward than the left legs. If a horse is loping in a circle to the right on the left lead, he is said to be on the wrong lead or is counter-cantering.

Lead feeding Gradually increasing grain fed cows to a level equal 1.0 to 1.5 percent of body weight beginning about three weeks prior to the predicted calving date. Following parturition, grain is increased until a cow reaches maximum feed intake. Also called challenge feeding.

Lead rope A rope usually having a snap on one end, used to lead or tie a horse.

Lead shank A webbing or leather strap with short length of chain and a snap, used to lead a horse.

Leash A chain, rope, or strap attached to the collar or harness of an animal, especially a dog, and used to lead it or hold it in check.

Leather The flap of the ear; the outer ear supported by cartilage and surrounding tissue.

Lecithin Phospholipids found widely in animals and plants,(e.g. egg yolk) that have emulsifying, wetting, and antioxidant properties.

Leg Bands Cloth or plastic strips of a bright color used for marking treated cows, fresh cows, or cows needing special handling.

Leg Yielding Exercises designed to teach the horse to move away from leg pressure

Legging up Conditioning a horse's muscle tone by gradually increasing his work.

Legume Any of thousands of plant species that have seed pods that split along both sides when ripe. Some of the more common legumes used for human consumption are beans, lentils, peanuts, peas, and soybeans. Others, such as clover and alfalfa, are used as animal feed. Legumes have a unique ability to obtain much or all of their nitrogen requirements from symbiotic nitrogen fixation.

Lemon Used to describe pointers, this color is a brilliant, medium-saturated yellow. Color definitions may vary by breed. Always check the breed standard for the definitive color description.

Lens Structure in the eye which functions to transmit and focus incoming light rays directly on the retina; this is facilitated by accommodation - the subtle change in lens shape brought about by contraction and relaxation of the ciliary body; the accommodative ability of the lens is limited in domestic species.

Lens capsule A clear elastic membrane surrounding the lens body.

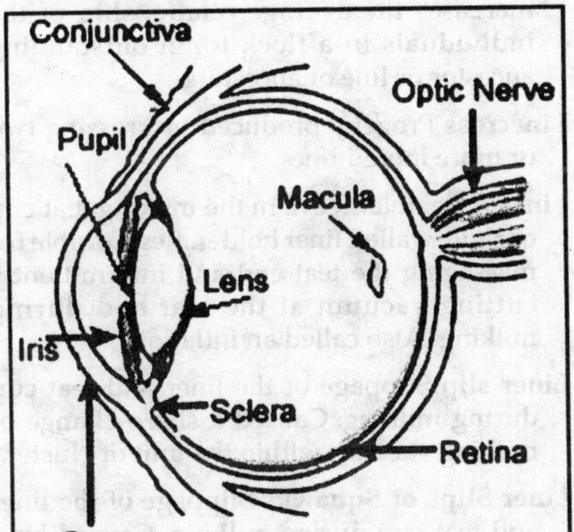

Fig. Lens capsule

Lens luxation Primary or secondary displacement of the lens either anterior into pupil or anterior chamber or posterior into the vitreous chamber.

Leptospirosis An infectious disease caused by various leptospira bacteria affecting most warm-blooded species.

Lesion An abnormal lump or bump.

Letdown The process in a cow where physical stimulation causes a release of oxytocin and the contraction of smooth muscles surrounding milk alveoli resulting in fluid pressure within the udder and milk flow.

Lethargy Malaise or inactivity.

Lethargy or lethargic An animal which is slow to react, lacks energy, and is often sick.

Leucocytes Leucocytes is the anatomical term for colourless corpuscles. (White blood cells).

Leukemia A cancerous proliferation of one of the subsets of White Blood Cells.

Leukocyte A general term for a white blood cell. Leukocytes include lymphocytes, monocytes, and polymorhonuclear leukocytes.

Leukocytosis High white blood cell count.

Leukopenia A condition in which the numbers of white blood cells in the blood are lower than normal.

Leukotriene Substances derived from arachidonic acid in cell membranes that mediate allergic responses.

Levator palpebrae superioris Muscle in the upper lid that elevates the upper eyelid. It is innervated by cranial nerve 3, the oculomotor nerve.

Level Bite When the front teeth (incisors) of the upper and lower jaws meet exactly edge to edge. Also called pincer bite, equal bite, or even bite.

Level Gait Dog moves without rise or fall of withers.

Levels This refers to the results from monitoring the AED serum concentration in the blood. Also called blood levels, serum levels.

LFA-3 Lymphocyte function-associated antigen-3 is a molecule found on many cells that is the ligand for CD2 (also known as LFA-2). It is a member of the immunoglobulin superfamily.

Lhasa Apso A breed of small dog originating in Tibet and having a long, straight coat.

Libido Usually refers to the male's sex drive.

Lichenification Thickening, hardening and often hyperpigmentation of the skin.

Licorice A commonly used medicinal herb from the plant called Glycyrrhiza glabra which has tiny violet flowers in the summer. Licorice root may be used as a cough suppressant or for digestive disorders. Large amounts of licorice over long periods of time may affect the body's electrolyte balance.

Lidocaine A drug used as a local anaesthetic and as an antiarrhythmic agent in treatment of certain cardiac arrhythmias such as ventricular fibrillation.

Lifetime production totals The production totals for milk and components for a cow since her first calving (or first time on DHI test). Totals will include production beyond 365 days in a lactation, production credits for an abnormally initiated record and any production from prepartum milking.

Ligaments Strong. fibrous bands connecting bone to bone.

Ligand Usually refers to a protein like BMP that is secreted and binds to a receptor (often on the surface of a cell.)

Lignin A compound which, with cellulose, forms the cell walls of plants. It is practically indigestible.

Limbic system A group of brain structures which exert an important influence on the endocrine and autonomic motor system's and which influence (emotion) mood states.

Limbus Junction between conjunctiva and cornea.

Limited Type of class with entry restrictions for the horse and/ or the rider, related to prior winnings at specified shows. May be based on number of blue ribbons (usually six) or monetary earnings.

Line The strap leading from the bit to the driver's hands in a driving harness

Linear immunoglobulin A dermatosis Clinically presents as subcorneal pustules, epidermal collarettes, etc. generally truncal in distribution. Most often seen in the dachshund.

Linear score (SCC) Linear scores for somatic cell counts (SCC's) convert SCC logarithmically from cells per milliliter to a linear score from 0 to 9. The linear score has a straight line, inverse relationship with milk yield. An increase of one in the linear score is associated with a 400-pound decrease in lactation milk yield or a 1.5 pound drop in daily yield.

Linebreed To mate together cats that have some of the same ancestors. For example, two cats that have the same grandfather.

Linebreeding A form of inbreeding which increases the average relationship of the individuals in a flock to an outstanding ancestor or line of ancestors.

Linecross Progeny produced by crossing two or more inbred lines.

Liner A flexible sleeve in the milking teat cup or rigid-walled liner holder. Responsible for massaging the teat end and intermittently cutting vacuum at the teat end during milking. Also called an inflation.

Liner slip Slippage of the liner and teat cup during milking. Caused a sharp change of milking vacuum within the unit or cluster.

Liner Slips or Squawks Slippage of the liner and teat cup during milking. Caused by a sharp change of milking vacuum within the unit or cluster by drawing in air alongside the teat. Generally creates a "squawking" sound.

Liniment A liquid applied externally to increase circulation to a part of the body.

Lip The lips are the fleshy edges of the opening of the mouth.

Lipase Digestive enzyme, produced by the pancreas, which breaks down fat.

Lipid Any one of a group of organic substances that are insoluble in water though soluble in alcohol, ether, chloroform, and other fat solvents, and have a greasy feel. They are rich sources of dietary energy.

Lipoxygenase 5-LOX5 lipoxygenase breaks down arachidonic acid to form the leukotrienes. The leukotrienes mediate activation and margination of neutrophils, altered vascular permeability, and promotion of gastric ulceration or degenerative joint disease.

Liquid protein supplement LPSA protein product usually containing molasses, urea, added vitamins and trace minerals; particularly useful in pasture feeding.

Liquid solid separation The process of passing a liquid-solid suspension, such as animal manure, over a screen or similar device to partially remove solids prior to storage or application.

Listeria monocytogenus A species of the genus Listeria that is aerobic, microaerophilic, motile peritrichous bacterium. The bacteria are found in the feces of humans and other animals, in vegetation and in silage, and are parasitic on poikilothermic and warm-blooded animals including humans.

Listeriosis A sporadic disease causing meningitis septicemia, endocarditis etc. Sometimes involved in infections of immunocompromised individuals and in neonatal infections.

Litter One or more kittens produced by a single pregnancy. Litter size averages three or four, but some litters may have six to ten kittens!

Litter registration The recording by a cat registering association of the birth of a litter, including the date of birth, number of kittens, sire and dam, and the breeder of the litter.

Live basis sale The most common method of selling lambs at private treaty and/or auction. The buyer makes an offer for the live lamb (per head or per pound) which the seller accepts or rejects.

Live vaccine A vaccine in which live virus is weakened through chemical or physical processes in order to produce an immune response without causing the severe effects of the disease. Attenuated vaccines currently licensed in the United States include measles, mumps, rubella, polio, yellow fever and varicella. Also known as an attenuated vaccine.

Live vector vaccine A vaccine that uses a non-disease-causing organism (virus or bacterium) to transport foreign genes into the body, thereby stimulating an effective immune response to the foreign products. This type of vaccine is important because it is particularly capable of inducing CTL activity.

Liver chestnut (n and adj.) A very dark red chestnut color, with mane, tail, and legs the same color as the body or flaxen.

Liver The largest organ in the abdomen, responsible for producing enzymes required for digestion of food, and bile that helps to digest fat. The liver also detoxifies the blood and may be damaged in the process.

Liver flukes Small leaf-shaped organisms that rolls up like a scroll in the bile ducts or liver tissue.

Liver The liver is the largest gland in the human body. The liver has three functions: it secretes bile, stores glycogen and converts waste products into urea and uric acid for excretion.

Loading Chute A chute used for loading animals into a truck or trailer.

Loafing (area) (alley) (barn) (shed) A resting area for cattle.

Loafing area Area of farm, often associated with free stalls and milking barn where animals are free to exercise and move voluntarily.

Lobate With lobes (toes).

Local Veterinary Inspector A private veterinary surgeon who carries out some work for the State Veterinary Service.

Lochia Green colored post-partum discharge. The appearance of lochia before delivery indicates placental separation and impaired blood flow to the fetuses.

Loin The part between the last rib and the hip bones.

Long bones In human anatomy, long bones are found in the limbs where they form levers. They have a hollow shaft.

Long feed Coarse or unchopped feed such as hay, as contrasted with short, or chopped, feed.

Long term care facility A long-term care facility is a facility that provides rehabilitative, restorative, and/or ongoing skilled nursing care to patients or residents in need of assistance with activities of daily living. Long-term care facilities include nursing homes, rehabilitation facilities, inpatient behavioral health facilities, and long-term chronic care hospitals.

Long test interval Routinely, tests are conducted each 15 to 45 days, or approximately one each month. An emergency or supervisor vacation schedules may extend the interval beyond 45 days. For herds on official plans, reasons for a long test interval (46 to 75 days) must be reported on the barnsheet by the supervisor. Official status of the record is lost if the interval exceeds 75 days.

Long trot An extended jog or trot. Or in the giated equine, a slang used to refer to the gait of a horse that is being pushed or over ridden in the fox trot. A horse that is long trotting will have some fly time on the front end, but may not have fly time on the back end. A long trotting horse will have at least three feet off the ground part of the time, and will not give as smooth a ride as a horse that is foxtrotting correctly.

Longe To work a horse in a circle usually on a 30-foot line around you at various gaits.

Longhair A cat with relatively long fur, often varying in length over different parts of the cat. Some longhairs have shortish fur on the body, but all longhairs have long fur on the tail, forming a "plume" or "brush," and most have long fur around the neck forming a "ruff."

Longus capitis The longus capitis is the human muscle which flexes the head.

Longus cervicis The longus cervicis is the human muscle which bends the cervical portion of the vertebral column forwards.

Loom A machine for producing cloth by weaving.

Loose Housing Facilities that allow cattle access to a large, open bedded area for resting (also known as free housing). Loose housing should provide at least 200 square feet per animal for feeding and resting (freestall housing uses only 90 square feet per animal).

Loose housing Facilities which allow cattle access to a large, open bedded area for resting. Also known as free housing. Loose housing provides at least 200 square feet per animal for feeding and resting while freestall housing uses only 90 square feet per animal.

Lope A three-beat gait 1. an initiating hind leg;

2. a diagonal pair including the leading hind leg and the diagonal foreleg; and

3. the leading foreleg. Also, to canter slowly.

Loratidine Claritan. An antihistamine.

Lore Area between eye and bill.

Low moisture silage Silage that contains 35 to 55 percent moisture. See haylage.

Low passage vaccine A low passage vaccine contains virus particles which have been attenuated, or weakened, less than those in the 'average' vaccine. Low passage vaccines can generally elicit an immune system response in young animals who have a maternal antibody level that would prevent them from responding to an 'average' vaccine.

Lowfat milk Milk containing at least 8.25 percent solids and from which sufficient milk fat has been removed to produce, within limits of good manufacturing practice, a milk fat content of 0.5, 1.0, or 2.0 percent.

Low set Having short legs.

LRS Used for adding body fluids to a dehydrated goat (known as Lactated Ringers Solution).

Lucerne Alfalfa (Medicago sativa) A legume of high feeding value for ruminants.

Lufeneron A benzoyl-phenylurea compound that inhibits chitin development. An insect growth regular.

Lumbar vertebrae In human anatomy, the lumbar vertebrae are the 5 vertebrae following the thoracic vertebrae.

Lumbricals The Lumbricals are muscles in the human fingers used in writing etc.

Lunate bone The lunate bone is one of the bones in the human wrist.

Lungs The lungs are organs used for respiration.

Lungworms Roundworms found in the respiratory tract and lung tissue.

Lupus A disease characterized by inflammation of the connective tissue (which supports and connects all parts of the body). Chronic swelling of the connective tissue causes damage to the skin, joints, kidneys, nervous system and mucous membranes. The disease begins with fever, joint pain and fatigue. Additional symptoms continue to develop over the years including nausea, fatigue, weight loss, arthritis, headaches and epilepsy. Problems with heart, lung and kidney function may also result. This condition is diagnosed most frequently in young women but also occurs in children.

Lutalyse (PGF2a or Prostaglandin) A hormone used for estrus synchronization, infected uteruses, and inducing abortion.

Luteinizing hormone LH LH causes ovulation of ovarian follicles. LH is also believed to be involved in testicular descent into the scrotum.

Luxating tarsus Dislocation of the 'ankle'

Lyme disease A bacterial disease transmitted by infected ticks. Human beings may come into contact with infected ticks during outdoor activities (camping, hiking). Symptoms include fatigue, chills, fever, headache, joint and muscle pain, swollen lymph nodes and a skin rash (in a circular pattern). Long-term problems include arthritis, nervous system abnormalities, irregular heart rhythm and meningitis. Lyme disease can be treated with antibiotics or prevented with the use of a vaccine recently licensed by the Food and Drug Administration.

Lymph A usually clear fluid similar to blood serum; it may be free in the tissues of the body, in lymph vessels, or part of the blood.

Lymph nodes Part of the immune system of an animal. Small masses of tissue that contain white blood cells called lymphocytes. Blood from the nearby area is filtered through the lymph node allowing foreign or infectious material to be recognized and destroyed if possible.

Lymphoblastoid Describing a peripheral blood lymphocyte immortalized by a virus such as Epstein-Barr virus (EBV).

Lymphocyte Any of the colorless mobile cells originating from stem cells and differentiating in lymphoid tissue (as of the thymus or bone marrow). Lymphocytes are the typical cellular elements of lymph (or tissue fluids), include the cellular mediators of immunity, and constitute 20 to 30 percent of the white blood cells of normal human blood.

Lymphoid organs Organs that regulate the production and differentiation of lymphocytes. The main lymphoid organ are the salivary glands, the thymus, the spleen, and the bone marrow.

Lymphokines Chemicals produced by T lymphocytes. Some lymphokines signal macrophages and other phagocytes to destroy foreign invaders.

Lymphoma A tumor of lymphocytes that grows in lymphoid and other tissues but do not enter the blood in large numbers. There are many types of lymphoma, which represent the transformation of various classes of lymphoid cell.

Lymphosarcoma Malignant tumor that arises from cells of the lymphoreticular system. Commonly presents with swollen lymph nodes, masses, enlarged liver or spleen, fevers, weight loss.

Lysosome A saclike structure within cells that contains various enzymes that break down other cellular products.

M

Mate The pairing of a rooster with one or more hens; a hen or rooster so paired.

MacKenzie Brush technique This technique employs a sterile toothbrush to comb the hair coat of an animal suspected to be a carrier of dermatophytes. The bristles of the brush are then embedded or shaken over agar for culture.

Macro minerals Minerals required in relatively large amounts by livestock. Includes calcium (Ca), phosphorus (P) magnesium (Mg), potassium (K) chlorine (Cl), sulfur (S) and sodium (Na).

Macrophages Modulate the inflammatory response and stimulate the immune system; are a critical part of the body's response to injury

Macule A circumscribed, flat (not raised or depressed) change in the color of the skin. Large macules are patches.

Magnetic resonance image MRIA ·diagnostic technique that produces computerized images of internal body structures. MRI uses a large magnet to polarize hydrogen atoms in the tissues and then monitors the spinning energies within cells.

Mahogany Used to describe several breeds, this color is a medium-saturated, dull, reddish brown. Color definitions may vary by breed. Always check the breed standard for the definitive color description.

Maiden Division open to a rider (or horse) who has not won a blue ribbon at specified shows.

Maiden ewe A female that has not been bred by a ram.The term is commonly applied to ewes that have not had their first lamb.

Maiden female A female that has not been bred.

Maiden mare Mare that has never been bred.

Maintenance phase A phase of acute renal failure following initiation during which oliguria persists. Whether an ARF patient is oliguric or polyuric reflects the severity of insult which caused ARF. The majority of ARF dogs and cats become oliguric although some ARF patients are never oliguric. In those patients which can repair the renal damage, the oliguric phase lasts 1-2 weeks. Many animals die or are euthanized during the oliguric phase because of the poor prognosis. The most life-threatening consequences of the oliguric phase include hyperkalemia and overzealous fluid therapy resulting in overhydration.

Maintenance solutions Maintenance solutions are hypotonic compared to extracellular fluid. They have more potassium than extracellular fluid and less sodium than extracellular fluid. Maintenance solutions can be purchased or "created" from other cystalloid solutions.

Making a Wheel Term given to the circling of the tail over the back.

Malabsorption syndrome Maldigestion syndrome: A condition involving the intestine in which food may not be properly digested or the nutrients not absorbed.

Malassezia pachydermatis A budding yeast considered part of the normal flora of the external ear canal. M ay become pathologic in certain situations. Formerly called Pityrosporum canis.

Malignancy Cancer.

Malignant A process that does harm to nearby tissues. Usually synonymous with cancer, a tumor that grows quickly and spreads into other tissues.

Malleus The malleus is a small bone in the middle ear which transmits sound vibrations from the tympanum to the incus.

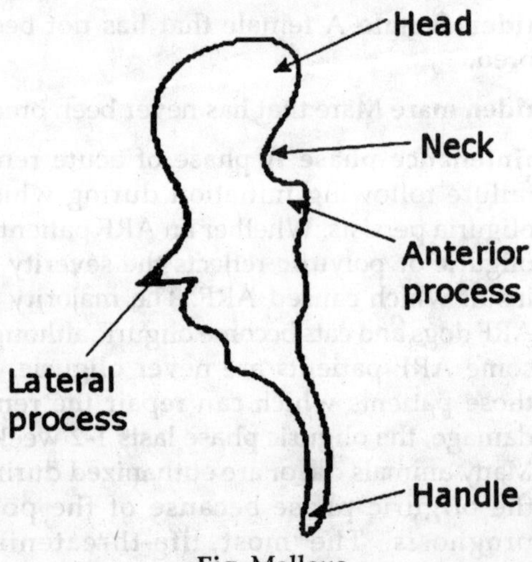

Fig. Malleus

Malnutrition Ill health due to dietary deficiency or imbalance.

Mammal A warm blooded vertebrate with hair; in the female milk producing glands; and give birth to live young.

Mammary gland The udder or breast.

Mandible In human anatomy, the mandible is the bone at the front and bottom of the skull (lower jaw).

Mandible The bone of the lower jaw.

Mane Long, thick hair on top and sides of neck.

Mange Any of several skin and ear conditions caused by a variety of mites.

Mange Mites Mites which infest and damage the skin and hair.

Manners The degree of training of a horse in his interactions with humans and other horses. The energetic yet cooperative attitude of a horse.

Mantle Dark-shaded portion of the coat on shoulders, back, and sides.

Manty A piece of canvas that encases the load tied on a pack animal.

Manubrium The first sternabra of the chest.

Manufactured milk products These include cheeses, butter, evaporated whole milk, condensed whole and skim milks, whole milk powder, nonfat dry milk, ice cream, frozen desserts, aerated cream, frozen and plastic creams, and milk used in candy, soup, bakery products, and animal feeds.

Manufacturing grade milk Milk produced under regulations less strict than those for grade A milk production.

Manufacturing milk Milk for the manufacture of dairy products.

Manure The fecal and urinary excretions of livestock.

MAOIs Monoamine oxidase inhibitors. Substances that inactivate the enzyme monoamine oxidase which regulates certain transmitter chemicals between nerves. These compounds include certain types of antidepressants and also insecticides containing amitraz (such as Mitaban and Preventic collars).

Marbling The fat within the muscle.

Marcel Effect Regular continuous waves (specified in the American Water Spaniel standard).

Mare Adult female or mother horse.

Mark To earn a score.

Marker In reining and horsemanship, a location for the pattern.

Market hog A hog that is ready for the market. Market hogs weigh from 200 to 400 pounds.

Market milk Milk produced and handled under conditions that qualify it for use as fluid milk in an organized marketing area. Grade A milk meets this requirement.

Marking An instinctual behavior in which male dogs urinate in certain locations to establish their territory.

Markings White on the face or legs of a horse.

Marsupial An order of mammals including kangaroos, opossums, and sugar gliders in which the female has a pouch on the abdomen which holds the young and has nipples for the young to nurse.

Martingale 1. Piece of training equipment designed to fix an animal's head position. Common types include running, standing, and German.

2. Strap from cavesson to girth to keep animal from throwing its head up, or from hames to girth to help back load.

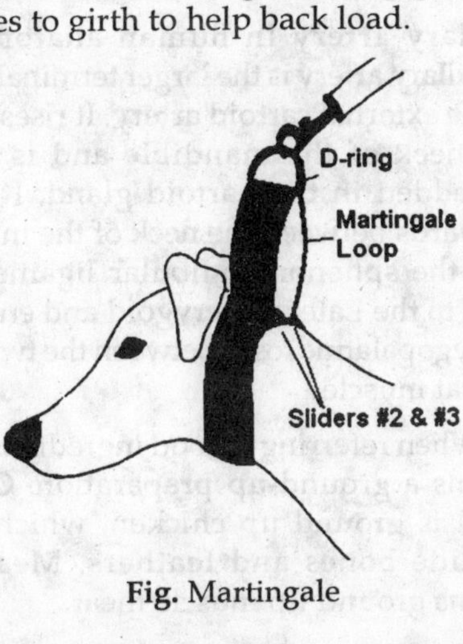

Fig. Martingale

Martingale Running- A strap that attaches to the girth, runs up between the front legs and splits into two straps with a ring at the end. The reins are run through the martingale rings. The martingale pulls down on the reins and the bit when the horse raises his head.

Martingale Standing- A strap which attaches to the girth and runs between the front

Masculinity Possession of well-developed secondary male sex characteristics in the head, neck and shoulder.

Mask Dark shading on the foreface.

Massage The systematic therapeutic stroking or kneading of the body or part. The manipulation of the soft tissues of the body in order to reduce tension and stress, increase circulation, aid the healing of muscle and other soft-tissue injuries, control pain, and promote overall well-being.

Masseter The masseter is the human muscle which moves the mandible for chewing.

Mast cell A large cell that exists mainly in connective tissue. Mast cells have a colorful granules containing substances (as histamine and heparin) that act as molecular toolkits to mediate allergic reactions and stimulate tissue repair.

Mast cell tumor A nodular growth, usually on the skin, which involves cells (mast cells) which contain large amounts of histamine and normally play a role in allergic reactions. All mast cell tumors in dogs should be considered potentially malignant.

Mastectomy Removal of the mammary glands.

Master problem list MPLA list of all the problems shown by a patient. The master problem list is dynamic and may expand over time.

Masticate Chew.

Mastiff An ancient breed of large strong dogs, probably originating in Asia and having a short, often fawn-colored coat.

Mastitis Inflammation of the mammary gland caused by bacterial infection, resulting in reduced milk production.

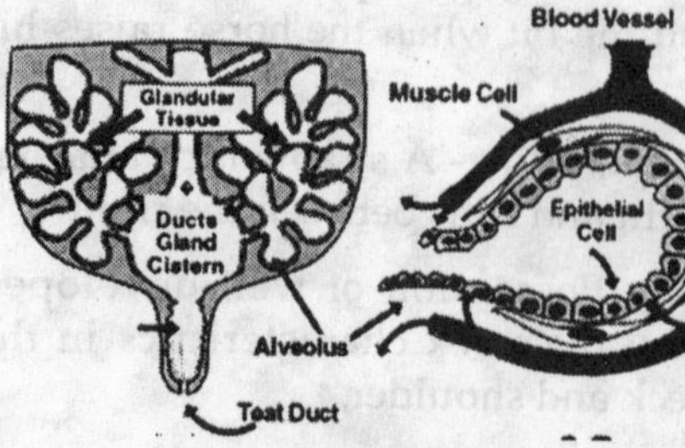

Fig. Mastitis

Mastocytoma, mast cell tumors A growth of mast cells (cells in the dermis which is directly beneath the outer skin layer, which release histamine to counter allergens). These tumors may become malignant.

Mate To breed a dog and bitch.

Maternal antibody Antibody in a newborn animal which the newborn acquired through the placenta or colostrum (the first milk).

Maternal Effect The effect that a dam's maternal ability may have on a trait. For example, the effect of milk yield on weaning weight.

Maternal Immunity A form of temporary immunity passed from a mother to her offspring while in the uterus and after birth in the colostrum and milk.

Maternal Pertaining to the mother or dam.

Maternal Sires Sires that are used in a crossbreeding program to sire replacement females for the flock. These sires have strong maternal traits to produce the next generation of productive ewes.

Maternity Barn A special needs facility where cows can be closely monitored during the period immediately before and after they give birth.

Matrigel A liquid preparation that is extracted from mouse tumor cells and is rich in extracellular matrix proteins. Its major component is laminin, followed by collagen IV, heparan sulfate proteoglycans, and entactin. At body temperature, the matrigel polymerizes to form a matrix of connective tissue proteins. It is often used as a carrier substance for the injection of proteins such as BMPs.

Mattress Bedding material compacted to 3 to 4 inches and sandwiched in a heavyweight polypropolene or other fabric. Possible fillers include: long or chopped straw, poor quality hay, sawdust, shavings, rice hulls and, most commonly, shredded rubber.

Mature equivalency (ME) Age-conversion formulas (provided by the USDA and dairy breed associations) applied to milk production records of young cows to predict their expected milk production potential as mature cows.

Mature follicle A large follicle on the ovary that secretes estrogens that make the female receptive and will be able to respond to mating by ovulating.

Maturities Those types of events for aged horses (five and older).

Maxilla The maxilla is the bone comprising the upper jaw in the human skull.

Maxilla Upper bill.

Maxillary artery In human anatomy, the maxillary artery is the larger terminal branch of the external cartoid artery. It rises behind the neck of the mandible and is at first imbedded in the partoid gland. It passes forwards between the neck of the mandible and the sphenomandibular ligament and then to the Lateral pterygoid and enters the pterygopalatine fossa between the two heads of that muscle.

Meal When referring to food ingredients, meal means a ground-up preparation. Chicken meal is ground up chicken, which might include bones and feathers. Meat meal means ground up muscle meat.

Mean The average value for a trait of a group.

Meat Breeds Breeds of chickens developed for their quick growth and heavy muscles. These breeds are developed for eating.

Meat Hygiene Service An Executive Agency of the Food Standards Agency. It enforces the regulations about hygiene and animal welfare at slaughterhouses, and carries out meat inspection in them.

Meat type Breeds of sheep that are used primarily for the production of meat.

Mecate Braided horsehair reins; knotted to a bosal.

Meconium Fecal matter that is passes a few hours after birth by a foal.

Medal Class AHSA equitation competition. National champions are chosen annually at Harrisburg, Pennsylvania, in hunter seat, saddle seat, and stock seat and a dressage class for juniors.

Median survival time Time at which 50% of the animals had died.

Medication administration recordA type of flow sheet on which one records drugs, doses and administrations.

Meditation The practice of sitting or resting quietly and performing mental exercises designed to relax the body and focus concentration.

Medium Gait Between collected and extended.

Megacalorie (Mcal) Equivalent to 1000 kcal or 1,000,000 cal. A megacalorie is equivalent to a therm.

Megacolon A condition in which the colon enlarges and dilates, which results in feces accumulating in the colon. Constipation then occurs. This condition is more common in cats than dogs.

Megaesophagus Overly enlarged esophagus causing buildup of food and saliva and regurgitation. Associated with aspirative pneumonia from an early age.

Megestrol acetate A progestin marketed for estrus control in the dog and commonly used for managemnet of severe pruritus in the cat.

Meibomian gland adenoma A benign tumor of the Meibomian glands.

Meibomian glands Glands thatline the margins of the superior and inferior eyelids and produce part of the tear film.

Meiosis The cellular process that results in the number of chromosomes in gamete-producing cells (eggs and sperm) being reduced to one half. One of each pair of homologous chromosomes passes to each daughter cell.

Melangestrol acetate MGAA hormone added to diets to suppress estrus cycling and improve feed efficiency and growth rate in feedlot heifers.

Melanoma A malignant cancer derived from pigment producing cells (melanin-producing) of the skin or any part of the body characterized by the ability to frequently metastasize widely.

Melena Darkening of the stool due to the presence of digested blood, which indicates bleeding is occurring in the stomach and/ or beginning of the small intestine. The feces generally look black and tarry.

Memory (Immunologic) Memory: When an animal mounts an immune response against a foreign substance, some cells are created to 'remember' the antigens on that substance. If the animal is again exposed to the substance, these cells will help the body respond much faster and to a higher degree.

Memory cell Memory cells are a subset of T cells and B cells that have been exposed to specific foreign substances (antigens) and can then proliferate (recognize the antigen and divide) more readily when the immune system re-encounters the same antigens.

Menace reflex Used to assess vision and the ability to close the eyelids.

Meningitis Inflammation of the brain and spinal cord that can result in permanent brain damage and death.

Meningitis Not a disease, but a symptom, the inflammation of the membranes covering the brain and spinal cord, the meninges. This can be caused by bacteria, virus, fungi, or chemical toxins. ? aseptic meningitis - is inflammation of the meninges for which no identifiable infectious agent can be cultured or tested for, and is probably genetic.

Mentalis The mentalis is a muscle in the human face, it raises and protudes the lower lip and wrinkles the skin of the chin.

Meridians In Chinese theory, these are the energy pathways which run through the body carrying the vital force or energy called chi.

Merino sheep Sheep, common in large numbers in Australia, South Africa, and South America, giving the finest wool.

Merozoite The form of the malaria parasite that invades human red blood cells; one of the organisms formed by multiple fission of a sporozoite within the body of the host during the asexual phase of reproduction of a malarial plasmodia and other sporozoa.

Metabolic acidosis A condition in which the pH of the blood is too acidic because of the production of certain types of acids.

Metabolic reactions to food An adverse reaction due to an effect of a substance upon the metabolism of the host, or as a result of defective metabolism of a nutrient by the host.

Metabolic weight The weight of an animal raised to threequarter power (W0.75).

Metabolism All of the chemical changes nutrients undergo following absorption from the digestive tract.

Metabolizable energy MEA measure of the useful energy in a feed. It represents that portion of the feed gross energy not lost in the feces, urine and belched gas.

Metabolize energy (ME) (ME) is the net energy available to an animal from a certain food.

Metabolize To have molecules transformed within the body tissue through chemical processes.

Metacarpus The front limb between the carpus and the phalanges (toes).

Metadata Metadata is often described as 'data about data'. It is like a set of labels about a source of information, similar to those on an everyday product in a supermarket. The supermarket labels describe the product in a way that is useful both to the consumer (e.g. the ingredients) and to the computer systems that control the store (e.g. the barcode). Similarly metadata "labels" can be included with documents or other data sources to give information such as what it is about, how it was collected and by whom etc. This makes it easier for people to find the data and allows computers to process the information effectively.

Metaphase Metaphase is the 2nd stage of mitosis cell reproduction. The chromosomes have become irregular V shaped and arrange themselves around the equator.

Metastasis Spread of a tumor from its original location to a remote one, by tumor cells that are carried in the blood.

Metatarsus The metatarsus are the 5 bones in the anterior part of the human foot. They are between the tarsus and the phalanges.

Methemoglobin An altered hemoglobin which does not carry oxygen.

Methemoglobinemia A condition of the blood in which there are large amounts of methemoglobin which is an altered hemoglobin which does not carry oxygen.

Methoprene Precor. An insect growth regulator. Present in rinses, sprays, collars, and household sprays/foggers. Recently added to a topical pour-on product containing fipronil (TopSpot Plus: Meriel).

Metritis Infection of the uterus. If the infection follows birthing, it is a postpartum metritis

MF (milk fat) The lipid or fatty acid components of milk.

MF59 adjuvant An oil-in-water emulsion of various particulate immunostimulators used in vaccines recently (e.g. Fluad vaccine licensed in Europe) that results in the recruitment of antigen presenting cells to the site of administration.

MHC (major histocompatibility complex) The gene cluster that controls certain aspects of the immune response. Among the products of these genes are the histocompatibility antigens, such as HLA class I antigens, which are present on every cell with a nucleus and serve as markers to distinguish self from non-self.

MHC class I these molecules present peptides generated in the cytosol to CD8 T cells.

MHC class II Molecules of MHC II present peptides degraded in intracellular vesicles to CD4 T cells.

MHV-68 A serotype of mouse herpes virus.

Miatake Mushroom Extract of this mushroom can stimulate the immune system by presenting unique macromolecules to the intestinal tract, where they alter the immune regulation by intestinal antigen processing systems. In addition, it has been shown to activate NK Killer cells which attack tumor cells and to prevent destruction of T-Helper cells.

Micro minerals Minor mineral elements required in very small amounts in the ration of animals. Includes manganese (Mn), copper (Cu), zinc (Zn), selenium (Se) iron (Fe), cobalt (Co), iodine (I) and fluorine (Fl).

Microarray Gene Expression Studies Used to quantitatively examine the expression of RNA for thousands of genes in the genome. Gene expression refers to the transcription of gene from the stable DNA code into the less stable RNA intermediate that is used by the cell to direct the formation of proteins. In order to identify abnormal gene expression, we use gene chips (a key component of this technology), which are sensitive to mRNA levels in a particular sample, to assay the expression level of >30,000 individual genes at one time. This strategy allows us to determine how these genes respond in any particular single situation. If a gene behaves differently in a disease state vs. a normal state, then it can be inferred to have something to do with the disease.

Microbes Organisms so small that a microscope is required to see them. Microbes are also called microorganisms.

Microencapsulated Surrounded by a thin layer of biodegradable substance referred to as a microsphere. A means of protecting a drug or vaccine antigen from rapid breakdown. Microencapsulation may also enhance an antigen's absorption and the immune response to that antigen.

Microencapsulation A process whereby an insecticide is packaged into small microspheres (polyurea, nylon, etc). This process increases the LD50 and decreases biodegradation (extends duration of action). Currently, microencapsulated products include pyrethrins, diazinon, and chlorpyrifos.

Microfilaremia The presence of microfilariae in the blood.

Microfilaria The larval form of some parasitic worms, for example heartworms. These worms do not lay eggs, they produce microfilariae (plural of microfilaria) instead.

Microfilaricide Compound which kills microfilaria, the immature forms of heartworms which circulate in the blood.

Micronutrient Aný ingredient, such as minerals, vitamins or drugs, added in very small amounts to a ration.

Microorganism A single-celled life form that is invisible to the naked eye and that may cause disease in man or animals.

Microphthalmos A small eye that has failed to develop properly.

Micturition A synonym for urination.

Milbemycin oxime A systemic treatment for demodectic mange.

Military dermatitis A cutaneous reaction pattern characterized by the formation of multiple, circumscribed crusted papules.

Military Small, resembling a seed.

Milk A white liquid secreted by special glands of female mammals for suckling their young.

Milk assignments The assignment of milk income to directly pay for purchase of farm, machinery, cattle or feed.

Milk composition Average composition of dairy cow milk includes the following constituents: 87% water, 3.25% protein, 2.5% casein, 5% sugar (lactose), 3.7% fat and 0.8% minerals and vitamins.

Milk equivalent The quantity of milk, as produced, required to furnish the milk solids in manufactured dairy products. For example, approximately 10 and 20 pounds of milk are required to manufacture 1 pound of Cheddar cheese and butter, respectively.

Milk fat A complex mixture of triglycerides containing numerous fatty acids. DHI laboratories use electronic photometry and infrared absorption for rapid milkfat tests. Milk fat also is referred to as butterfat or fat.

Milk fat test The percentage of fat in the milk. To be legal, whole milk must contain at least 3.25% fat.

Milk Fever Substantial reduction in plasma calcium which interferes with nerve transmission, causing partial or almost total paralysis occurring at or just giving birth and initiation of lactation.

Milk Handlers Processors or dealers of milk who commonly purchase raw milk and sell pasteurized milk and milk products.

Milk House The area near a milking parlor where the bulk milk tank, cleaning units, and equipment are located.

Milk House Waste Water having been used in cleaning the milking equipment and washing the parlor.

Milk meter A device between the cluster or milking unit and the milkline for measuring a cow's milk yield in either mass or volume.

Milk only (MO) Record Type of testing plan where only milk weights are recorded and no milk samples are collected for component sampling. This plan is intended for management use only. The records made are not official and DHI rules need not be followed.

Milk preservative A compound used to stabilize and to prevent decomposition of milk samples sent to DHI laboratories for component analysis. See bronopol.

Milk replacer A substitute for fresh whole milk, fortified with vitamins, minerals and sometimes antibiotics; used as a nutrient source for young animals.

Milk serum The nonfat components of milk.

Milk shed A geographical area in which milk is produced for a given milk-marketing area.

Milk soil Residue on equipment, utensils, or containers after emptying.

Milk Solids-not-fat (SNF) The solids portion of the milk minus the fat component represents about 8.5 to 9.2 percent of the total milk solids.

Milk Thistle A plant that is used to treat liver disorders. The plant, Silybum marianum, grows wild and in gardens and may reach five feet in height.

Milk vouchers Statements provided by the dairy company or cheese factory once or twice a month: May be used to verify income.

Milk well The opening in the abdominal wall through which milk veins (subcutaneous abdominal veins) enter to join the vena cava and return blood from udder to heart.

Milking parlor This is the building in which the dairy cows are milked twice a day. This building houses the milking equipment, storage equipment, and provides feed for the cows as they are being milked.

Milking Pit A sunken area that houses both the milker and some milking equipment during milking. This places the milker at shoulder level with udders and reduces physical demands.

Milkstone Residue on equipment, utensils, or containers used for handling milk. It is characterized by a high mineral content, especially calcium. It is normally soluble in acid.

Milliliter (ml) A metric volume measurement that is identical to cubic centimeter (cc).

Mineral Inorganic substance found naturally in all body cells, tissues and fluids.

Mineral supplement A rich source of one or more mineral elements.

Mineralization The process in which minerals are laid down within tissue in an abnormal pattern causing a hardening of the tissue.

Mineralocorticoids Hormones produced by the adrenal gland which regulate the amounts of sodium, potassium, and chloride in the blood.

Minimum data base A minimum data base is the minimum amount of information collected for a medical record and includes: the chief complaint(s), history, patient signalment and physical examination.

Mink farming Raising mink for pelts. Mink produce one litter of kits per year and average 3 1/2 kits per litter. Kits are generally born in spring and pelted out in late fall. Pelts are usually sold at fur auctions in New York or Minneapolis.

Minnesota Wisconsin price The average price paid for manufacturing grade milk in about 400 plants in Minnesota and Wisconsin, an area in which about 50 percent of the U.S. manufacturing grade milk is produced. The price often used as the basis for classified pricing in Federal Milk Marketing orders.

Mirroring A process where seizures which start on only one side of the brain can in time 'mirror' themselves on the other side of the brain thus increase the frequency of the seizures. This is one reason for obtaining early control of the seizures.

Mismate A drug given in attempt to prevent pregnancy.

Mite A tiny jointed-legged body parasite.

Miticide An agent that kills mites.

Mitochondria Any of various round or long cellular organelles that are found outside the nucleus, produce energy for the cell, and are rich in fats, proteins, and enzymes.

Mitosis Mitosis is cell reproduction by indirect division. It is the common method of division in the higher animals. It is characterised by a series of complex changes in the nucleus leading to its subdivision. The process takes between 30 minutes and a few hours, and is comprised of 4 stages: prophase, metaphase, anaphase and Telophase.

Mitotic Recombination Any process of cell division that generates a diploid daughter cell with a re-assorted combination of genetic information (alleles).

Mitral valve defect A defect in the heart valve that separates the left atrium and the left ventricle.

Mixed breed A cat of unknown or mixed parentage. Mixed breed cats can be shown in the household pet (HHP) competitive class.

Mixing pen A confined area where several ewes and their lambs are co-mingled after being removed from jugs.

ML Milliliter, same as CC; 3CC and 3ML are the same thing in shots.

MLK A multimodal analgesic administration technique combining lidocaine, ketamine and morphine in IV fluids such as LRS.

Modified live vaccine Vaccines which are made by taking the real, disease-causing virus and altering (attenuating) it in a laboratory to a non-disease causing virus. Compare with 'killed vaccine' and 'recombinant vaccine.'

Modified live virus MLV A vaccine which contains an antigenic agent that has been altered chemically of physically so it stimulates cell-mediated and humoral response without evoking disease. The altered virus can still replicate in the host.

Moggy The UK term for mixed breed.

Molt The annual shedding and renewing of a bird's feathers.

Monoamine oxidase inhibitor (MAOI): Substances that inactivate the enzyme monoamine oxidase which regulates certain transmitter chemicals between nerves. These compounds include certain types of antidepressants and also insecticides containing amitraz (such as Mitaban and Preventic collars).

Monoclonal antibody The term used to describe a homologous Ig produced by a clone of B cells. This occurs naturally in neoplasia of B cells resulting in myeloma.

Monoclonal Derived form a single cell.

Monoclonal Originating from a single precursor cell.

Monocyte A large white blood cell in the blood that ingests microbes or other cells and foreign particles. When a monocyte passes out of the bloodstream and enters the tissues, it develops into a macrophage.

Monorchid An adult male cat which has only one descended testicle. This is a disqualification in all associations.

Monovalent vaccine A vaccine that is manufactured to stimulate the body to produce protection against only one disease, e.g., rabies vaccine. Compare with 'multivalent vaccine.'

Moon blindness Periodic opthalmia, or uveitis (inflammation of internal eye that comes and goes).

Morbidity Incidence of disease; morbidity rate is the proportion or percentage of individuals in a group that become ill during a specified time.

Morphogen A diffusible protein that exerts control over tissue formation especially by forming a concentration gradient.

Morphology The form and structure of an organism

Mortality Percentage killed by a disease.

Mortality rate Proportion or percentage of individuals that die from a disease during a specified time, usually 1 year.

Motility Movement, e.g., intestinal motility is the muscular contractions of the intestines which move the food from the stomach to the anus.

Motivational affective dimension of pain This is the disruption of the feeling of well-being that results in suffering to the degree that it triggers an active response from the animal in response to pain.

Motoneurons Neurons that make contact with and send messages directly to muscles

Mount To climb onto, as demonstrated by females in heat and by males in natural service.

Moxibustion A technique using various applications of heat by burning the herb

Artemesia vulgaris to stimulate acupoints. Burning moxa gives off mild and constant heat which effectively penetrates the tissues. It has a pungent smell.

MUC-1 Abnormally glycosylated mucin found in breast and pancreatic tumors.

Mucin Mucin is a protein and the principal constituent of mucus.

Muco purulent A discharge that is a combination of pus and mucus.

Mucolytic Breaks down mucous.

Mucopolysaccharide A carbohydrate which also contains a hexosamine molecule and is a component of mucous.

Mucosa Specialized membrane which covers various passages and cavities exposed to the air such as the mouth, nose, inner portion of the eyelids, vagina. Examination of the mucous membranes can provide important information: if they are dry, the animal is likely dehydrated; pale, and the animal may be anemic or in shock; yellow, and the animal is said to jaundiced due to accumulation of waste products which should be eliminated by the liver. Mucous membranes.

Mucosal immunity A form of local immunity on the body surfaces of the respiratory, intestinal and genital tracts.

Mucous membranes Specialized membrane which covers various passages and cavities exposed to the air such as the mouth, nose, inner portion of the eyelids, vagina. Examination of the mucous membranes can provide important information: if they are dry, the animal is likely dehydrated; pale, and the animal may be anemic or in shock; yellow, and the animal is said to be jaundiced due to accumulation of waste products which should be eliminated by the liver.

Mucus Mucus is a thick fluid secreted by mucus membranes in animals. It acts as a protective barrier, lubricant and a carrier of enzymes.

MÜeller cells Cells responsible for support and nutrition of the retina.

Muff The feathers (always found in association with a beard) sticking out from both sides of the face, under the beak, of such breeds as Ameraucana, Faverolle, and Houdan; also called "whiskers."

Mule A cross between a jack and a mare. With rare exceptions, the mule is sterile.

Muley A polled cow.

Muller's muscle Smooth muscle in the eyelids which provides tone to the lids. Innervated by sympathetic fibers.

Multi modal Using more than one method.

Multiple Sclerosis Multiple sclerosis is a disease of the central nervous system characterized by the destruction of the myelin sheath surrounding neurons, resulting in the formation of "plaques." MS is a progressive and usually fluctuating disease with exacerbations (patients feeling worse) and remissions (patients feeling better) over many decades. Eventually, in most patients, remissions do not reach baseline levels and permanent disability and sometimes death occurs. The cause of MS is unknown. The most widely held hypothesis is that MS occurs in patients with a genetic susceptibility and that some environmental factors "trigger" exacerbations. MS is 3 times more common in women than men, with diagnosis usually made as young adults. Also see demyelinating disorders.

Multiple Trait Selection Selection for more than one trait at the same time.

Multipotent stem cells Multipotent cells can only become some types of cells, for example nervous system or muscle.

Multivalent A vaccine containing multiple antigens.

Multivalent vaccine A vaccine that combines two or more components to stimulate the body to produce protection against all the components. Most 'distemper' vaccines for puppies are of the multivalent type, and commonly include distemper, parvovirus, adenovirus cough, hepatitis, and parainfluenza. Compare with 'monovalent' vaccine.

Mummified fetus A shriveled fetus that has remained in the uterus instead of being aborted or expelled. Fluids from the fetus have been partially reabsorbed by the mother.

Mupriocin Bactoderm: Pfizer. Topical antibacterial ointment effective against staphylococci.

Murmur An abnormal heart sound associated with the opening or closing of a heart valve. This may indicate a structural or functional abnormality.

Musculoskeletal Pertaining to the muscles and skeleton.

Mustard Mustard contains ingredients which improve digestion and bowel function.

Mutation A change in the DNA sequence that usually leads to a disease.

Mutein A genetically engineered protein arising as a result of a laboratory-induced mutation.

Mutton The meat from sheep older than 12 months of age.

Mutualistic A relationship where both participants or parties benefit.

Muzzle The end of a horse's face, including the nose, nostrils, and lips.

Myasthenia gravis Myasthenia gravis is a neuromuscular disease in which there is a failure of the nerves' ability to stimulate and control the actions of certain muscles.

Mycobacteriosis Feline leprosy caused by Mycobacterium lepraemurium.

Mycoplasma These are a group of bacteria that have lost their cell walls.

Mycosis Disease caused by a fungus such as blastomycosis, histoplasmosis, and ringworm.

Mycotoxin A substance produced by fungi and toxic to animals, e.g., vomitoxin, zearalenone and aflatoxin.

Mycotoxin Toxic compounds, produced by fungi, that contaminate plants.

Mydriasis Small pupil size.

Myelin Fatty substance that provides insulation in the CNS, wraps around axons to allow for electrical conduction

Myelitis Inflammation or infection of the spinal cord.

Myelogram Radiograph (x-ray) of the spinal cord taken after a contrasting dye has been injected into the space around the spinal cord.

Myelosuppression A suppression of the bone marrow so that it does not produce normal numbers of red blood cells, white blood cells and platelets.

Myocardium The middle layer of heart muscle.

Myopathy Inflammation of muscle.

Myosin A fibrous protein of muscle that can split ATP, an energy molecule, and that reacts with actin to form actomyosin (not to be confused with Actinomycin : A type of drug that has the capability of inhibiting the transcription of mRNA from DNA).

N

N.A.E.T. Nambudripad's Allergy Elimination Technique is an approach to detecting and eliminating allergies. N.A.E.T. combines Kinesiology and Oriental Medicine to clear allergic reactions. The technique used involves stimulation of specific acupuncture points along the spinal column which are associated with the individual organs of the body. A surrogate may be used when testing animals.

NAAB stud code An identification number composed of a one-or two-digit prefix indicating the AI stud and a letter indicating the breed of bull. The remaining numbers identify the bull within a stud.

NaBr Sodium bromide. An AED.

Naked DNA Antigen encoding DNA plasmid molecules that result in de novo production of correctly folsded antigen at the site of delivery.

Naloxone An antagonist of morphine and other opiods.

Nanny A mother goat; infrequently used depending upon your location.

Nares (sing., naris) Nostrils.

Nasal Nasal is a classification of human skull shape found in primarily in Negroes.

Nasolacrimal system The route of drainage of tears from the eye to the nose.

National animal disease information service An independent, privately-organised network of about 40 veterinary practices and the six UK veterinary schools. They collect and publish information about animal diseases.

National Association of Animal Breeders (NAAB) The national organization made up of representatives from the artificial insemination (AI) industry.

National cooperative dairy herd improvement programs (NCDHIP) The national, industry-wide cooperative framework within which all DHI-related activities function.

National Park Service A bureau of the U.S. Department of the Interior, created in 1916, that manages the natural, cultural, historical, and recreational areas of the federal government.

National Research Council (NRC) A division of the National Academy of Sciences established in 1916 to promote the effective use of scientific and technical resources. This private, nonprofit organization of scientists publishes bulletins periodically giving nutrient requirements of domestic animals.

National/international award An award given to cats that earn enough points during a show year to be ranked among the highest scoring cats in the entire association for that year. Some associations add a title to the registered name of each award winner. The number of high scoring cats receiving national/international awards depends on the association and the competitive class (e.g. Kitten, premiership, championship, household pet, etc.). For example, CFA gives national awards to the top 25 cats in Championship each year.

Natural Breed A breed of dog which occurred naturally without the interference of much selective breeding. This is usually a result of geographical and environmental conditions.

Natural Immunity Inherited resistance to disease that varies between breeds, strains within breeds and individuals.

Natural Mutation A genetic accident which permanently alters certain genetic characteristics.

Natural Selection The process in nature by which, according to Darwin's theory of evolution, only the organisms best adapted to their environment tend to survive and transmit their genetic characteristics in increasing numbers to succeeding generations while those less adapted tend to be eliminated.

Natural Service Breeding of a cow utilizing a bull rather than artificial insemination.

Nauplii Newly hatched brine shrimp.

Nausea A feeling of sickness in the stomach characterized by an urge to vomit.

Navicular Tiny bone, part of coffin joint; disease of this bone causing lameness.

NDHIA, Inc. The national DHI organization, made up of member state DHI organizations and administered by an executive secretary and an elected board of directors.

Neapolitan Mastiff A large, powerful breed of dog characterized by it's massive head and wrinkled face.

Near side The horse's left side.

Nebulize Convert into a fine spray form.

Neck rein Movement of the rein against the horse's neck cues him to turn. Also called a "brace rein" or "bearing rein."

Neck The neck is the part of the body which connects the head with the shoulders.

Neck Well Set On Good neckline, merging gradually with withers, forming a pleasing transition into topline.

Neck yoke Wooden device that holds end of pole up and is attached to hames with chain or strap on a draft harness.

Necropsy The animal equivalent to human autopsy, and means evaluating an animal after death for signs that might indicate the cause of death.

Necrosis The death and breakdown of cells.

Necrotic Decaying tissue. Often the tissue is black, decomposed, and has a foul odor.

Nematodes A common name for any roundworm of the phylum Nematoda.

Neonatal Pertaining to a newborn animal.

Neonate Refers to a young puppy or kitten shortly after birth.

Neoplasia Any type of cancer in the body. This term is usually associated with some type of mass or lump.

Neoplasm New growths that should not be where they are. A tumor. An FOP lesion.

Neoprene A synthetic rubber or closed cell foam.

Nephritis Inflammation of the kidney(s).

Nephropathy Any disease or abnormal functioning of the kidney.

Nephrotoxic A drug or chemical that causes damage to the cells of the kidneys.

Nerve root signature Lameness due to nerve root involvement

Nerve The nerves are a part of the body which generate and transmit electrical impulses.

Nest egg A wooden or plastic egg placed in a nest to encourage hens to lay there.

Nest run Ungraded eggs.

Nesting Behavior Behavior of a pregnant female who prepares a place to give birth and nurture young.

Net energy NEThe amount of feed energy actually available for animal maintenance and production. It represents the energy fraction in a feed left after fecal, urinary, gas and heat losses are deducted from the gross energy value of a feed.

Neural plasticity Ability of the brain, spinal cord and neurons to adapt to change, as when changes are seen in these structures after learning or injury

Neuralgia Pain along the distribution of nerves.

Neuritis Inflammation of the nerves.

Neuroblastoma A malignant neoplasm characterized by immature, only slightly differentiated nerve cells of embryonic type, i.e. neuroblasts.

Neurogenesis The process of forming new nerve cells. Neurogenesis occurs through the process of cell division.

Neuroleptanalgesic A combination of a tranquilizer and an opiate which provides a synergistic effect for sedation and analgesia.

Neuron / nerve cell A cell that send electrical and chemical signals from one part of the body to another

Neuropathic pain Pain originating in peripheal nerves and nerve roots.

Neuropathy A general term for any dysfunction in the peripheral nervous system. Symptoms include pain, muscle weakness, numbness, loss of coordination and paralysis. This condition may result in permanent disability.

Neurotransmitter A substance released from a neuron of the central or peripheral nervous which excites or inhibit the target cell. Examples include: acetylcholine, norepinephrine, epinephrine, dopamine, substance P, enkephalins, endorphins and serotonin.

Neuter To castrate a male cat. A "neuter" is a male cat which has been neutered. Sometimes the term "neuter" is also used to refer to spaying female cats.

Neutral detergent fiber NDF The insoluble fraction containing all plant cell wall components left after boiling a feed sample in a neutral detergent solution. NDF is of low digestibility, but can be broken down somewhat by the digestive tract microorganisms. NDF value is used to predict ruminant feed intake.

Neutralize To change from acidic or alkaline to a neutral pH.

Neutralizing antibody A type of antibody that specifically blocks virus receptor sites on the virus preventing attachment to target cells in the body.

Neutrophil The most common type of white blood cell observed in the blood stream.

Newfoundland A breed of large, strong dog developed in Newfoundland and having a thick, usually black coat

Niacin A water-soluble vitamin of the B complex found in various animal and plant tissues. It is essential for normal carbohydrate metabolism.

Niche The unique way of life of an organism where it lives and what it does in the community.

Nick A cross of two different bloodlines that consistently produces superior offspring.

Nictitans The third eyelid which is a fold of tissue covered by conjunctiva and containing a lacrimal gland on the inner (bulbar) surface.

Nictitating membrane "Third eyelid" drawn over the eye to clean it.

NIDDM Non-insulin dependent diabetes mellitus (NIDDM): A type of diabetes mellitus in which although the blood glucose levels are higher than normal, they are not immediately life-threatening, and the animal can survive without supplemental insulin. Also called Type II diabetes.

Nigropallidal encephalomalacia A specific brain lesion seen in horses with yellow star thistle poisoning. The clinical sign is an inability to swallow.

Nikolsky sign The epidermis may be rubbed off with slight trauma. Named after a Russian dermatologist.

Nitrate A final decomposition product of organic nitrogen compounds. A nitrogen-oxygen ion (NO3-) available as a plant nutrient and soluble in water.

Nitrate Poisoning Condition in which toxic levels of nitrates accumulate in plants.

Nitrification The biochemical transformation by oxidation of ammonium (NH4) to nitrite (NO2) or to nitrate (NO3).

Nitrogen balance Nitrogen in the food consumed minus nitrogen in feces and nitrogen in urine (nitrogen retention).

Nitrogen free extract (NFE) Consisting of carbohydrates, sugars, starches, and a major portion of materials classed as hemicellulose in feeds. When crude protein, fat, water, ash, and fiber are added and the sum is subtracted from 100, the difference is NFE.

NK cells Natural killer cells, a type of lymphocyte that is large, usually granular, non-T, non-B lymphocytes that can kill certain microbes and cancer cells. NK cells are important in innate immunity to viruses and other intracellular pathogens, as well as in antibody-dependent cell-mediated cytotoxicity (ADCC).

NMDA receptor Glutamate dependent N-methyl-D-aspartate (NMDA)receptors. This type of receptor develops in the central nervous system in response to sustained pain and appears to be responsible for amplifying pain, and causing opioid tolerance.

NOAH Network of Animal Health (on-line veterinary community through the AVMA).

Nociception The detection of noxious stimuli by the nervous system.

Nociceptors Peripheral receptors for pain which sense painful stimuli and transmit signals to the central nervous system where the sensation of pain is perceived.

Nocturnal Animals that are active during the night and sleep during the day.

Nodule Solid bump or lump in the skin that is over 1/3 inch in diameter.

Noggin The name of a specific secreted BMP antagonist (like gremlin). If BMP is a bone making signal, noggin is a "stop making bone" signal.

Nogo A small protein that prevents nerve cells from regrowing after injury, called an inhibitory molecule

Noil The short and tangled fibers which are separated from the long fibers, known as top, on a worsted comb.

Nomenclature of Units for Territorial Statistics The European Office for Statistics has produced a set of definitions of administrative areas, so that statistics from different member states can be related to comparable sized human populations. For instance, in England a NUTS level 3 area is equivalent to a county.

Non essential amino acids Acids Amino acids that can be synthesized by the animal.

Non protein nitrogen NPN Nitrogen not derived from true protein, but can be used by rumen microbes to build microbial protein.

Non ruminant herbivore Animals with simple stomachs able to digest roughages and other fibrous feeds because of the microbial population in their hindgut. Examples: horse, rabbit.

Non steroidal anti inflammatory drug NSAID A drug such as aspirin that has anti inflammatory properties but that is not a corticosteroid.

Non structural carbohydrates NSC Simple carbohydrates, such as starches and sugars, stored inside the cell which serve as a cellular energy source. Non-structural carbohydrates are rapidly and easily digested by the animal.

Non terrestrial rabies Rabies in mammals that do not walk on the ground: bats.

Nonadditive Gene Effects Favourable effects produced by specific gene combinations in which the members of the gene pairs are not equally expressed. This is the primary cause of heterosis.

Noncontagious Disease A disease that cannot be spread between animals by direct contact.

Noncore vaccine Vaccine which should only be given to animals at increased risk of exposure to a disease, example, leptospirosis in dogs or feline leukemia in cats.

Nonepileptic Seizures Seizures that can be identified as either nonneurogenic (ie:cardiac, metablic disturbances, recurrent abdominal problems) and neurogenic (ie narcolpesy, vestibular disease, myasthenia gravis) in origin.

Nonpathogenic Not causing disease. Some bacteria, such as those that normally live in an animal's intestines, are nonpathogenic.

Nonpro An amateur or nonprofessional by specific definition from each association such as **NRHA, NCHA,** and **AHSA**.

Nonprotein nitrogen (NPN) Feed ingredient that is not a protein but which contains nitrogen (an example is urea).

Non Return Dip Cup A dip cup that does not allow the liquid to reenter and potentially contaminate the storage container.

Nonreturn The breeding efficiency of bulls expressed as the percentage of cows that conceive on first service. Also called nonreturn rate.

Nonseptic A condition not caused by an infection. For example, septic arthritis is caused by an infection with bacteria, yeast, or other agent; a case of nonseptic arthritis may be caused by injury or cancer.

Non steroidal anti-inflammatory NSAIDS Agents which reduce inflammation, but are not in the class of drugs known as steroids. Examples include aspirin, Rimadyl, and phenylbutazone.

Normal Distribution (Bell Curve) A graph of all possible performance levels for a trait. The number of individuals displaying each performance level usually forms a normal distribution.

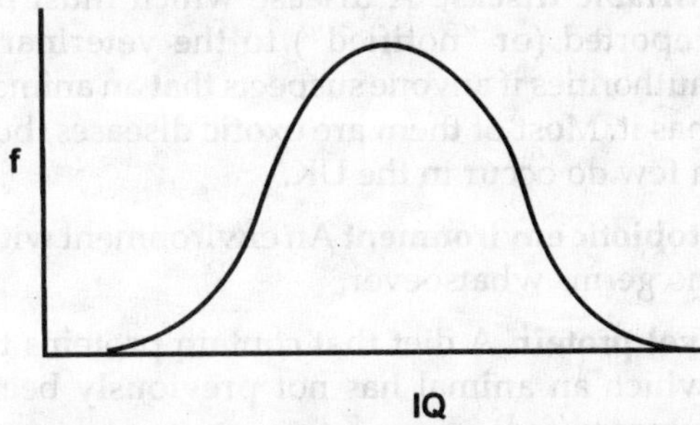

Fig. Normal Distribution (Bell Curve)

Normal saline 0.9% sodium chloride. It is isotonic. It contains only sodium and chloride. Sodium chloride is used when blood sodium is decreased; such as in Addison's disease because it has a higher concentration of sodium than does lactated Ringer's. It may be used in lieu of lactated Ringer's for rehydration in patients with lymphoma. It is used as a rehydration solution when a patient has an increased potassium or calcium, and the administration of additional calcium or potassium are contraindicated.

Norwegian catheter A stainless steel catheter protected by a plastic sheath used for transcervical intrauterine AI.

Nose Bots Tiny larvae that crawl into nasal passages.

Nose clamp Humane twitch.

Nose The nose is an animal's organ of smell.

Nosocomial Referring to an infection acquired by a patient while in a hospital.

Nosodes Products prepared from infected tissues, infected discharges, or a pathogenic organism, which are processed and administered orally in attempt to "vaccinate" against an infectious agent.

Not for breeding A cat that has been designated by the breeder as not to be used for breeding. Such a cat cannot have registered offspring.

Notched With a notch, like a pointed bite taken out of it (bill, tail).

Notifiable disease A disease which must be reported (or "notified") to the veterinary authorities if anyone suspects that an animal has it. Most of them are exotic diseases, but a few do occur in the UK.

Notobiotic environment An environment with no germs whatsoever.

Novel protein A diet that contain proteins to which an animal has not previously been exposed(fed).

Novice In general, an inexperienced horseman; a division for horse (or rider) who has not yet won three first-place ribbons at specified shows.

Noxious stimulus A stimulus that is potentially or actually damaging to tissue. A stimulus that is of adequate intensity to trigger a nociceptive reaction in an animal (the feeling of pain).

NSAIDS (Nonsteroidal anti-inflammatory drugs) Drugs that decrease inflammation, swelling, and pain. These drugs reduce inflammation and are not steroids.

Nuclear sclerosis Compression of older lens fibers in the nucleus of the lens which results in light-scattering that clinically appears as a gray, homogenous, perfectly round area in the center of the lens which is bilaterally symmeterical; a normal aging change and does not interfere with vision or visualization of the fundus

Nucleated erythrocytes Immature form of red blood cells.

Nucleated Having a nucleus or nuclei.

Nucleus The central controlling body within a living cell, usually a spherical unit enclosed in a membrane and containing genetic codes for maintaining life systems of the organism and for issuing commands for growth and reproduction.

Number averaged molecular weight The mean of the molecular weight of all the polymers in a solution. The number-averaged molecular weight tells you how quickly a fluid will exert an effect. The smaller the number-averaged molecular weight, the quicker the initial oncotic response.

Nurse cow A dairy cow used to supply milk for nursing calves, commonly other than her own.

Nutmeg A spice native to Indonesia which is mostly used in cooking. Nutmeg comes from the nut of the nutmeg apple which grows on an evergreen tree. It may also be used to treat diarrhea, insomnia, indigestion, and flatulence.

Nutraceutical A very broad term describing certain components in food (plant or animal) or nutritional supplements, which contain substances normally present in the body that aid in the proper functioning of body systems.

Nutrient allowances Recommendations of nutrient amounts necessary for maintenance, growth, gestation, lactation or performance that include a safety margin to account for variability in feeds and animals (e.g., environment, health, storage losses).

Nutrient Compounds in foods which are essential for life. Nutrients include protein, fats, vitamins, minerals, etc.

Nutrient requirements The minimal amounts of nutrients (energy, protein, minerals and vitamins) necessary to meet an animal's minimal needs for maintenance, growth, reproduction, lactation or work.

Nutrients Feed components required for the maintenance, production and health of animals (water, carbohydrates, lipids, proteins, minerals and vitamins).

NY-ESO-1 A cancer-testis antigen.

Nymph A young stage of insects and ticks that have incompletely developed sex organs.

Nystagmus Constant involuntary movement of the eye, often from side to side.

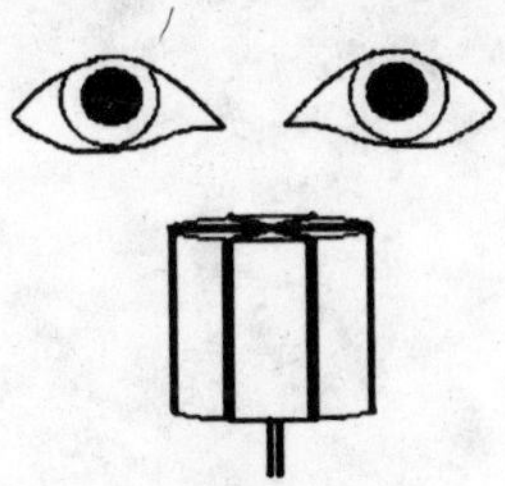

Fig. Nystagmus

O

Obedience Trial An event held under AKC rules at which a leg toward an obedience degree can be earned.

Obesity The condition of being obese; increased body weight caused by excessive accumulation of fat.

Objective information Any information that can be quantified such as the size of a mass, a laboratory value or the grade of a heart mumur.

Obligate carnivore An animal that requires in its diet nutrients that are found in sufficient quantities only in meat or other animal products.

Obligate pathogen Parasite that generally will cause disease – e.g. Brucella abortus (Brucellosis); Yersinia pestis (Plague); and Mycobacterium bovis (Tuberculosis).

Oblique Shoulders Shoulders well laid back.

Obliquely Placed Eyes Eyes with outer corners higher than their inner ones.

Obsessive compulsive A behavioral condition in which a pet repeatedly performs an action out of context. It is thought that the behavior is an expression of stress, frustration and/or conflict. Certain breeds are more prone to these behaviors. The behaviors include tail-chasing, some cases of excessive barking, continual licking, and biting the air as if snapping at an invisible fly.

Obtuse Not very sharply pointed.

Occipital bone The occipital bone is the plate forming the back of the human skull.

Occipital Protuberance A prominently raised occiput characteristic of some sporting and hound breeds.

Occipitofrontalis The occipitofrontalis is the broad muscle of the human scalp.

Occiput Dorsal, posterior point of the skull.

Occult Indicating a disease or condition that is clinically not apparent.

Ocular Relating to the eye.

Odd-Eyed Eyes of different color, such as one brown eye and one blue eye.

OEGs Olfactory ensheathing glia, or OEGs, are cells that aid in the regeneration of smell neurons, the only adult neurons we know of that regenerate as part of normal functioning

Oesophageal Oesophageal is a secretion from the membrane of the oesophagus. It is a mucus lubricant to assist peristalsis.

Oestrogen Oestrogen is a hormone produced in the ovary of a vertebrate.

Off billet The strap (or straps) on the off side that buckle one end of the girth in place.

Off feed Having ceased eating; without a healthy and normal appetite.

Off label Term used to describe the use of a medication for a condition for which it was not FDA approved. A large number of medications used in veterinary medicine are used 'off label.' If veterinarians only used FDA approved medications, options for treatments of certain conditions would be severely limited or nonexistent. The safety and efficacy of off-label uses of medications is often determined in university research settings, but the manufacturer of the drug does submit the results or go through the elaborate FDA approval process.

Off side The horse's right side.

Offal Animal organs rejected at slaughter as unfit for human consumption, e.g., spleen, intestine, brain, lungs.

Office International des épizooties The world organisation for animal health. It collects and publishes information on animal diseases from 167 countries. To help control the spread of diseases it develops standards for health certificates for the international movement of animals.

Official production record Standard DHIA and DHIR Records pertaining to milk production made under the supervision of an unbiased individual. Such records are used for management purposes (e.g., feeding, breeding, and culling), genetic evaluation (sire summaries), publicity, and sales. See DHIR.

Official Veterinary Surgeon The Veterinary Surgeon who is the team leader of the Meat Hygiene Service hygiene and inspection teams in slaughterhouses and other licensed meat production premises. The OVS is fully responsible for ensuring compliance with the structural, hygiene, inspection, health marking and animal welfare requirements at licensed premises.

OFV The Organization of Future Veterinarians (Pre Vet Club).

Old English Sheepdog An English breed of sturdy dog having a docked tail and a thick, shaggy, bluish-gray and white coat with fur that hangs over the eyes.

Oligodendrocytes Glial cells that wrap around axons in the CNS and create insulating myelin.

Oliguria A small volume of urine produced. In adult dogs and cats oliguria is defined as urine production of less than 0.5 ml/lb/hr (1 ml/kg/hr).

Omasum The third part of a ruminant stomach located between the reticulum and the abomasum.

Omega 3 fatty acids Omega-3 fatty acids like eicosapentaenoic acid (EPA) and docosahexaenoic acid (DHA) are the constituents of fish oils that act as anti-inflammatory agents. These may be worth trying for a dog that has an autoimmune disorder or arthritis. Omega-3 fatty acids come in varied forms from salmon oil to capsules of concentrated EPA. Alternatively, flax seeds, flax oil, or hemp oil can be used as a dietary supplement rather than fish oils. These materials reduce the platelet function for a brief period in dogs, but it seems that dogs compensate for this within about eight weeks. Omega-3 fatty acids replace the 2-series fatty acids over time, and cellular stimulation will instead produce 3-series prostaglandins and thromboxanes. The 3-series do not cause inflammation and reduce blood flow like the 2-series thromboxanes.

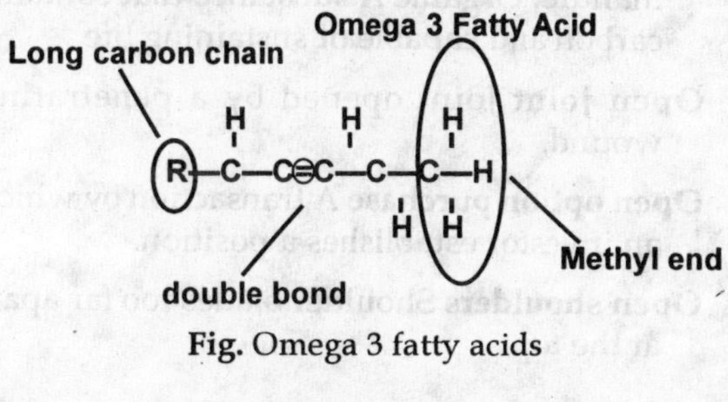

Fig. Omega 3 fatty acids

Omentum The omentum is a long fold of the peritoneum. It is loaded with fat and lies in front of the bowels in the abdominal cavity. It protects the bowels and keeps them warm.

Omnivore A person or animal that feeds on both animal and vegetable substances.

On deck Next to go in the pen.

On the hoof Designating a living meat animal.

Oncology The field of medicine concerning the diagnosis, treatment and study of cancer.

Oncotic The pressure or pull of fluids created by colloids in solution. In blood, the oncotic pressure created by particles such as plasma proteins offsets the hydrostatic pressure created by the pumping of the heart that acts to drive fluid out of vessels into the extravascular space. The oncotic pressure of the plasma proteins holds fluid in the blood vessels.

On Dog Identification A system of tagging, tattooing, or microchipping used to uniquely identify a dog.

Onychomycosis Fungal infection of the nailbed.

Oocyst A stage in the life of coccidia (a protozoal parasite) that is shed in manure. Goats become infected by ingesting oocysts from contaminated pastures.

Open A term commonly used for nonpregnant farm mammals.

Open Barns/Tromp Sheds/Loose Housing Open spaced shelter in which cattle are free to move about or rest wherever they might prefer, usually on a pack of bedding and manure. Organic A substance that contains carbon and capable of sustaining life.

Open joint Joint opened by a penetrating wound.

Open option purchase A transaction by which an investor establishes a position.

Open shoulders Shoulder blades too far apart at the top.

Openness A quality in dairy cattle associated with length of body and width and length of rib.

Operculum Fleshy partial covering over nostril.

Ophthalmic Of or relating to the eye; ocular.

Opioid Synthetic compounds with effects like opium but which are not derived from opium.

Opportunist A bacteria that causes clinical disease in animals that are some how weakened and can not fight off the infection.

Opportunistic pathogen Parasites that are usually harmless commensals in their normal habitat, but can cause disease when they gain access to other body sites – e.g. Pasteurella haemolytica (pneumonia) and Staphylococcus aureus (mastitis). Impairment of animal's immune defense is the principle factor leading to opportunistic infections.

Opsinizing antibody A type of antibody that coats particles, such as bacteria to promote phagocytosis.

Optic Type of antimicrobial agent made from a mold or a bacterium that kills, or slows the growth of other microbes, specifically bacteria. Examples include penicillin and streptomycin.

Optic nerve Formed by axons of the ganglion cells of the retina.

Optic nerve hypoplasia Incomplete development of the optic nerve.

Optic neuritis A medical condition where vision deteriorates rapidly over hours or days. One or both eyes may be affected. This condition results for the demyelination of optic nerves. In most cases, the cause of optic neuritis is unknown. Patients may regain their vision or be left with permanent impairment.

Oral Giving something by mouth or refering to the mouth.

Oral hypoglycemic A medication, given by mouth, which lowers the level of glucose in the blood. Example: glipizide.

Oral transmission Common route of animal-to-animal exposure due to contact with infected placenta, fetal fluids, milk.

Orange Belton Color definitions may vary by breed. Always check the breed standard for the definitive color description.

Orbicularis oculi muscle Muscle that encircles the eye and acts to closes the eye. It is innervated by cranial nerve 7, the facial nerve.

Orbit In human anatomy, the orbits are a pair of roomy cavities in the skull which contain the eyes.

Orbital fascia The connective tissue sheath that lines the orbit and envelopes all the structures within the orbit.

Orbital opening The orbital openings are the eye-sockets in the human skull.

Orbital Orbital is a classification of human skull shape and refers to the skulls of Tasmanians.

Orbital rim techniqueA surgical technique that is no longer recommended for correction of prolapse of the gland of the third eyelid. This technique fixed the gland so it could no longer sweep across the eye speading tears.

Orbitotomy Surgical procedure to access the back of the globe for a biopsy.

Orchitis A complication of mumps infection occurring in males (who are beyond puberty). Symptoms begin 7-10 days after onset of mumps and include inflammation of the testicles, headache, nausea, vomiting, pain and fever. Most patients recover but in rare cases sterility occurs.

Organ system A group of organs that function together. For example the digestive system includes the esophagus, intestinal tract, liver and pancreas because they all function to absorb and digest food.

Organic Material Substances containing plant or animal substance. In the context of milking equipment this usually refers to manure.

Organic nitrogen Nitrogen bound in organic compounds, such as protein or amino acids. Requires microbial decomposition prior to nitification as a plant nutrient.

Organism Any living thing. Organisms include humans, animals, plants, bacteria, protozoa and fungi.

Orifice The hole in the end of a teat.

Os calcis The Os calcis is the heel bone of the human foot.

Os penis A bone in the penis of a dog. This is a structure unique to the dog.

Osis A condition or a process, especially one that is abnormal.

Osmolality A property of fluids determined by the number and size of particles in the fluid. Fluids with large numbers of small particles have a high osmolality.

Osmolality The concentration of osmotically active particles in a solution expressed in as osmoles of solute per kilogram of solvent.

Osmolarity The concentration of osmotically active particles in solution expressed in as osmoles of solute per liter of solution.

Osmotic diuretic A compound that increases the amount of urine formed and rids the body of excess fluid by being filtered through the kidney into the urine in concentrated amounts and carrying water with it.

Osteochondritis dessicans, OCD A piece of cartilage tears away forming a flap. The flap may reattach to the bone on its own, or it may tear away, becoming a joint mouse in the joint cavity. Symptoms include pain and limping.

Osteoclast A large multinucleated cell whose sole responsibility is to resorb (eat up) bone.

These cells are derived from blood-forming stem cells in the bone marrow.

Osteogenesis The development and formation of bone.

Osteomyelitis An inflammation and infection of the bone.

Otic Pertaining to the ear.

Otitis externa Inflammation of the external ear canal.

Otitis Media A viral or bacterial infection that leads to inflammation of the middle ear. This condition usually occurs along with an upper respiratory infection. Symptoms include earache, high fever, nausea, vomiting and diarrhea. In addition, hearing loss, facial paralysis and meningitis may result.

Otobius megnini The spinous ear tick may induce otitis in dogs and occasionally cats.

Otodectes cynotis Ear mite.

Ototoxic Destructive to the structures of the ear.

Out of Terminology for mothered by in animal breeding.

Out side tie When the male ejaculates with the bulbus glandis engorgement outside of the vagina. Females bred with an 'out side tie' usually don't get pregnant.

Outbreak Sudden appearance of a disease in a specific geographic area (e.g. neighborhood or community) or population (e.g. adolescents).

Outcross Mating an individual to another in the same breed who is not closely related to it.

Outcrossing Mating of individuals within a breed that are not closely related.

Outside In a pen, the side of the horse toward the fence.

Ovarian bursa A structure that surrounds the ovaries and collects eggs released from the ovary and channels those eggs to the uterus.

Ovariohysterectomy OVHThe removal of the female reproductive organs. Spaying, spayed, (NOT SPADE).

Ovary The female reproductive gland in which the eggs are formed and progesterone and estrogenic hormones are produced.

Over shot or parrot mouth When the lower jaw is shorter than the upper jaw and the teeth hit in back of the dental pad.

Over the counter Can be purchased without a prescription, like aspirin and vitamins.

Over the counter (OTC) Products that do not require a veterinary prescription to purchase.

Overconditioned An animal with excess flesh and patchy fat deposits, especially over the shoulders, back, hips, and thighs.

Overo A Paint or Pinto coat pattern of spots that are irregular, scattered, or splashy. The horse usually has a large white facial marking as well.

Over stride If the rear foot of a horse passes the track of the same side front foot as it is set down, the distance between the front of the front track and the rear of the rear track is the amount of over - stride.

Oviduct The tube inside a hen through which an egg travels when it is ready to be laid.

Ovine Pertaining to sheep.

Ovine progressive pneumonia OPPA chronic inflammatory disease of the lung leading to eventual suffocation.

Ovulate The release of an egg from the ovary of the female.

Ovulation When the follicle ruptures and the ovum, or egg, is released into the oviduct.

Ovum Egg.

Owner sampler (OS) An unofficial milk production record system, the records of which originate with the breeder (owner) through a local DHIA. This type of testing plan allows dairy farmers to weigh and sample milk from their cows. Records are intended for management use only and are not official.

Oxer Parallel bar-type fence with two rails. A square oxer has even rails. A step or ascending oxer has a lower front rail.

Oxidize To combine with oxygen.

Oxyglobin A red blood cell substitute made from polymerized bovine hemoglobin.

Oxytocin A naturally secreted hormone that is important in milk letdown and the contraction of smooth uterine muscles during parturition.

P

P.O.P Purified oxytocin principal.

P - Q Parasite An organism that lives on or inside a host animal and derives food or protection from the host without giving anything in return.

P3 The third phalanx, or the third bone in a digit.

Pace The pace is a two-beat lateral gait in which a horse moves both right feet and then moves both left feet. In a pace the front and rear foot are picked up and then set down simultaneously making only one beat. A pacing horse will move its head side to side to counter the motion of its feet.

Pace walk The pace-walk is a lateral four-beat gait in which the horse will pick up both the front and rear foot simultaneously, then moves the rear foot faster than the front foot and sets the rear foot down before the front foot. This allows the pace-walker to have an up and down head shake, and have a four-beat cadence. The pace-walk is much closer to a flat foot walk than a pace, having both a head shake and a four beat cadence.

Pacing Continuous stall or pen walking. Often an unhappy horse's reaction to confinement.

Pack Multiple hounds cast at one time.

Packed cell volume (PCV), hematocrit: A laboratory test to monitor the relative number of red blood cells present in the blood. A blood sample is placed in a tiny glass tube and spun in a centrifuge. The cells are heavier than the plasma and are compacted at one end of the tube. After the tube is spun, it is examined and the packed cell volume is determined as the percentage of the red cellular portion relative to the total amount of blood in the tube (i.e., remainder being the plasma). The normal for dogs is 40-59 and cats is 29-50.

Packed RBC's Red blood cells from which much of the plasma has been removed. Used to provide RBCs to patients that may not be able to handle a large fluid load, for example patients with cardiac disease. Separation of cells from plasma also allows for early freezing of the plasma to preserve labile coagulation factors.

Packing plant Place where hogs are slaughtered, cleaned, and cut into pork chops, bacon, and roasts for the supermarket.

Pacy Slang term that is used to refer to a horse that is moving in a fashion that is between the gait desired at the time and a pace. Most common when referring to a horse that is walking with a rhythm that is more lateral than a correct flat foot walk.

Padding A compensating action to offset constant concussion when a straight front is subjected to overdrive from the rear; the front feet flip upward in a split-second delaying action to coordinate the stride of the forelegs with the longer stride from behind.

Paddocks Subdivision of a pasture designed to provide short-duration grazing followed by an appropriate (related to species, soil type and weather conditions) rest period for regrowth and stand maintenance.

Pads Tough, shock-absorbing projections on the underside of the feet. Soles.

Pain An unpleasant sensory and emotional experience which may cause tissue damage.

Pain, chronic Persisting for a long time.

Paint (1). A breed of horse with large blocks of white and black or white and brown.

Paint (2). Coat pattern on any breed of horse that is similar to that on a Paint Horse.

Paint Sticks Contain liquid or chalky paint used for marking treated cows.

Palatability The appeal and acceptability of feedstuffs. Affected by the taste, odour, texture and temperature of the feed.

Palatable or palatability The taste and texture of forage. A forage that is highly palatable has a pleasant taste and texture.

Palatable Tasty; refers to food that is readily accepted.

Palatine bones The palatine bones are part of the floor of the nasal cavity and the roof of the mouth in the human skull.

Palliative treatment Palliative treatment is given to patients with untreatable diseases in order to make them more comfortable. Includes a combination of supportive and symptomatic treatments.

Palmate Completely webbed (3 toes connected).

Palpation To examine something by touching and feeling it.

Palpebrae Eyelids.

Palpebral fissure The opening between the eyelids.

Palpebral or blink reflex Used to assess sensation and the ability to close the eyelids.

Palpebral Pertaining to the eyelids.

Pamprodactyl All four toes in front, as in swifts.

Pancreas The pancreas is an elongated secreting gland which secretes pancreatic juice and insulin.

Pancreatitis Inflammation of the pancreas due to a variety of causes such as infections and drugs. The pancreas produces enzymes and bicarbonate important in digestion and absorption of nutrients as well as insulin. Chronic, severe pancreatitis can result in malabsorption and diarrhea as well as diabetes mellitus.

Pandemic An epidemic occurring over a very large area.

Panic snap A safety snap often used in horse trailers and cross-ties. The design allows the snap to be released even if there is great pressure on it.

Panniculitis Inflammation of subcutanious fat. Several proposed causes and is sterile in some breeds such as the Dachshund.

Pannus A chronic condition of the eye in which blood vessels grow across the cornea (the clear surface of the eye). The cornea looks hazy and sometimes reddened; it may eventually take on a dark pigment. This condition is also called chronic superficial keratitis.

Panosteitis, pano Inflammation of the bone, particularly the long bones in growing dogs. Causes pain and limping.

Pantothenic acid A vitamin of the B complex group that is present in all living tissues as part of the coenzyme A (CoA) molecule or the acyl carrier protein.

Pants See Breeches.

PAO2 The concentration of oxygen in the blood.

Pap smear Vaginal or cervical cells obtained for cytological study.

Paper Foot A flat foot devoid of arch to the toes.

Papers The pedigree and registration slip for a cat.

Papillon A breed of small dog related to the spaniel, having a long silky coat, a bushy tail that curves over its back, and large ears shaped like the wings of a butterfly.

Papule Solid bump on the skin, less than 1/3 inch in diameter.

Parabasal cell A small and round cell with a large and distinct nucleus. Parabasal cells, along with red blood cells (RBCs), are present during proestrus.

Parade horse A horse trained to carry ornamented tack in parades.

Paradoxical CSF acidosis Paradoxical CSF acidosis is a condition caused by the administration of a large amount of bicarbonate to an acidotic patient, which will result in neurologic dysfunction. When one gives bicarbonate, the equation is shifted towards the left of the screen, towards the generation of CO2. CO2 is very diffusible, and will diffuse across the blood brain barrier and then shift the equation in the cerebral spinal fluid towards the right with a generation of hydrogen ions. Even though additional bicarbonate is being generated in the CNS, the neurons perceive the increase in hydrogen ions and malfunction. The bicarbonate that was administered IV cannot cross the blood brain barrier.

Parainfluenza In canines, a disease characterized by fever, vomiting and diarrhea.

Parakeratosis Any abnormality of the stratum corneum (horny layer of epidermis) of skin, especially a condition caused by edema between the cells, which prevents the formation of keratin.

Parallel milking parlor A raised milking area or platform where the cow stands perpendicular to the operator and milking units are attached between the rear legs. Also called side-by-side.

Paralysis Loss of motor function (movement) in a certain part of the body. Paralysis may be flaccid, in which muscles are weak and have little or no tone; or spastic, in which the muscles are tight.

Paraphimosis Paraphimosis is when the penis is extruded from the prepuce and cannot be returned to its normal position. This may occur following breeding or sexual excitement such as being kenneled next to a bitch in heat, or by a traumatic fracture of the os penis.

Parasite An organism that grows, feeds, and is sheltered on or in a different organism while contributing nothing to the survival of its host.

Parasites Any organism that lives in or on another organism without benefiting the host organism; commonly refers to pathogens, most commonly in reference to protozoans and helminthes.

Parasiticide A substance that kills parasites.

Parasitism Denotes organisms which survive and persist on or within another living organism. The parasite usually does not harm the animal. The most successful parasites achieve a balance whereby both the parasite and host animal survive.

Parasympathetic The portion of the nervous system which stimulates the pancreas to produce digestive enzymes and stimulates many of the smooth muscles in the body including those of the stomach and intestine. It also tends to slow the heart rate.

Parasympathomimetic effects A drug that produces effects similar to the effects produced by stimulation of parasympathetic nerves.

Parathyroid Glands The parathyroid glands are two small glands in the neck concerned with the use of calcium in the body.

Parenteral Administered intravenously or by injection. For example, medications or vaccines may be administered by injection into the fatty layer immediately below the skin (subcutaneous), or into the muscle (intramuscular). Medications, but not vaccines, can also be administered into a vein (intravenously).

Parenterally A term used to describe the administration of a drug by means other than by mouth.

Paresis Slight or incomplete paralysis.

Parietal bone The parietal bone is the plate on the top of the human skull, comprising most of the dome of the skull.

Parity price A level of farm prices intended to provide the same approximate purchasing power for farmers as enjoyed during a preceding base period.

Park horse A horse with a brilliant performance, style, presence, finish, balance and cadence and usually animated gaits.

Parlor The specialized area on the dairy farm where milking is performed. Parlors come in many types:

Flat Barn,

Walk-through,

Herringbone,

Parallel,

Swing and Rotary.

Paronychia Inflammation of the nail fold.

Parous Females that have produced young.

Paroxysmal The sudden onset of a symptom that reoccurs. For example paroxysmal seizures begin suddenly and occur more than once.

Parrot mouth A malformed mouth of an animal in which the upper jaw abnormally protrudes beyond the lower.

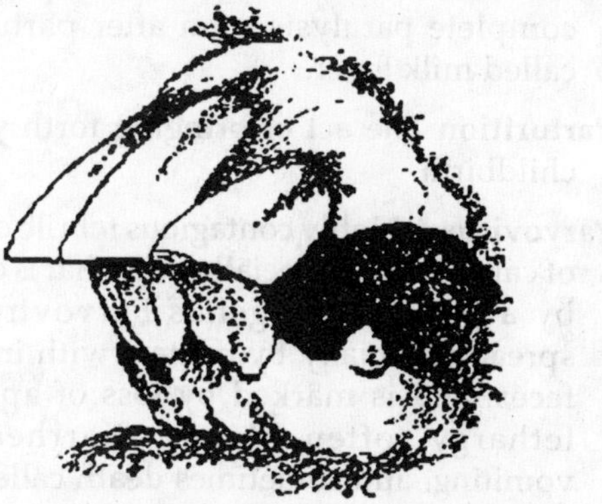

Fig. Parrot mouth

Parsley The leaves of parsley, which are often used in salads and cooked foods, are a source of vitamin C and vitamin A. It may be used as a digestive aid, a diuretic, or a mild laxative.

Parthenogenesis A form of reproduction in which the egg develops into a new individual without fertilization by sperm. Parthenogenesis has been observed in many lower animals, including some snails and insects.

Partial parenteral nutrition ppnProviding energy and nutritional supplementation to a patient at 50 to 70% of the patient's nutritional needs.

Partial Seizure See Focal seizure.

Particle size Measure of the diameter of granular feed materials and/or the length of roughage fragments. Particle size can affect mixing of feed ingredients and digestion rate.

Parti Color Two or more definite, well-broken colors, one of which must be white. For example, black parti-color would be black and white. Color definitions may vary by breed. Always check the breed standard for the definitive color description.

Parturient paresis A condition (observed especially in highproducing dairy cows) characterized by a low blood calcium concentration which results in partial to complete paralysis soon after parturition called milk fever.

Parturition The act of bringing forth young; childbirth.

Parvovirus A highly contagious febrile disease of canines and especially dogs that is caused by a parvovirus (genus Parvovirus), is spread especially by contact with infected feces, and is marked by loss of appetite, lethargy, often bloody diarrhea and vomiting, and sometimes death called also parvo.

Passage Very collected, elevated, and cadenced trot characterized by a pronounced engagement of the hindquarters, more exaggerated flexion of the knees and hocks, and a graceful elasticity of movement.

Passive immunity Protection against disease through antibodies produced by another human being or animal. Passive immunity is effective, but protection is generally limited and diminishes over time (usually a few weeks or months). For example, maternal antibodies are passed to the infant prior to birth. These antibodies temporarily protect the baby for the first 4-6 months of life.

Passive transfer Acquiring protection against infectious disease from another animal. This commonly occurs when a newborn consumes antibody-rich colostrum from its mother. Failure to have sufficient passive transfer increases the risk of disease.

Passport A document which contains information about the identity and sometimes the health status of an animal. Cattle passports contain information specified by EU law, and are used to record cattle movements and notify them to the Cattle Tracing System. Horse passports show whether or not the animal's carcase may be used for human consumption. EU passports for cats, dogs and ferrets under the Pet Travel Scheme show whether the animal is qualified to enter or re-enter the country without going into quarantine.

Pastern Area and joint between fetlock and hoof.

Pasteurization The process of heating milk to at least 62.8øC. (145øF.) and holding it at that temperature for not less than 30 minutes (holding method); to 71.7øC. (161øF.) for 15 seconds (HTST); to 88.3øC. (191øF.) for 1 second, to 95.5øC. (203.9øF.) for 0.05 second, or to 100øC. (212øF.) for 0.01 second (ultrapasteurization).

Pasteurized Milk Ordinance (PMO) Regulations approved by FDA governing the design and maintenance of dairy farms and processing plants to make sanitation and milk quality uniform across state lines.

Pasting Loose droppings sticking to vent area, also known as "pasting up" and "sticky bottoms".

Pasture Plants, as grass, grown for feeding or grazing animals. Also to feed cattle and other livestock on pasture.

Pasture breeding When a stallion is pastured with mares and breeding takes place as in the wild.

Patella The patella is the largest of the sesamoid bones. It is situated in front of the knee-joint. It is a flattened, triangular bone.

Patellar luxation Dislocation of the 'knee' cap, causing mild to severe, continuous or intermittent pain.

Patent ductus arteriosus, PDA The normal opening between the aorta and pulmonary artery, which allows blood to bypass the unoxygenated lung in utero, fails to close after birth.

Patent period The parasites are producing eggs with in the host.

Paternal Pertaining to the father or sire.

Patho pathy Abnormality.

Pathogen Any microorganism that produces disease (bacteria, viruses, yeasts, molds, and parasites).

Pathogen/pathogenicity Capacity of parasite to produce disease.

Pathogenesis The origin and development of disease. More specifically, it's the way a microbe (bacteria, virus, etc.) causes disease in its host.

Pathogenic Capable of causing disease.

Pathogens Bacteria, viruses, parasites, or fungi that can cause disease.

Pathologist A specialist in veterinary medicine who examines the changes in body tissues and organs caused by disease.

Pathology a : The study of the essential nature of diseases and especially of the structural and functional changes produced by them. **b** : Something abnormal. **c** : The structural and functional deviations from the normal that constitute disease or characterize a particular disease.

Pathology The study of tissues for signs of disease.

Pathophysiology The physiology of abnormal states; specifically, the functional changes that accompany a particular syndrome or disease.

Pattern A prescribed order of maneuvers in a particular class such as reining or trail.

Paunch (rumen) The large, first stomach compartment of a ruminant.

Pavletic A surgical technique used to repair lid defects using skin from the lip.

Pawing A bad habit usually caused by nervousness and/or improper ground training; can also be a sign of colic.

PB Phenobarbital. An AED.

PCR Polymerase chain reaction is a technique for amplifying a specific sequence in DNA by repeated cycles of synthesis driven by pairs of reciprocally oriented primers.

PCV Packed cell volume. PCV, hematocrit: A laboratory test to monitor the relative number of red blood cells present in the blood. A blood sample is placed in a tiny glass tube and spun in a centrifuge. The cells are heavier than the plasma and are compacted at one end of the tube. After the tube is spun, it is examined and the packed cell volume is determined as the percentage of the red cellular portion relative to the total amount of blood in the tube (i.e., remainder being the plasma). The normal for dogs is 40-59 and cats is 29-50.

Peak Level Either the results from or the testing of the AED blood serum values when it is at its highest in the dog's blood. This value is of concern where toxicity might be an issue. For PB levels, the peak is taken 4-6 hours after PB dosing. Giving the PB with food can add another 2 hours to the peak time.

Peak milk Maximum daily milk yield during lactation. Good peak yield is 100-120 lbs and occurs between 60-90 days in milk.

Pecking order Social rank of each horse in a group; one horse is the boss and the others find their place.

Pectinate Comblike (structure on one side of central toenail).

Pectineus The Pectineus is a muscle in the human thigh.

Pediatric administration set An adminstration set for intravenous fluid administration. The set has a spike to penetrate the container of fluids, a drip chamber and a long flexible tube that connects to the patient's catheter. The drip set drips 60 drops to deliver one ml of fluid. The drops form in the drip chamber through a rigid needle-like structure. This needle-in-the-drip chamber identifies a pediatric drip set.

Pediculicide An agent that destroys lice.

Pediculosus Lice infestation.

Pedigree A document recording the ancestors of a cat. Pedigrees may show few or many generations. A "3 generation pedigree" shows the cat itself plus three generations back. Most pedigrees show three to five generations.

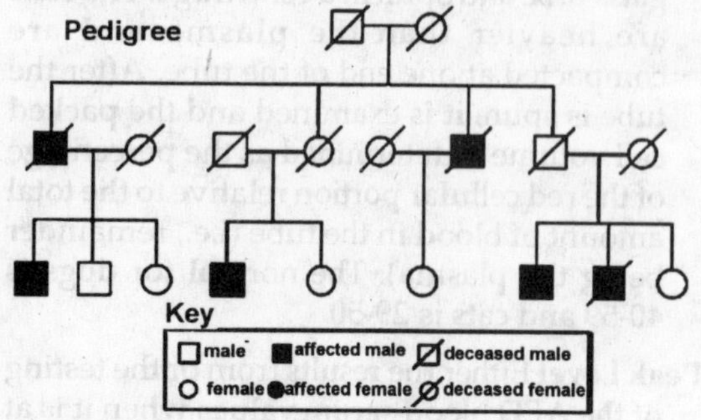

Fig. Pedigree

Pedigree A record of an animal's ancestors, usually only those of the five closest generations. A complete pedigree may include milk production, type classification, and other information pertaining to dairy cattle.

Pedigreed cat A cat with a pedigree. Note that this does not necessarily mean that the cat is purebred or registered!

PEG tubes Feeding tubes placed percutaneously using endoscopic guidance.

Pelham bit A combination of snaffle bit and curb bit requiring two reins, used in English riding.

Pelodera dermatitis Rhabditic dermatitis. Larvae of the free living nematode, Pelodera strongyloides which penetrate the skin of animals.

Pelt The skin of a sheep including the wool.

Pelvis The pelvis is a bony girdle in vertebrates that connects the body with the lower extremities.

Pemphigus erythematosus PEPossibly an abortive form of pemphigus foliaceus. The clinical presentation is as a facial dermatitis.

Pemphigus foliaceus A generalized scaling disease, with hair loss, and sometimes with the formation of heavy crusts. Involvement of a nail bed leads to loss of the nail.

Pemphigus foliaceus PF The most common form of pemphigus recognized in the dog. Also seen in the horse and other species.

Pemphigus vegetans PVU A benign variant of pemphigus vulgaris with two classifications: the Neumann type which may begin and end as PVU and Hallopeau which is thought to be more of a benign form.

Pen The show ring or an outdoor living space that is at least 24 feet long and 24 feet wide. Also to corral cattle, as in team penning.

Pen mating A small number of females are penned with a male at regular intervals and are supervised during breeding.

Pencil shrink A percentage adjustment in lamb live weight, generally between 2 and 4 percent, which is subtracted to insure that responsibility for weight loss during transport are shared by the buyer and seller.

Pendulous Udder A loosely attached udder.

Pendulous udders Loosely attached mammary glands are collectively referred to as pendulous udders.

Penetration The penis entering the female reproductive tract.

Penicillinase An enzyme produced by some bacteria which inactivates certain types of penicillin thus making the bacteria resistant to them.

Penis The male organ used to deposit semen in the female.

Percentile (%ILE) For bulls, percentile (%ILE) is a ranking based on the Active AI bull population; for cows, %ILE is a ranking based on cows with recent lactations. With the Animal Model, PTA$ Protein is used to determine percentiles.

Perch The place where chickens sleep at night; the act of resting on a perch; also called a "roost."

Perforate Continuous with other side (nostrils).

Performance Exhibition of gaits or other required routines.

Performance horse A horse especially accomplished in showing, jumping, and dressage.

Peri Around.

Perianal fistula A deep infection around the anus which often results in ulcers and deep draining tracts, most commonly seen in German Shepherds.

Perianal The region around the anus.

Pericardium A very thin tissue surrounding the heart. Abnormal fluid can accumulate between the heart and the pericardial membrane causing pericardial effusion.

Perineal The area between the anus and the genital organs.

Periodic opthalmia See moon blindness.

Periople External covering of the hoof wall.

Periparturient hypocalcemia Low serum calcium associated with calving which can result in loss of motor function. (See also parturient paresis.)

Periparturient The time around calving.

Peripheral Blood The fluid that circulates in the heart, arteries, capillaries, and veins of an animal. Peripheral blood carries nourishment and oxygen to and brings away waste products from all parts of the body.

Peripheral IV catheter A catheter placed in a smaller vein in a limb (cephalic or saphenous). These catheters are relatively short in length.

Peritoneal cavity The abdominal cavity between the viseral and parietal peritoneum.

Peritoneal dialysis A process used to remove waste products from the body. Electrolyte fluids are administered into the abdomen, waste products of the body enter the fluids, and then the fluids are removed.

Peritoneal The abdominal or belly cavity.

Peritoneum The membrane lining the wall of the abdominal cavity.

Peritonitis Nflammation of the internal surface of the abdomen. This condition is often the result of infections and certain diseases.

Perivascular Cells Cells surrounding a blood vessel.

Permanent identification Identification that stays with the animal for its lifetime and cannot be lost. Examples are tatoo, color markings (sketch or photo) and hot or freeze brand.

Permethrin Defend, Coopers) a topical antiparasitic agent.

Peroxidase antiperoxidase staining This technique uses an immunohistochemical procedure designed to demonstrate the presence of Ig or complement in a tissue section.

Persistency of lay The ability of a hen to lay steadily over a long period of time.

Persistency The quality of being persistent, as in the ability of lactating animals to maintain milk production over a period of time.

Persistent pupillary membranes PPMs Remnants of a blood vessels that once filled the anterior chamber and nourished the developing lens.

Pet quality A cat that does not meet the breed standard closely enough to be valuable to a breeding program. Of course, pet quality cats are just as healthy and friendly as other cats.

Pet Travel Scheme A scheme which allows cats, dogs and ferrets from certain countries to enter the UK without having to go into a quarantine kennel. It also allows animals from the UK to visit certain countries and return home without quarantine. Details of vaccination and rabies blood tests must be shown on a PETS certificate or EU passport.

PETA People for the Ethical Treatment of Animals, an animal rights organization.

Petit-Mal Seizure See Absence Seizure.

pH How much acid or how much base is in a sample. The lower the pH of a substance, the more acidic the sample. Conversely, the higher the pH, the more basic the sample. Normal rumen pH should be around 6-7, depending on the ration being fed.

Phaeohyphomycoses Subcutaneous nodules, granulomatous lesions and draining tracts caused by Pythium sp.(Hyphomyces sp.), Dreschlera sp and other species.

Phagocyte Cell in the body which 'eats' damaged cells and foreign substances such as virus and bacteria. A macrophage is a type of phagocyte.

Phagocytosis The process of capture and destruction of foreign material. The two leading cells in this process are neutrophils and macrophages (Phagocytes).

Pharmaco Pertaining to drugs.

Pharmacodynamics The behavior (e.g. quick, slow, short term, long term, etc.) of an antimicrobial at its receptor site (i.e. where it initiates its effect).

Pharmacologic reactions to foods An adverse reaction to as a result of a naturally derived or added chemical that produces a drug-like of pharmacologic effect.

Pharynx Back of the mouth. Throat.

Phase II clinical trial A scientifically controlled study carried out in, usually to test the effectiveness of a new treatment.

Phase III clinical trial These are pilot efficacy studies aimed at generating statistically relevant data.

Pheasant A species of gamebird that comes in many breeds and varieties. They are raised for meat, feathers, ornamental value or to be released into the wild.

Phenotype Manifestation of genotype or the combined manifestation of several different genotypes.

Phenotype The phenotype of an animal is the composite of all its tangible features. The phenotype includes an animal's external appearance, measures of its productivity, and its physiological characteristics.

Phenotypic Correlation A correlation between two traits caused by genetic plus environmental factors influencing both traits.

Pheromone Chemical secreted by an animal and sensed by another animal of the same species, and often causing behavior change in that animal.

Phimosis The penis cannot be extruded from the prepuce. Phimosis may be congenital due to a small preputial orifice or a persistent frenulum. Acquired inflammation or neoplasia can reduce the size of preputial orifice or increase the size of the penis causing phimosis.

Phosphate An ion of phosphorus and oxygen (H2PO4- or HPO4-2). May exist as an ion in solution or as an ester or salt of phosphoric acid.

Phosphorylation The process of adding a phosphate group to a molecule. This often activates the molecule by altering its shape or charge and allows it to participate in a chemical reaction.

Photoperiod Length of day (or length of period artificial light is provided). Also expressed as a ratio of daylight to darkness.

Photoperiod The number of hours of light per 24-hour period.

Photoreceptor layer Layer of the retina composed of the rods and cones.

Photosensitivity A condition in which the skin reacts abnormally to light, especially ultraviolet light or sunlight. It is usually caused by the interaction of light with certain chemicals in the skin such as antibiotics, other medications, hormones, or toxins.

Photosynthesis The process by which plants, using energy from the sun, combine carbon dioxide and water to form sugar, from which the plants obtain nutrition.

Phthisis bulbi An eye that has degenerated after injury.

Physiology The science dealing with the functions of animals.

Phytochemical Substances in plants which affect a body system and may promote health and decrease the risk of a disease such as cancer.

Phytoestrogen Substances which have an activity similar to estrogens and are produced by plants.

Piaffe(R) Highly collected and cadenced trot in place.

Pica A craving for unnatural articles of food such as is observed in phosphorus-deficient animals; a depraved appetite.

Picket line Rope tie rail.

Pickout Vent damage due to cannibalism.

Pig Swine up to 120 pounds.

Piggin string A short, narrow rope used to hogtie a calf or steer.

Piglet Young new born pigs.

Pigmentary keratitis The accumulation of pigment in the cornea in response to inflammation.

Pigmentation The color of a chicken's beak, shanks, and vent.

Pinfeathers The tips of newly emerging feathers.

Pink eye (conjunctivitis) An inflammatory disease of the eye of cattle of all ages. The eye may become pearl colored and opaque leading to blindness.

Pinkeye A highly contagious disease that affects the eyes of goats (also contagious to humans).

Pinking upA lay term used to indicate pink nipples in a queen which indicates increased blood flow to the nipples under the influence of progesterone.

Pinna femoral" reflex "When the ear is rubbed, the dog scratches aggressively with the hind leg! Not a "real" reflex but is highly suggestive of scabies.

Pinnae The flap of the ear.

Pinnal dermatitis Skin lesions on the ears.

Pinworms Oxyuris equi; parasites.

Pip 1. The hole a newly formed chick makes in its shell when it is ready to hatch.

2. The act of making the hole.

Pipeline A stainless steel or glass pipe used for transporting milk.

Pipeline A stainless steel or glass pipe used for transporting milk by gravity to storage. May be above the milking units (high line) or below the level of the units (low line).

Piriformis The Piriformis is a muscle in the human hip.

Pirouette Circle executed on two tracks with the radius equal to the length of the horse, with the forehand moving around the haunches and maintaining the exact rhythm and sequence of footfalls of the gait being used.

Pisiform bone The pisiform bone is one of the bones in the human wrist.

Pit A contained unit usually with concrete walls in which liquid or semi-liquid manure is stored.

Pitch To loosen the reins abruptly and completely, or to toss a rope.

Pituitary gland A hormone secreting (endocrine) gland at the base of the brain; it regulates growth as well as regulating the proper functioning of many other glands and processes.

Pituitary gland A small gland located in the brain. Several hormones are produced in this gland.

Pituitary gland The pituitary gland is a gland within the brain concerned with regulating growth and regulating other ductless glands.

Pivot Crisp, prompt turn on the hindquarters.

Pizzle Prepuce.

Placebo A substance or treatment that has no effect on human beings.

Placebo A substance which is given that has no therapeutic value; often called a 'dummy pill' or 'sugar pill.' Often given to half of the patients in a trial of a new drug, to better assess the effectiveness of the new drug.

Placenta (afterbirth), the membrane attached to the inside of the uterus which takes nutrients from the mare's blood to the fetus through the umbilical cord.

Placenta After birth. An organ that allows for the mother to provide nutrition and remove wastes from the developing baby in the uterus.

Placentitis Abnormal inflammation of the placenta, usually due to infectious disease.

Plain A term suggesting general inferiority; coarse; lacking the desired quality or breed character.

Plans In a problem oriented record there are diagnostic plans, therapeutic plans and plans to inform the client.

Plantais The Plantais is a muscle in the leg.

Planter Used to plant seeds.

Plantigrade stance Standing and walking with the hocks on or almost touching the floor.

Plaque A flat surfaced, raised skin lesion.

Plasia Growth

Plasma The clear part of blood that remains after blood is separated into cells and fluid before the blood clots. If the blood is allowed to clot then separated into cells and fluid, the fluid is then called serum.

Plasma cell pododermatis Swelling and ulceration of the foot pads. Seen most frequently in cats.

Plasmodium The genus of the parasite that causes malaria. The genus includes four species that infect humans Plasmodium falciparum, Plasmodium vivax, Plasmodium malariae, and Plasmodium ovale.

Plastron The lower hard shell-like structure which protects the abdomen of a turtle or tortoise.

Plate Cooler A heat exchanger in which water at ground temperature or chilled water is used to cool milk prior to its movement to the bulk milk tank.

Platelets Cellular components found in the blood which help clots to form. In the body, microscopically small vessels often break in the normal course of events. Platelets and a protein called fibrinogen 'plug' the break in the vessel and prevent blood from leaking out.

Pleasure Rail class designed to showcase smooth movers.

Pleura One of the two thin, smooth membranes lining the interior of the chest and covering the surface of the lungs.

Pleural effusion Increased amounts of fluid within the pleural cavity usually due to inflammation.

Plow Used to help break the soil so that it is ready for planting.

Plumage The total set of feathers covering a chicken.

Pluripotent stem cells Pluripotent cells can become many types of cells but not all types of cells.

Pluronic gel Topical application of an analgesic.

Pneo Pertaining to a. Breathing. b. Breath.

Pneumonia Inflammation of the lungs characterized by fever, chills, muscle stiffness, chest pain, cough, shortness of breath, rapid heart rate and difficulty breathing. Polysaccharide vaccines- Vaccines that are composed of long chains of sugar molecules that resemble the surface of certain types of bacteria. Polysaccharide vaccines are available for pneumococcal disease, meningococcal disease and Haemophilus Influenzae type b.

Pneumothorax The abnormal accumulation of air in the chest cavity outside the lungs.

PNS Peripheral nervous system, the nervous system of the body

Pocket A comfortable, secure place in the saddle. In timed events, the area where you collect the horse and start your turn around a barrel or pole.

Pocket technique Surgical technique for replacing a prolapse of the gland of the third eyelid.

Points Units of achievement awarded to a cat in a show that are accumulated towards a towards a title, a regional award, or a national award. Each association has its own way of determining how many points are awarded for a particular type of show win, and may have several different point scales for different titles or awards. In European associations such as fife, certificates are awarded and accumulated towards titles instead of points.

Poison Any substance that can cause an adverse effect when introduced into a biological system (not acting mechanically).

Pole barn A barn built on poles set in the earth.

Poliosis Whitening of the hair.

Poll The junction of the vertebrae with the skull located between a horse's ears; an area of great sensitivity and flexion.

Pollakiuria Frequent passage of small amounts of urine. Pollakiuria is indicative of diseases of the lower urinary tract and genital tract.

Polled Breed where there has been a genetic selection for no horns. Some sheep breeds are horned in both sexes, in others only the males are horned and in yet others (the majority of breeds) neither sex is horned.

Polled Naturally hornless cattle or cattle with horns cut off.

Pollution Made dirty or impure due to the presence of waste or garbage in the air, water, or on land; the contamination of natural system.

Poly Means several or too much such as polydactyly means having too many toes.

Polyarteritis nodosa An inflammatory disease of small and medium sized arteries.

Polyarthritis Arthritis which involves two or more joints.

Polyarthropathy Inflammatory joint disease that involves multiple joints.

Polyclonal antibodyA term used to describe a mixture of Ig to a wide array of antigens.

Polycystic kidney disease PKD A disease in which kidney tissue is replaced by multiple cystic stuctures. There is an inherited form of polycystic kidney disease in Persian cats.

Polycythemia Polycythemia is an increased number of circulating RBC. Most animals with increased PCV have relative polycythemia due to hemoconcentration. Splenic contraction can increase PCV by 10 to 15%. Absolute polycythemia is an increased total hemoglobin/RBC mass with normal plasma volume. Absolute polycythemia can be a primary myeloproliferative disorder called polycythemia vera. The signs of polycythemia vera can include polyuria and polydipsia, bleeding from small capillary rupture, neurologic disturbances caused by increased viscosity of blood.

Polydactyl The presence of extra toes.

Polydipsia Drinking large amounts of water.

Polydipsia Excessive thirst - a possible side effect of being on some AEDs.

Polyestrous During one sexual season, continuing to come into heat if not bred. Cats are polyestrous, dogs are not.

Polygastric Possessing more than one stomach compartment, as does the cow and other ruminants.

Polymer A molecule made of repeating units (monomers). For example starch is a polymer of glucose molecules.

Polymerase chain reaction PCRA technique to rapidly produce many copies of a fragment of DNA.

Polymyositis Inflammation of several muscles at one time.

Polyp A small growth from mucous membranes such as those lining the nasal cavity and intestinal tract.

Polyphagia excessive hunger - a possible side effect of being on some AEDs.

Polysaccharide A carbohydrate containing a large number of sugar groups. Starch is an example of a polysaccharide.

Polyurethane A type of plastic used to make, among other things, IV catheters.

Polyuria Excessive urination - possible side effect of being on some AEDs.

Polyvalent A vaccine containing several antigens (multivalent).

Pommel The wide uplifted front of the saddle (forming the fork in the western saddle).

Pony Club A national organization that teaches youngsters to care for and ride horses.

Pony Technically, a horse under 14.2 hands, but for practical purposes, individuals of one of the classic pony breeds such as Shetland, Welsh, Connemara, Pony of the Americas (P.O.A.), etc.

Pool, cooperative Each producer who belongs to a cooperative receives a common blend price calculated on the basis of use of all milk sold through the cooperative.

Pool, individual handler A pool in which each producer selling raw milk to a single handler (dealer) receives the same blend price for milk regardless of the use made of any individual producer's milk.

Pool, marketwide A pool in which each producer supplying a market receives the same uniform price for milk calculated on the basis of use of all milk received by handlers in the market.

Population This usually means the total number of animals of a defined type being considered in a specific area or as a group. Examples of animal populations are "all the lambs in a county", or "all the badgers in a wood", or "all the dairy cows in the UK". Sometimes it refers to a number of farms instead of a number of animals. So the "population" might be "all the pig farms in Scotland".

Pork Meat from pigs.

Portosystemic shunt PSS abnormal blood vessels in the liver preventing normal circulation and functioning of the liver.

Position An interest in the market, either long or short, in the form of one or more open contracts.

Positional cloning A technique used to identify genes, usually those that are associated with diseases, based on their location on a chromosome.

Post ictal The period after a seizure. Can last for minutes or days. The dog can be temporiarily blind, restless, confused, disoriented, confused. Sometimes this is the only indication that the dog has had a seizure.

Post Mortem After death.

Post mortem examination Tests carried out on the carcases of animals which have died in order to find out the cause of death.

Post mortem inspection The checks carried out by the Meat Hygiene Service on the carcases of animals slaughtered for human consumption.

Post partum After parturition. After giving birth.

Post renal azotemia An increase in nitrogen containing wastes in the blood due to an inability to excrete urine as a consequence of an obstruction to urine passage or to a ruptured bladder.

Post renal azotemia An increase in nitrogen containing wastes in the blood due to an inability to excrete urine as a consequence of an obstruction to urine passage or to a ruptured bladder.

Post To rise from the saddle in rhythm with the horse's trot.

Posteriad Toward the rear.

Posterior chamber Space between the iris and lens.

Posterior pituitary extract Hormone produced by the pituitary gland causing milk letdown and contraction of the uterus at foaling.

Posterior Positioned in back of another body part, or towards the rear half of the animal. Opposite of anterior.

Posterior synechia Occurs when the inflamed iris sticks to the lens.

Post-legged A condition in which the hind legs are too straight, so that the springy quality of the hock and pastern is lost.

Post-Milking Teat Dip A product applied after milking to protect the teat from contagious pathogens that may have come into contact with the teat during the milking process.

Postmortem Pertaining to or occurring after death.

Postoperative After surgery.

Postprandial The period of time immediately after eating.

Potash An oxide of potassium (K2O) used as a plant nutrient or fertilizer.

Potato dextrose agar A fungal growth media that promotes rapid sporulation making identification possible at an earlier time than when using standard culture media.

Potomac fever Disease caused by a rickettsia (Ehrlichia equi), with acute projectile diarrhea, laminitis, and usually death its means of spread from animal to animal has not been determined.

Poult A turkey chick.

Poultry Domesticated birds typically including chickens, turkeys, ducks, geese. Occasionally ratites will be classed with poultry.

Poultry grower Farmer that raises poultry.

Poultry Term for all the different birds that are raised on farms. Examples turkeys, ducks, geese, and chickens.

Povidine iodine Betadine. A topical antibaterial available as a shampoo or in solution.

Ppb Parts per billion. It equals micrograms per kilogram or microliters per liter.

Ppm Parts per million. It equals milligrams per kilogram or milliliters per liter.

Pre anesthetic A drug given before general anesthesia; usually a sedative or tranquilizer which is given to reduce apprehension and to allow the use of lower doses of the more potent anesthetic agents.

Pre breeding evaluation Examination of potential breeding animals to assess their capability to produce offspring.

Pre emptive analgesia Refers to the prophylactic administration of analgesics to reduce the requirements for pain medication. Administration of an analgesic before an injury or surgery, lessens the amount of analgesic (or anesthetic) required later on.

Pre erythrocytic Prior to entering red blood cells.

Pre ictal The period prior to the start of the seizure. Sometimes called aura. Some of the signs are restlessness, nervousness, whining, trembling, salivation, affection, wandering, hiding, hysterical running and apprehension.

Precaution A condition in a recipient, which may result in a life-threatening problem if the vaccine is given, or a condition, which could compromise the ability of the vaccine to produce immunity.

Predator One animal that hunts another for food.

Predicted Producing Ability (PPA) An estimation of the amount of milk and/or components that a cow will yield above or below herdmates based on the cow's pedigree information and performance, if available.

Predicted Transmitting Ability (PTA) An estimation of an animal's potential to transmit yield productivity to its offspring based on pedigree information and the animal's performance, if available.

Predicted transmitting ability PTA Genetic merit of parent transmitted to its progeny.

Preemptive analgesia The administration of analgesic drugs before the onset of a painful stimulus, administered to reduce the perception of pain.

Prefix The cattery name at the beginning of the cat's name, indicating the breeder's cattery. For example, in the name "CH Sheenah's Ashley of Ashmanor, DM" the prefix is "Sheenah's" ("CH" is a title).

Pregnancy Toxemia A metabolic disease of pregnant does generally caused by diet deficient in energy during late pregnancy.

Preliminary milking The first milking of a three-milking verification test for herds milked twice daily.

Premature calving Termination of pregnancy during the last trimester.

Premiership The premiership class at a North American show is open to altered adult cats that are purebred and registered and meet the standard for their breed. In some associations, this class is called the "alter class."

Pre Milking Teat Dip A product applied in preparation for milking to clean the teat and reduce the spread of disease and maintain healthy teats.

Premix A uniform mixture of one or more microingredients and a carrier, used to facilitate uniform dispersion of micronutrients into a larger mixture.

Premolars The teeth that are located in front of the molars.

Preosseous Tissue that is at an intermediate stage between undifferentiated connective tissue and bone.

Prepartum Occurring before birth of the offspring.

Prepotent A cat who has such a strong genetic influence on its offspring that the offspring consistently resemble the parent. Most prepotent cats are linebred on one or more outstanding ancestors.

Prepotent Designating an animal that transmits its own character to its progeny to a marked or highly uniform degree.

Prepotent The ability of a parent to pass traits to it's progeny so that they resemble the parent more than usual. Inbred sheep are usually more prepotent than outbred sheep because more homozygous gene pairs are present.

Prepuce The tissue that covers the penis. Sometimes called the sheath.

Prerenal azotemia An increase in nitrogen containing waste products in the blood caused by reduced renal blood flow as a consequence of hypovolemia or dehydration. Untreated prerenal azotemia can progress to intrinsic renal disease.

Prerenal azotemia An increase in nitrogen containing waste products in the blood caused by reduced renal blood flow as a consequence of hypovolemia or dehydration. Untreated prerenal azotemia can progress to intrinsic renal disease.

Prescribing practices The behavior of licensed medical or veterinary practitioners regarding their prescription of medicines, including such aspects as high or low propensity to prescribe such medicines, and procedural aspects such as readiness to delegate to non-medically-qualified staff decisions on repeat prescriptions and other routine demands.

Prescription Drugs Drugs that the FDA has determined must be used only under the direction and supervision of a licensed veterinarian.

Prescription-only medicines Medicines that are only legally available to the "end user" if he/she obtains a prescription from a licensed professional (e.g. veterinarian, Medical doctor, dentist).

Presence Personality, charisma. A proud carriage and alert attitude that causes the individual to stand out in the crowd.

Prevalence The proportion of sampled animals that display a condition of interest at a given point in time. It is a single measurement of each animal in a group. It is usually a static measure in which the time is short (1-7 days).

Prey An animal that is taken by a predator as food.

Primal cuts Also called wholesale cuts. The original cuts resulting from the first division of the fore and hindsaddle of lamb or mutton.

Primaries 9-10 or more outermost flight feathers, attached to hand.

Primary abnormality Morphologic abnormalities of sperm that occur while the sperm are being produced in the testes.

Primary closure Suturing the raw edges of the wound together.

Primary Epilepsy See Idiopathic Epilepsy. Also known as genetic, inherited or true epilepsy.

Primary oocyte The form of an ova which has not released the first polar body and is inpenetrable by spermatozoa.

Primary uterine inertia Ineffective or absent uterine contractions during parturition. Primary uterine inertia should be considered when a bitch is not able to start uterine contractions. This condition occurs most often in older bitches and/or bitches with hypocalemia and/or hypoglycemia.

Primary waste treatment Usually, the initial treatment of waste water to reduce pollution potential or health hazard. With animal manure an example would be liquid-solid separation.

Prime boost Administration of one type of vaccine, such as a live-vector vaccine, followed by or together with a second type of vaccine, such as a recombinant subunit vaccine. The intent of this combination regimen is to induce different types of immune responses and enhance the overall immune response, a result that may not occur if only one type of vaccine were to be given for all doses.

Priming Giving one vaccine dose(s) first to induce certain immune responses, followed by or together with a second type of vaccine. The intent of priming is to induce certain immune responses that will be enhances by the booster dose(s).

Prions Proteinaceous infectious particles associated with transmissible neurodegenerative diseases of humans and animals.

Private veterinary surgeon A veterinary surgeon who is "in practice" – in other words, who is available to be consulted by the general public for a fee.

Probiotics A live microbial feed supplement which beneficially affects the host animal. Claims include reduced early mortality, increased growth rate, improved feed conversion, egg quality and animal health.

Problem A problem is anything that interferes with the patient's well being and requires further management or evaluation.

Problem list A list of what is wrong with a patient based on the information that is gathered from history, physical examination and the results of disgnostic tests.

Problem oriented medical records POMR The POMR system is a logical system centered around the identification and resolution of the patient's problems. The problem oriented approach differs from other approaches in which a list of differential diagnoses are generated in the exam room, without giving much consideration to the possibility that not all the patient's problems are due to the same cause. Although the problem based approach is also intended to lead to a diagnosis, the problem based approach prevents the clinician from "jumping to a diagnosis" with tunnel vision and potentially overlooking important aspects of the patients disease(s).

Problem specific data base The minimum amount of information that is planned to be collected for patients with specific types of problems. For example, a chest radiograph may be recommened to be preformed on all patients that were hit by a car.

Procerus The procerus is a muscle in the human nose.

Prodrome The period (hours to days) before a seizure. Extra AEDs given during this period might help reduce the severity of the seizure or eliminate it.

Produce A female's offspring The produce of dam commonly refers to two offspring of one dam.

Producer settlement fund (equalization fund) A fund maintained by the market administrator into which some processors pay money, because they use above average proportions of milk as Class I, and from which other processors receive money, because they use below average proportions of milk as Class I. This fund is used in conjunction with a marketwide pool.

Production and type index (PTI) Combines genetic merit measurements for production and type in a ratio thus ranking sires on their ability to transmit a balance of these traits.

Production I.E. production Rhode Island Red would be a bird that has many characteristics of a Standard Rhode Island Red, but is bred for utility purposes and is not appropriate for poultry shows or 4-H showing.

Production report The computer report of production and management data which is returned to the dairy producer 5 to 7 days following the test day and after component sampling is completed at the laboratory. The records are processed at one of the DRPC's.

Proestrus Proestrus is the beginning of the bitch's 'season'. The owner notices spotting or bleeding from the bitch's vagina. The stage of the estrous cycle of the bitch during which she attracts males but will not allow the male to breed her.

Professional The definition varies among associations but most term professional the following activities of a person over eighteen being paid for riding, driving, or showing at halter; for training or boarding; for instructing; for conducting seminars or clinics; in some situations for being employed as a groom or farrier; for use of name or photo in connection with advertisement; for accepting prize money in classes.

Profiles A set of information about a disease, arranged under a series of standard headings, and intended to be held on a computer database.

Progenitor cells A cell that, upon dividing, gives rise to a particular type of cell, for example, oligodendrocyte progenitor cells give rise to oligodendrocytes.

progeny Offspring.

Progeny testing Evaluating the genotype of an individual by a study of its offspring. An evaluation of the transmitting ability of an individual based on the performance of offspring.

Progeny Testing The evaluation of an individual's genotype using the performance records of it's progeny.

Progesterone The hormone produced by the corpus luteum, which helps to maintain pregnancy and control the estrus cycle.

Prognosis The chances of an animal having a normal quality of life following a disease or problem. This is reported using the words poor, fair, good, or excellent.

Progress notes A written description in a patient record that summarizes data; plans; treatment; rationelle for diagnostics and treatments; and the patient response to treatment.

Progressive retinal atrophy, PRA Any of a number of inherited diseases of the eye leading to blindness. Generally starts with difficulty seeing in the dark followed by a loss of vision in the daylight. In the BMD it is an autosomal recessive trait.

Projected 305-day lactation A calculation for predicting a cow's total yield in 305 days based on the information from a lactation in progress.

Prolactin Hormone secreted by the pituitary gland that stimulates the growth of mammary tissue and the production of milk.

Prolapse An interior organ pushing outside of the body.

Prolapsed rectum Because of irritation or injury, the inner part of the rectum is pushed out so that it is visible as a pink mass protruding from the anal opening.

Prolapsed uterus A condition in which the uterus is partially or completely turned inside out, outside the animal's body, usually following parturition.

Prolific Tendency to produce many offspring.

Prolificacy (fecundity) The number of offspring actually produced by a female.

Prop In timed events, a pole or barrel.

Prophase Prophase is the 1st stage in mitosis cell reproduction. The nucleolus disappears and a number of chromosomes become apparent.

Prophylactic use The administration of an antimicrobial to healthy animals prior to an unexpected exposure to an infectious agent or, following such an exposure prior to onset of laboratory-confirmed clinical disease. Generally such usage is in a herd or flock situation and not an individual animal.

Prophylaxis Prevention of disease.

Proprietary handler A milk processing company owned privately or publically by investors other than milk producers. The business differs from a cooperative.

Proprioception Maintenance of posture and movement through stimuli originating in the receptors in the joints, tendons, muscles, and labyrinth.

Proptosis Bulging of the eye out of the socket.

Prostaglandin analogs DRugs used in the treatment of glaucoma. They cause extreme miosis and may have an influence on the unconventional outflow of aqueous. Lantoprost (trade name Xalatan) is available as a 0.005% topical solution.

Prostaglandin F2 alpha A hormone that destroys the corpus luteum which in turn causes progesterone to decrease.

Prostaglandin Several types of chemicals made by cells which have specific functions such as controlling body temperature, stimulating smooth muscle, and influencing heat cycles.

Prostaglandins A type of fatty acid that is made from the enzymatic breakdown of cell membranes that perform a variety of hormone-like actions (as in controlling blood pressure or smooth muscle contraction).

Prostate A gland in the male reproductive system that lies just below the bladder and surrounds part of the canal that empties the bladder.

Prosthesis An artificial eye placed after enucleation for cosmetic purposes.

Protease Enzyme which breaks down protein.

Protected fat A fat that has been treated or combined with another substance to prevent breakdown in the rumen.

Proteins Any of numerous naturally occurring, extremely complex substances that consist of amino-acid residues joined by peptide bonds. Proteins include many essential biological compounds (as enzymes, morphogens, growth factors, structural proteins, hormones, or immunoglobulins).

Protein equivalent A term indicating the total nitrogen content of a substance in comparison with the nitrogen content of protein (usually plant). For example, the nonprotein nitrogen (NPN) compound, urea, contains approximately 45 percent nitrogen and has a protein equivalent of 281 percent (6.25 x 45 percent).

Protein nitrogen units PNU Unit of stength for antigens used in intradermal skin testing. 100,000 PNU - 1 mg protein.

Protein Supplement Feedstuff that contain a high level of protein. Fed to animals in addition to their base diet.

Proteoglycans Any of a class of high molecular weight protein-sugar polymers that are found especially in the extracellular matrix of connective tissue.

Prothrombin time PT Measurement of clotting time of plasma in the presence of excess tissue thromboplastin. Factors measured are fibrinogen, prothrombin, and factors V, VII, and X.

Protocol The detailed plan for a clinical trial that states the trial's rationale, purpose, vaccine dosages, routes of administration, length of study, eligibility criteria and other aspects of trial design.

Protozoa Single-celled microscopic animals.

Protozoans Single-celled animals invisible to the naked eye. Most are free living and a few are parasites in animals or man.

Proud flesh Excessive granulation tissue, seen especially on wounds on horse's lower legs that are allowed to heal themselves.

Proven sire A bull whose genetic transmitting ability has been measured by comparing the milk production performance of his daughters with that of the daughter's dam and/or herdmates under similar conditions. Plus-proven sires are those whose daughters exceeded their dams and/or herdmates in milk production.

Proximal A structure that is nearer the main body. For example, the three bones in the foot are designated by the terms proximal, middle, and distal depending on their location relative to the main body.

Proximate analysis Tests for nitrogen (crude protein), crude fiber, ether extract (lipids), and ash which, with nitrogen-free extract, represent the gross composition of feed.

Prudent use of antimicrobials Usage of antimicrobials, which maximizes therapeutic effect and minimizes the development of antimicrobial resistance.

PSA antigen A glycoprotein found in normal seminal fluid and produced by the prostatic epithelial cells. Elevated levels in blood serum are associated with prostatic enlargement and prostatic adenocarcinoma, and this allows detection of cancer in many cases.

Pseudohyperparathyroidism Pseudohyperparathyroidism causes hypercalcemia and most commonly occurs in patients with lymphoma or tumors of the apocrine anal sac. Pseudohyperparathyroidism has been reported associated with other tumor types.

Pseudomycetomas Deep dermal or subcutaneous infections by dermatophytes. They present as nodules and draining lesions, that histologically are pyogranulomatous to granulomatous panniculitis. M. canis is the causative organism in the cat.

Pseudopregnancy Giving the appearance of being pregnant when not really pregnant. Signs may include weight gain, enlarged abdomen, mammary gland enlargement, and nesting behavior. Pseudopregnancy is considered a normal occurrence in the bitch.

Psittacine Birds that belong to the order Psittaciformes. Common psittacines include budgies, cockatiels, lories, cockatoos, conures, amazons, African greys, lovebirds, senegals, and jardines.

Psychrophilic Cold loving It refers to microorganisms that grow best at refrigerated temperatures, that is, 4 to 15øC.

Psychrotrophic Cold tolerant It refers to microorganisms that grow at low temperatures, 4 to 15øC., but may have an optimum temperature above this range. These organisms especially affect the shelf life of refrigerated dairy products such as cottage cheese.

Psyllium The ground up seeds of the plant Plantago psyllium are rich in fiber and are used as a safe, gentle, bulk-forming laxative. It is used to treat both constipation and diarrhea because the herb absorbs excess fluid in the bowel and increases stool volume.

PTA See predicted transmitting ability.

Pteryla Feather tract.

Pterylae Plural of pteryla.

Puarter Usually refers to the portion of the wall of the hoof such as inside rear quarter, inside front quarter, outside rear quarter, etc.

Puberty When an animal becomes sexually mature.

Pullet A female chicken (sometimes applied to other species) under 1 year of age.

Pulmonary arteries The large vessels leading from the heart to the lungs.

Pulmonary Artery The pulmonary artery opens out of the right ventricle in the human heart and conveys venous blood to the lungs for collecting oxygen.

Pulmonary edema Fluid accumulation in the lungs.

Pulmonary emboli Pulmonary embolism: Blood clot that travels to the blood vessels in the lung and obstrucis them.

Pulmonary Relating to the lungs.

Pulse Heart rate. Normal adult resting heart rate varies among horses but is usually 40 beats per minute.

Pulseless electrical activity PEA A new term for electrical-mechanical disassociation in which an ECG shows electrical activity of the heart but there is no associated mechanical activity (heartbeat).

Punctum Holes in the edges of the eyelids through which tears enter the nasolacrimal ducts.

Pupa A dormant form of an insect (plural pupae). A larva spins a cocoon to protect itself, and becomes a pupa. The pupa does not feed, but gradually changes form and becomes a new adult.

Pupae The stage of development between the bot egg and the bot fly.

Pupillary light response PLR The ability of the pupil to constrict in response to light.

Purebred A cat whose ancestors are all of the same breed, or whose ancestry includes crossbreeding that is allowed in the breed standard. For example, a purebred Bombay may also have Burmese cats in its background.

Purebred Dairy Cattle Association (PDCA) An organization made up of members of the six purebred dairy cattle registry associations: Ayrshire, Brown Swiss, Guernsey, Holstein, Jersey and Milking Shorthorn.

Purebred The offspring of purebred parents of the same breed. Ancestors of purebreds can be traced to foundation stock in the original herdbook. An animal with two registered parents of the same breed. Purebreds are not all registered.

Purulent A term describing pus-like discharge or infection.

Pus A liquid product of inflammation consisting of leukocytes, lymph, bacteria, deadtissue cells, and fluid derived from their decomposition.

Pustule Small elevated area on the skin filled with pus.

Put down To euthanize.

Pyelonephritis Inflammation of the kidney, beginning at the "pelvis." (The pelvis is the enlarged hollow area inside the kidney where urine pools before entering the ureter.) Pyelonephritis is generally due to a bacterial infection.

Pyloroduodenal An obstruction in the area where the stomach and small intestine meet.

Pyoderma Skin infection with bacteria. Pyodermas involve coagulase positive bacteria, most commonly Staphylococcus intermedius.

Pyometra Pyometra is infection of the uterus that occurs during diestrus, 3-6 weeks after ovulation. It is commonly seen in bitches older than 5 years. Pyometra is also referred to as cystic endometrial hyperplasia (CEH) which is the term descriptive of the morphological changes occurring in the uterus. Hormones, primarily progesterone which is secreted from the corpus lutei (CLs) of the ovaries during diestrus stimulate CEH.

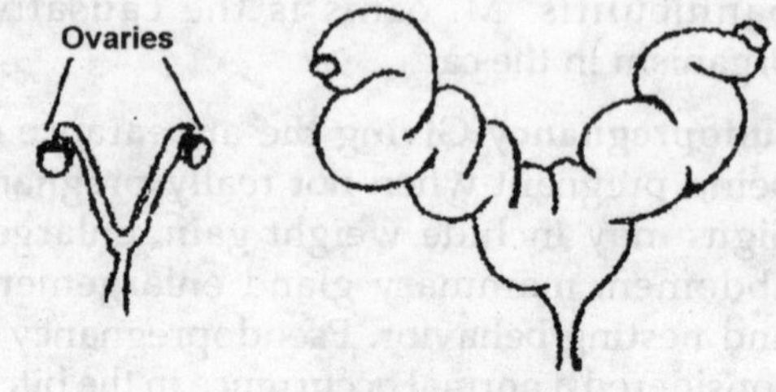

Fig. Pyometra

Pyrexia Elevated temperature, fever.

Pyridoxal A form of vitamin B_6. Pyridoxal phosphate is a major coenzyme involved in amino acid metabolism.

Pyridoxamine One of the three active forms of vitamin B_6. Pyridoxamine phosphate is a coenzyme involved in amino acid metabolism

Pyridoxine One of the forms of vitamin B_6.

Pyriproxyfen An insect growth regulator. Available combined with permethrin in a spray for use on adult dogs and a fogger or spray for household treatment (Knockout: Virbac).

Pyuria White blood cells in the urine.

Q

Qi Qi is an idea of the smooth interaction of the rhythmic patterns or biorhythms within the body.

Qigong A Chinese discipline which emphasizes breathing, meditation, stationary and moving exercises to enhance the flow of chi.

Quadrate Bone The Quadrate Bone is a bone developed in reptiles and birds by means of which the lower jaw is articulated to the skull.

Qualitative Traits Traits which show a sharp distinction between phenotypes. For example, polled and horned. Usually only one or few gene pairs are involved.

Quality Overall degree of merit flat bone and clean joints, refined features and fine`skin and hair coat.

Quantitative Traits Traits that do not show a sharp distinction between phenotypes. There is a gradual variation from one phenotype to another, for example, birth weight. Usually, environmental effects as well as many gene pairs are involved.

Quarantine To confine and keep an animal from contacting other animals or people. This is essential to stop the spread of infectious diseases that are potentially transmissible to other animals or humans.

Quarter crack A split starting at the lower edge of the hoof and running up to the coronet.

Queen A female cat. When used as a verb, "to queen" describes a cat giving birth.

Queening The birthing process (parturition) in a cat.

Quick Mix A pre-made solution used in partial parenteral solution.

Quick The vein running through a dog's claw.

Quidding Spitting out pieces of partially chewed hay.

Quirt A riding whip with a short handle and a rawhide lash.

Quittor Infection of the lateral cartilage of the hoof.

R

Rabies A fatal virus disease of warm blooded animals including man, that affects the brain and is spread in the saliva of infected animals. Rabid animals have a temperament change. Wild creatures become bold enough to attack human beings, and docile domestic animals may turn on their owners.

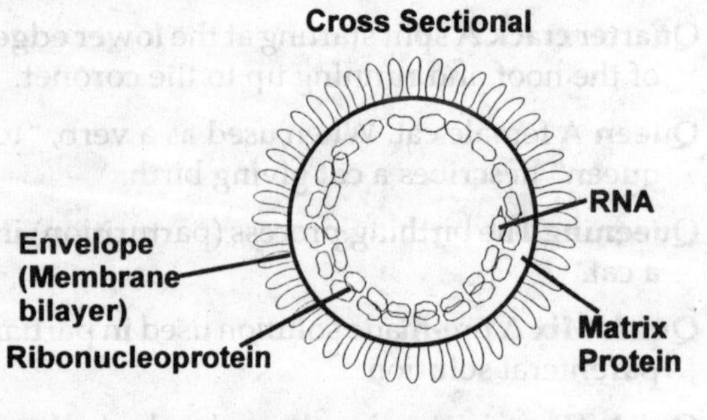

Fig. Rabies Virus

Race sulky Light two-wheeled vehicle used in Standardbred racing.

Rack Racking in the world today includes both the slow rack, and the fast rack. The gaits used are the rack and the stepping pace. In both the rear of the horse provides the most of the forward motion and support while the front end does little pulling. Both have an even four beat cadence without any head shake. In the slow rack the feet are picked up one foot at a time with the front end moving up and down with little forward extension. The fast rack or stepping pace is performed by picking up the feet like a pace, but holding the front foot up for an extra half step. The front feet are picked up and held in the up position for a split second then lowered as the other front foot is picked up meeting at a point near knee high. This means the front end is not supported at all some of the time. However, the horse gives a very smooth ride because the rear foot is up under the horse far enough to support its center of gravity at that moment. A horse doing a fast rack will seem low in the rear because of the extra reach under the horse.

Racy Tall, of comparatively slight build.

Raddle Paint or crayon applied to a ram's chest to mark females he mates.

Radial Iimmunodiffusion RID A test used to evaluate whether the newborn has received antibodies in colostrum.

Radio allergosorbent test RAST Test to measure specific serum IgE levels.

Radiograph The image generated by an x-ray. Often the term x-ray is used incorrectly to refer to a radiograph.

Radioimmunoassay A method to measure the amount of a substance using an antibody against the substance for specificity and a radioactive label for detection and measurement.

Radiology X-ray.

Radius The radius is one of the two long bones which form the human lower arm.

Ragged Muscles appear ragged rather than smooth.

Rail The fenceline, as in a "rail" class.. Also, Western term for a flat class.

Ram A male sheep of any age. Sometimes a ram may be called a buck.

Rambouillet A large bodied Merino sheep developed under French Government care from animals imported from Spain in 1786. Hardy sheep yielding good mutton and fine quality wool.

Ramp up A period of time during which effective blood levels of a drug are building up.

Rams (bucks) Male sheep which are part of the breeding herd for raising lambs.

Random Mating A mating system where all ewes have the same chance of being mated to any ram used.

Randomized trial A study in which participants are assigned by chance to one of two or more intervention arms or regimens. Randomization minimizes the differences among groups by equally distributing people with particular characteristics among all the trial arms.

Range fed Chickens that are allowed to graze freely.

Rangy Tall, long in body, high on leg, light-framed; gangly.

Rapid Analysis and Detection of Animal related Risks RADAR is a new information management system which collects veterinary surveillance data from many different sources around the UK and makes sure they can be used together. It will make it possible to analyse this information and publish reports highlighting threats to public health and animal health and welfare, the risks they pose and the areas at risk.

Rapid Exit Panels or rails that raise to release all cows on one side of the milking parlor at once.

Raptorial Feet with long, strong toes and long, sharp, curved claws.

Rat Tail The root thick and covered with soft curls; at the tip devoid of hair, or having the appearance of being clipped.

Rate of Genetic Improvement Depends on:

1. Number of traits being selected at one time
2. Heritability of the traits
3. Genetic correlations between the traits selected
4. Selection differentials
5. Generation interval in the flock. The rate of improvement is usually expressed per year.

Rate of passage The time taken by undigested residues from a given meal to reach the feces.

Rating Means of classifying the size of a show, sometimes done beforehand according to prizes offered, and sometimes after according to number of entries.

Ration The food allowed an animal for 24 hours. See balanced ration.

Ratite The family of birds including Ostriches, Emus ad Rheas.

Raw milk Fresh, unprocessed milk as it comes from a cow, goat, or other mammal.

Reabsorb Possible absorption of an early embryo back into the mare's system.

Reach of Front Length of forward stride taken by forelegs.

Reactogenicity The capacity of a vaccine to produce adverse reactions.

Reagent Any chemical used in a laboratory test or experiment.

Reagent grade A compound with the purity and quality that allows it to be used in a laboratory.

Rear Pastern The metatarsus; the region of the hindquarters between the hock and the foot.

Rearing A bad habit in a horse, of raising up on his hind legs when he is being led or ridden. An extremely dangerous habit that should be dealt with by a professional only.

Reata A braided leather rope; coiled and fastened to a Western saddle.

Recalcitrant In plant nutrition, refers to that portion of a nutrient in the soil that is unavailable for biochemical activity or plant uptake.

Receptive The female is accepting of being mounted and bred by a male.

Receptivity When the female starts becoming receptive to the male and is ready to breed.

Receptor A molecule on the surface of a cell that serves as a recognition or binding site for antigens, antibodies or other cellular or immunology components.

Receptor Signaling The process in which the binding of signaling molecules to cell surface receptors leads to activation of particular proteins that turn-on and turn-off genes.

Receptor Trafficking The movement of receptors from one part of the cell to another (often associated with receptor activation at the cell surface and/or degradation within the cell.)

Recessive Genes Recessive genes only affect the phenotype when present in a homozygous condition. Therefore, the recessive gene must be received from both parents before the recessive phenotype will be observed.

Recombinant DNA technology The technique by which genetic material from one organism is inserted into a foreign cell in order to mass-produce the protein encoded by the inserted genes.

Recombinant vaccine There are certain antigens on viruses and bacteria which are better at stimulating an antibody response by the animal than others. The genes for these antigens can be isolated, and made to produce large quantities of the antigens they code for. A recombinant vaccine contains these antigens, not the whole organism. Compare with 'modified live vaccine' and 'killed vaccine.'

Recombinant-Genetically Engineered A term used to describe the manufacture of a protein by "genetic engineering"; usually by using a cloned gene as a template for making a specific protein.

Reconstituted milks The product resulting from the mixing together and rehydration of a dried product of milk with water. For example, NDM and water yield reconstituted skim milk.

Record (2x, 305-day, ME) Estimates how much the cow would have produced during the present lactation when milked twice daily in the first 305 days of her lactation if she had been a mature cow calving in an average month.

Record in progress (RIP) A cow's production from her calving date until the most recent test day.

Record plan Specific DHI program that provides a particular service to dairy farmers. The plans are either official or unofficial according to rules of the program.

Rectal prolapse When a portion of the rectum protrudes past the anus.

Rectrices Plural of rectrix.

Rectrix Tail feather.

Rectum The rectum is the lowest portion of the large intestine, terminating at the anus.

Rectus muscles There are 4 rectus muscles that allow for movement of the globe: dorsal, ventral, lateral, and medial.

Recumbency Lying down.

Recurved Curved upward toward tip.

Recycle To extract and reuse substances found in human and natural products.

Red A reddish orange color of dog.

Red roan A mixture of red and white hairs all over a horse's body, with red, black, or flaxen mane and tail. Also called strawberry roan.

Red Sesame Red with a sparse black overlay (Shiba Inu). Color definitions may vary by breed. Always check the breed standard for the definitive color description.

Red The color also known as "orange," "ginger," or "marmalade."

Redefined A problem is redefined if a more specific lable can be applied. For example vomiting is redefined or updated to acute pancreatitis as laboratory results become available that support the diagnosis of pancreatitis.

Redefined problem A patient's problem is redefined if it is updated to a higher level..for example, vomiting may be updated to uremia as the results of diagnostic tests become available and show an elevated BUN.

Refinement Quality appearance, indicating good breeding.

Reflex ovulator Only ovulating after being bred. Cats are reflex ovulators, dogs are not.

Reflexology A system of therapy which involves manipulation of specific areas of the feet. Different regions of the feet are believed to correspond to particular body systems. It is believed that stimulation of these areas can eliminate energy blockage which produces disease in the associated organs.

Region A geographic area that makes up some of the territory of an association. Each region typically has its own regional director, awards its own year-end regional awards, and may operate under slightly different rules. For example, CFA has nine regions seven in the US, one in Japan, and one in Europe.

Regional award An award given to cats that earn enough points during a show year to be ranked among the highest scoring cats in the region for that year. Some associations add a title to the registered name of each regional award winner. The number of high scoring cats receiving regional awards depends on the association and the competitive class (e.g. Kitten, premiership; championship, household pet, etc.). For example, CFA gives regional awards to the top 25 cats in Championship in each region.

Register The act of enlisting a dog, puppy or litter with a dog association.

Registered A horse of purebred parents that have numbered certificates with a particular breed organization.

Registered cat A cat whose ancestry is documented and recorded with a cat registering association.

Registered cow Cow that has a pedigree and is registered at the Breed Association. There are 6 major dairy breeds within associations: Ayrshire, Brown Swiss, Guernsey, Holstein, Jersey, and Milking Shorthorn.

Registered name The official name of a registered cat. This name is often quite long, and may include one or more titles and cattery names.

Registered Purebred animal registered in the herdbook of the proper breed association. Certain associations (for example, the Red and White association) will register non-purebred cattle providing they satisfy certain other criteria.

Registration (Licensing, Authorization, Approval) The process of approving a drug for marketing in a country/region. Includes assessment using particularly the criteria of safety, quality, and efficacy. As a consequence of inadequate local capacity many developing countries rely on "third party certification", i.e. granting market authorization to products approved in certain developed countries.

Registration certificate Proof that the parentage of an animal is known and is recorded in the Breed Registry Herdbook.

Registration Papers Documents showing proof of registration, date of birth, parents, breeder and owner issued by a dog association for a particular dog.

Registries Organizations that keep official records on specific subjects. With respect to dogs, there are registries of purebred dogs for tracking lineage and health registries for rating certain health conditions (e.g., Canine Eye Registry Foundation, Orthopedic Foundation for Animals, etc.).

Regression or remission In relation to cancer, regression refers generally to the shrinking of a tumor by other than surgical means. A complete regression occurs when a tumor that was at one time measurable disappears completely. Partial regression describes the condition where the measurable tumor is reduced by at least 50 percent in size.

Regulation Using insulin to maintain the blood glucose level of an animal within the acceptable range.

Regulatory authority A government agency responsible for codifying and enforcing rules and regulations as mandated by law.

Regurgitate To cast up undigested food from the stomach to the mouth, as done by ruminants.

Regurgitation Backward movement of food from the esophagus out the mouth.

Rehydrate The addition of body fluids which have been lost from fever, illness, heat, etc.

Rehydration solution A solution administered to a dehydrated animal to return it's hydration state to normal. Most dehydrated dogs and cats have isotonic dehydration and are rehydrated with iostonic, iso-ionic solutions such as LRS or RS.

Rein The long strap that passes from the bit to the riders hands, by which the rider maintains control of the horse.

Rein-back To back up; a two-beat diagonal gait in reverse.

Relaxin A hormone which is detectable when a fertilized egg is implanted, which usually occurs around day 21 following fertilization. Marketed as ReproCHEK by Synbiotics.

Reliability (REL) The term used in dairy cattle breeding to indicate the precision with which genetic merit is estimated. Reliability, then, is a confidence factor which increases with the

1. number of daughters,

2. number of herds in which daughters are located,

3. number of lactations per daughter, and

4. information of relatives used.

Remex Large flight feather.

Remiges Plural of remex.

Ren Renal.

Renal blood flow RBF The blood presented to the kidneys. The kidneys receive about 20 to 25% of cardiac output each minute. Renal blood flow is determined by blood volume, blood pressure and cardiac output. The kidneys can also autoregulate their blood flow within certain ranges of blood pressure.

Renal insufficiency The decreased ability of the kidneys to rid the body of wastes.

Renal Of, relating to, or in the region of the kidneys.

Rennet An extract of the stomach of certain mammals containing rennin. It is used in the coagulation of milk proteins in the manufacture of most cheeses.

Renvers Haunches-out. The opposite movement to travers, with the tail instead of the head to the wall.

Replacement A calf kept and/or raised at the dairy as a future replacement for a cow in the herd. Replacement rate should average between 25%-33% of the herd/year.

Replacement females New females that have recently been introduced to a herd.

Replacements Heifers Often ones being raised to replace the cows currently in the herd.

Reproductive cycle Events that happen in the female such as ovulation, hormone production, receptivity, etc. In camelids the cycle does not follow regular time periods as it does in horses or cattle.

Rescue Remedy A homeopathic remedy from Bach Flower Essences (available at most Health Food Stores) that can help lessen the effects during the post-ictal or the actual seizure if given during the pre-ital period. No scientific studies have been done on this, however for many it DOES work .

Resection Surgical removal of tissue.

Reservoir Where a disease causing organism lives and multiplies. Therefore the reservoir may not be the source of the organism, that is only where it lives and multiplies.

Reservoirs of the contagious mastitis The cow herself, humans, flies, and other.

Residual Seizure Disorder (RSD) See seizures.

Resistance A term used to describe bacteria which have mutated or changed so they are not affected by an antibiotic that previously killed them or slowed their growth. As more bacteria become resistant to various antibiotics, there are fewer antibiotics which will have an effect on them, thus newer and stronger antibiotics will need to be developed. Inappropriate use of antibiotics (using them too often, for too short a duration or in insufficient dose) may promote the development of resistance.

Resolved problem A patient's problem is resolved if it no longer exists either due to the intervention of the veterinarian or Mother Nature's.

Resolved Problems are resolved if they no longer exist either because they were treated or reolved spontaneously with the passing of time.

Resorption In pregnancy, a condition in which the fetus dies, and instead of being aborted, the fetal tissue dissolves within the uterus and is absorbed by the mother. The mother will show no outward signs of a fetal resorption.

Resources The goods and services that ecosystems provide, especially for humans.

Respiration Normal adult respiration rate varies among horses but is usually twelve to fifteen breaths per minute. One breath consists of an inhalation and an exhalation.

Respiratory depression Decrease in the rate or depth of respiration.

Respiratory Relating to breathing or the lungs.

Respiratory transmission The most common route of human exposure in countries where infection is controlled in animals and where there is pasteurization of milk.

Resting membrane potential RMP The electrical charge of resting myocardial cells. Normally the RMP is -90 mV. Hyperkalemia elevates the RMP to a less negative state.

Resuscitative fluid A fluid used in cardiopulmonary resuscitation (CPR) in an attempt to restore circulation.

Retained placenta Placental membranes not expelled normally at parturition.

Reticular activating formation A collection of neurons in the brain that mediates many aspects of consciousness.

Reticulate With small netlike scales (tarsus).

Reticulo rumen Section of the ruminant gastrointestinal tract consisting of the reticulum and the rumen that is the primary site for microbial fermentation of feedstuffs.

Reticulum The second compartment of the ruminant stomach, also known as the second stomach. The lining has a honeycombed appearance to increase the surface are for absorption.

Retina The rear interior surface of the eyeball is called the retina. The retina contains nerve cells referred to as rods and cones. The rods are sensitive to light and the cones to color. The retina receives the light and color and converts them into nerve impulses which go to the brain.

Retinal dysplasia A congenital anomalous development of the retina.

Retinoids Synthetic derivatives of vitamin A.

Retractor bulbi muscle The muscle that pulls the eyeball back into the orbit.

Retrobulbar Located behind the globe.

Retropulsion Pushing on the orbit to evaluate the ability to compress the soft tissue structures behind the orbit.

Return Alley The alley through which cows must pass when moving from the milking parlor back to the cow housing area after milking.

Revolution Generic name is Selemectin.

Reye Syndrome Encephalopathy (general brain disorder) in children following an acute illness such as influenza or chickenpox. Symptoms include vomiting, agitation and lethargy. This condition may result in coma or death.

Rhamphotheca Horny covering of bill.

Rheumatoid factor An antibody that is usually found in the blood of adults who have rheumatoid arthritis is rarely present in children who have juvenile arthritis. Rheumatoid factor is more likely to occur in girls who have had many affected joints.

Rhino Short for rhinopneumonitis.

Rhinopneumonitis Herpes, a viral disease of horse causing respiratory problems ("snots") in young and abortion in pregnant mares.

Rib In anatomy, the ribs are elastic arches of bone which are connected behind with the vertebral column and form a large part of the skeleton of the thorax.

Riboflavin Also known as vitamin B_2. It is a component of FAD and FMN, which are coenzymes or prosthetic groups for certain enzymes that catalyse many oxidation-reduction reactions.

Rictal Referring to the corners of the mouth.

Ride To be transported in a mounted position, as one cow mounted on another during estrus.

Rigging On a saddle, straps that connect the cinch and the saddle tree.

Rigor Mortis The permanent contraction of skeletal muscle associated with death.

Ring An area at a show where one judge examines cats and awards prizes. A show may have several simultaneous rings.

Ring bone Arthritis of coffin joint and/or pastern joint causing excessive bone growth.

Ring Feeder A steel hoop with individual head gates that may be placed over a large round bale of hay when feeding it.

Ring sour A poor attitude in a horse who does not enjoy working in an arena and looks for ways to leave the arena or quit working.

Ring test A test for brucellosis performed by mixing stained Brucella bacteria with raw milk. If antibody to Brucella is present, the stained cells agglutinate (clump) and rise to the surface with the cream to form a blue ring.

Ringer's solution Ringer's solution does not contain lactate. It contains a higher concentration of chloride compared to lactated Ringer's solution. Ringer's solution is considered an acidifying solution. This does not mean that it can cause metabolic acidosis, but it can assist a patient who has a metabolic alkalosis correct their own acid base abnormality.

Ringworm A type of fungal infection of the skin.

Risk based evaluation Evaluation of scientific and other relevant information with the aim of obtaining a qualitative and/or quantitative estimation of the probability of occurrence and severity of known or potential adverse public health effects.

Risk The chances (or probability) of a hazard actually happening. Veterinary surveillance aims to find and use information to help us work out which are the most important risks. International disease surveillance tells us when and where there are outbreaks of diseases abroad. By using this information we can assess the risk to our animals from importing animals or animal products from other countries, or the chances of migrating wild birds introducing diseases.

RNA Any of various nucleic acids that contain ribose and uracil as structural components and are associated with the control of cellular chemical activities. RNAs may be intermediaries between DNA and proteins (as in messenger RNA) or may have specific structural or enzymatic activities as in ribosomal RNA, transfer RNA or inhibitory RNA.

Roached A mane or tail that has been clipped to the skin.

Roan A close mixture of red and white colors such as is often found in Milking Shorthorn cattle.

Roaring A breathing disorder.

Roaster A cockerel or pullet, usually weighing 4 to 6 pounds, suitable for cooking whole in the oven.

Robotic Parlor A completely automated system for milking cows that requires limited human contact.

Rolling Horse lying down and rolling over, may be normal or result of pain; possible sign of colic.

Rolling herd average (RHA) The average milk production per herd per year based on the 12 months just past. Upon completion of a new test record, the record for the same period of the previous year is deducted and the new record is added, then a new rolling 365-day average is calculated. RHA's are updated with each new test.

Rolling herd The most recent 12 month herd mild production average.

Romal A leather quirt, attached to braided leather or rawhide reins, or "closed" reins.

Rompun Brand of xylazine, an analgesic sedative mixture used as a painkiller, pre-anesthetic, etc.

Roost The place where chickens spend the night; the act of resting on a roost; also called "perch."

Rooster A male chicken (sometimes applied to other species) over 1 year of age.

Rope A running noose. To catch a cow with the noose.

Rose Hip Rose hips are the cherry-sized, bright red fruits that remain after the rose petals have fallen off. These contain vitamin C and flavonoids. The herb is used for colds and flu. Most of the vitamins may be lost if the herb is dried.

Rosemary An aromatic evergreen perennial which is used as a culinary spice and has many medicinal uses.

Rotary milking parlor A raised, round rotating platform or carousel on which cows ride while being milked.

Rotary Parlor A raised, round rotating platform or carousel on which cows ride while being milked.

Rotational Crossbreeding Systematic crossing of two or more breeds in which the crossbred ewes are mated to rams of the breed contributing the least genes to that ewe's phenotype.

Rotavirus A group of viruses that cause diarrhea in children.

Roughage Consists of pasture, silage, hay, or other dry fodder. It may be of high or low quality. Roughages are usually high in crude fiber (more than 18 percent) and relatively low in NFE (approximately 40 percent).

Route of administration The way a drug is administered to an animal; i.e. orally, intramuscularly, intravenously.

Route of infection The manner by which an infectious agent gains access to the animal.

Rowel A small wheel with points, attached to the shank of a spur.

Rubella Acute infectious disease resembling both scarlet fever and measles, but differing from these in its short course, slight fever, and freedom from sequelae. German measles.

Rubeola Measles. Acute contagious disease marked by fever, catarrhal symptoms, and a typical cutaneous eruption.

Rug Horse blanket, most times describing winter blankets.

Rugged When referring to an animal, it means large and strong.

Rule out R/O A possible cause for a patient's problem. Also called a differential diagnosis.

Rule outs R/O Rule-outs are also known as differential diagnoses and are possible causes for the problems displayed by a patient. For example, kidney failure is one rule out (or possible cause) for polyuria in a dog or cat.

Rumen The large fermentation compartment of the ruminant animal's stomach in which bacteria and protozoa break down fibrous plant material and other feedstuffs, and synthesize essential proteins and vitamins.

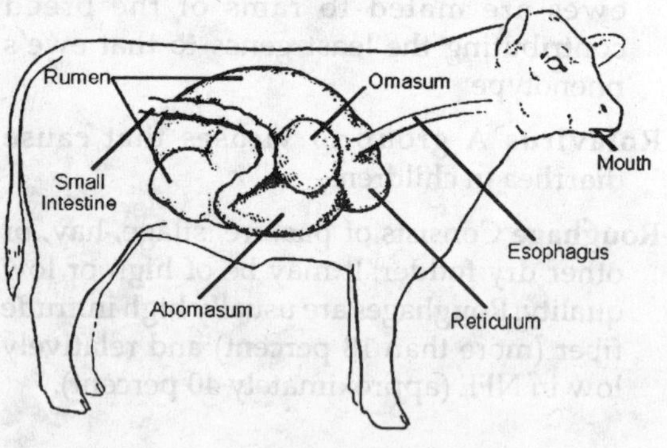

Fig. Rumen

Rumenocentesis (rumen tap) When rumen contents are collected by inserting a needle into the rumen.

Rumen reticulum Pregastric fermentation chamber that host a large microbial population.

Ruminant Animals having four stomach compartments rumen, reticulum, omasum and abomasums through which food passes in digestion. These animals chew their cud or regurgitate partially digested food for further breakdown in the mouth. Ruminant animals include cattle, sheep, goats, deer and camels.

Rumination The casting up or regurgitation of food (cud) to be chewed a second time, as cattle do; a chewing of the cud by ruminants.

Rump The area between the hip bones and the tail head.

Run A long, narrow fenced-in area usually attached to a stall.

Run on To graze or pasture on, as for cattle to run on the range.

Runners Leather loops which slide up and down and are used to keep the straps of a bridle in place.

Running walk Like the flat foot walk, the running is a four-beat gait in which each foot is picked up and set down in an even cadence. The rear end movement should be smooth and close to the ground without any snap or pop. Each stride should reach forward and slide in as it is set down, over striding the track of the front foot. The head shake is in time with the rear feet and should be smooth. The tail should set still and flow. The flat foot walk and the running walk have the same general movements and look alike in many ways. In a true flat foot walk at least one front foot is touching at all times, and as a flat foot walk is pushed faster, the front end of the horse will leave the ground for a split second each step. At that point it has become a running walk.

S

Sable Coat color produced by black-tipped hairs on a background of silver, gold, gray, fawn, or brown.

Sabouraud's dextrose agar The standard media for fungal culture.

Sacrum In human anatomy, the sacrum is the large triangular bone inserted like a wedge between the two hip bones. It is formed by the fusion of the five sacral vertebrae.

Saddle Back Overlong back, with a dip behind the withers.

Saddle Markings in the shape of a saddle over the back. Color definitions may vary by breed. Always check the breed standard for the definitive color description.

Safety (Sharps) Box A puncture proof/liquid proof container designed to hold used sharps during disposal and destruction.

Safety syringe Modified, disposable plastic syringe designed so that the healthcare worker can disable it is such a way that the needle is protected and cannot be re-used.

Saffron An expensive herb derived from the three tiny, orange stigmas within the flower of the plant Crocus sativus. To produce one ounce of saffron, it is necessary to harvest about 5,000 flowers.

SAGE Abbreviation for Serial Analysis of Gene Expression.

Sagittal Longitudinal view.

Sagittal suture The sagittal suture is the fissure running along the length of the top of the human skull dividing the parietal bone into two hemispheres.

Saint Bernard A breed of large strong dog developed in Switzerland, having a thick brown and white coat, originally used by monks of the hospice of Saint Bernard in the Swiss Alps to help patrol the snow-covered region.

Saline A saline solution, especially one that is isotonic with blood and is used in medicine and surgery.

Saliva Saliva is a secretion from the salivary glands in the oral cavity. It contains mucus to lubricate food and enzymes.

Salmonella A genus of bacteria in the family of enterobactreriaceae pathogenic to man and other animals. Several species exist causing various diseases such as typhoid, enteric fever, and food poisoning.

Salmonella DT104 An enteric bacteria that causes bloody diarrhea, has resistence genes in its genome, and is zoonotic.

SALT Serum alanine aminotransferase (SALT)or alanine aminotransferase (ALT). An enzyme found in hepatocytes (liver cells) released with cellular injury including cellular hypoxia.

Saluki An ancient breed of tall slender dog developed in Arabia and Egypt and having a smooth, silky, variously colored coat.

Samoyed A breed of medium-sized dog originally developed in northern Eurasia, having a thick, long, white or cream-colored coat.

Sample The normal meaning of a sample is a small quantity of blood, urine or other substance taken from an animal to test for a disease. However, it also has a special meaning in surveillance. We cannot usually study the whole of a given population, so we choose a certain number of animals, groups of animals, herds etc from the population. The ones we choose are known as the sample. So a survey for a disease in dairy cows may study all the animals in, say, 100 herds selected from all the dairy herds in the country: we say that we have studied a sample of 100 herds. In order for the results to be meaningful, it is important that the herds in the sample are selected so that they are truly representative of the dairy population as a whole.

Sand colic A digestive disorder that occurs when a horse eats sand or dirt with his feed.

Sand Separator A mechanical device or series of course ways used to settle sand from sand-laden manure.

Sandy Used to describe several breeds, this color is a dull, yellowish gray of medium saturation. Color definitions may vary by breed. Always check the breed standard for the definitive color description.

Sanitize To kill or remove injurious, microorganisms but not necessarily to sterilize. Dairy equipment is commonly sanitized with heat or chemicals.

Sanitizer A disinfectant of low toxicity used to reduce microbial contamination of food handling equipment.

SAP Serum alkaline phosphatase. Also known as AP. An enzyme found in many tissues but most often elevated in serum in response to cholestasis and bone remodeling and glucocorticoid excess.

Saprophytism Organisms survive and persist in non-living or decaying organic matter. They are not usually parasitic, although may cause disease under certain circumstances – e.g. Aspergillus fumigatus and bovine abortion (fungal abortion).

Sarcoid A tumor that occasionally occurs on the eyelids of horses.

Sarcoma A connective tissue neoplasm, usually highly malignant, formed by proliferation of mesodermal cells.

Sarcoplasmic Reticulum The specialized endoplasmic reticulum of cardiac muscle and skeletal striated muscle that functions especially as a storage and release area for calcium.

Sarcoptic mange Skin disease characterized by extreme itching, hair loss, and secondary infection. Usually widespread, but often seen on the belly and inner thighs. Can be treated, but spreads easily.

Satellite Cells A reserve cell population located in skeletal muscle fibers that is responsible for growth, healing, and regeneration of skeletal muscle.

Saturated fat A completely hydrogenated fat. Saturated fats are solid at room temperature. Example: animal tallow.

SAVMA Student American Veterinary Medical Association (a national group).

SC Abbreviation for subcutaneous.

Sc or sq See subcutaneous.

Scale Accumulation of loose fragments of the top layer of the skin.

Scales The small, hard, overlapping plates covering a chicken's shanks and toes.

Scan A process for the rapid isolation and functional characterization of tumor infiltrating and tumor associated T-cells.

Scanning surveillance All the work involved in keeping a continuous watch over the diseases which occur in animals. It includes inspections at markets and slaughterhouses, monitoring the diagnoses made by private vets and laboratories, and following up reports or information from farmers or the public. The main purpose is to detect anything unusual so that it can be investigated.

Scaphoid bone The scaphoid bone is one of the bones in the human wrist.

Scaphoid The scaphoid is a small bone in the human hand.

SCAVMA Student Chapter of the American Veterinary Medical Association (local group).

Schiff Scherrington posture A condition, caused by a lesion in the spinal cord, in which the front legs are held rigid and straight, and the rear legs are weak or paralyzed. Sometimes, the neck may be hyperextended, with the head held up and over the back.

Schiotz tonometer An indentation tonometer used to measure intraocular pressure based on how readily the cornea is "indented" Schiotz tonometer indentation tonometer - IOP is calculated from how readily the cornea is "indented"

Schirmer tear test A test of the ability to produce tears.

Schistosomiasis A parasitic disease due to infestation with blood flukes belonging to the genus Schistosoma, q.v. The disease is endemic throughout Asia, Africa and tropical America. Infestation occurs by wading or bathing in water containing cercariae that have issued from snails. SYN bilharziasis.

Schooling show Warm-up or practice show early in the season.

Schwann cells Neuronal insulation makers of the peripheral nervous system, myelin makers of the PNS

Sciatic The sciatic is a nerve in the leg.

SCID mice Severe combined immunodeficiency is an immune deficiency disease in which neither antibody nor T-cell responses are made. It is usually the result of T cell deficiencies. The SCID mutation causes severe combined immune deficiency.

Sclera The white part of the eye beneath the upper eyelid. The sclera normally has small blood vessels running across the surface.

Sclerosis A hardening of tissue, usually the result of chronic inflammation.

Sclerous tissue Sclerous tissue provides the stiffening which is essential for the formation of the general framework of the body. There are two varieties of sclerous tissue: cartilage and bone.

Score In roping, to break quickly to overtake the cow.

Scotch In reining, to anticipate a stop by slowing the gallop.

Scottish Agricultural College A higher education institution in Scotland which specialises in agriculture and other land-based industries. As well as education, it carries out research and provides services and advice. The Veterinary Science Division of SAC carries out post-mortem examinations, laboratory tests and on-farm investigations of disease problems.

Scours The discharge of more fluid than normal fecal matter from the bowel; often more frequently than normal.

Scratch. 1. The habit chickens have of scraping their claws against the ground to dig up tasty things to eat.

2. Any grain fed to chickens.

Scrape and Haul Manure handling system in which manure is scrape manually or with a skidloader, placed in a solid manure spreader and directly applied to appropriate crop land.

Screening Testing all or some of a population to check for evidence of a disease which may not otherwise be apparent.

Scrotal hernia The abnormal protrusion of part of an organ or tissue through the structures that normally contain it. An animal may be born with a hernia in which case it is congenital or it can get it can be acquired after birth.

Scrotum The purse or bag containing the testicles of a male animal.

Scrub An animal from nonpurebred parents not showing the predominant characteristics of any breed.

Scurs A rudimentary horn. A small rounded portion of horn tissue attached to the skin of the horn pit of a polled animal.

Scute In turtles and tortoises, the plates which cover the bony portion of the shell. In snakes, the larger, thicker scales on the underside of the body which provide support, protection, and traction.

Scutellate With large transversely oriented scales (tarsus).

Season A lay term used to refer to the beginning of proestrus.

Seasonally polyestrous Estrous cycles which are under the influence of light. The queen is a seasonally polyestrous animal.

Seat The part of the saddle where the rider sits, or the way a rider sits in a saddle.

Sebaceous adenitis Inflammation of a sebaceous (oil-producing) gland. In dogs, sebaceous glands are found on the top of the tail near its base, and at the junction of mucous membranes with skin. In cats, these glands are found on the chin, lip margins, and the top of the tail.

Sebaceous adenitis inflammation of the sebaceous glands (found at the base of hair follicles).

Sebaceous glands The sebaceous glands are ducts in the skin which secrete oil to lubricate the skin and hair.

Seborrhea Abnormal secretion of the sebaceous glands at the base of hair follicles causing anything from dandruff to greasy scales and crust.

Seborrhea, primary Metabolic seborrhea. Scaling caused by endocrine disorders, aberrations in lipid availability, nutritional imbalances.

Seborrhea, secondary Scaling due to allergies, ectoparasite infestation, mycotic infections, immune-mediated disease.

Sebum Formed of diester waxes, cholesterol and free fatty acids in sebaceous glands, which empty into the hair follicle or onto the skin.

Second cross Progeny resulting from the mating of true half-breeds and a distinct breed.

Second cuts The short portions of wool staples that result when the shearer makes two "blows" over the same area.

Second generation A description of medications developed from an earlier form of the medication. First generation medications were developed from the original form of the drug; second generation medications are adaptations of first generation drugs; third generation drugs are adaptations of second generation, etc.

Secondaries Flight feathers attached to forearm (ulna).

Secondary abnormality Morphologic abnormalities of sperm that develop while sperm are moving through the epididymus or occur as a result of handling sperm.

Secondary closure Do not suture the wound and let the tissue granulate in.

Secondary degeneration Tissue damage that occurs in the hours/days after injury; thought to be in part mediated by the immune response

Secondary Epilepsy Epilepsy for which a cause can be determined. Usually found in dogs under 1 year of age and over 5 years of age.

Secondary infection Infection which occurs because the tissue and its natural defenses have been damaged by another condition.

Secondary oocyte An ovum that has released its polar body and is ready to be penetrated by sperm.

Secondary response The faster and greater immune response produced by an animal who has previously encountered that specific antigen. Memory cells are responsible for this more efficient response. Also called 'anamnestic response.'

Secondary uterine inertia Ineffective or absent uterine contractions during parturition. Secondary uterine inertia may occur when a bitch is tired or exhausted from pushing to deliver and "gives-up" on delivering puppies.

Secondary waste treatment Usually, a second treatment of waste water to reduce pollution potential or health hazard. With animal manure an example would be storage in an anaerobic treatment lagoon and sprinkler field application.

Secretin Secretin is a hormone produced by the small intestine in vertebrates that stimulates the production of digestive secretions.

Seizure Also called convulsion, ictus, fit. The brain cells work together, communicating by means of electrical signals. When there is an abnormal electrical discharge from a group of cells, the result is a seizure. Seizures are either epileptic or nonepileptic.

Seizure Threshold The level at which dogs will have a seizure. It is suggested that this level is inherited. Lowering the threshold (though drugs like acepromazine, or through kindling), makes seizures more likely to occur. Raising the threshold (using drugs like phenobarbital or KBr) will make seizures less likely to occur.

Seizure threshold The level of stimulation at which a seizure is produced. Raising the seizure threshold makes it less likely a seizure will occur.

Selection Differential The difference between the average for a trait in replacement animals and the average of the group from which the replacements were chosen. The expected response from selection equals selection differential times heritability of a trait.

Selection intensity The margin of true genetic superiority of those animals selected in comparison to all those from which the choices were made.

Selection The causing or allowing of certain individuals in a population to produce the next generation. Artificial selection is that practiced by man; natural selection is that practiced by nature.

Selective IgM deficiency A deficiency in the production of the IgM antibody, one of the body's five classes of immunoglobulins, the proteins produced as antibodies to fight infection and toxins.

Selective serotonin reuptake inhibitor (SSRIs), Selective serotonin reuptake inhibitors: Medications which slow down the ability of nerve cells to absorb serotonin, a neurotransmitter (chemical that serves as a messenger between nerves). Example: Prozac.

Selemectin Trade name is Revolution, marketed by Pfizer. A neurotoxin recommended as a monthly topical "pour'on" insecticide. This product is also labeled for use as against scabies, ear mites, internal parasites, and for tick control.

Selenium A chemical element, atomic number 34, atomic weight 78.96, symbol Se. It is an essential mineral nutrient and a very potent poison. Selenium has antioxidant properties similar to vitamin E. Vitamin E can replace the requirement for selenium in the body, but selenium cannot substitute for vitamin E. In addition, selenium does not cross the blood-brain barrier like vitamin E. On the other hand, selenium may help vitamin E to be more effective. Many plant sources are low in selenium and supplementation may be important; however, selenium can create a toxicity if given at too high a level. Never give more than 200 µg of selenium per day in large dogs nor more than 100 µg per day to small dogs.

Self-feeder A feeding system that allows animals to eat at will. See ad libitum.

Semen extender A substance added to semen to provide an appropriate environment and energy for the sperm to survive in vitro.

Semen The fluid that contains sperm and fluid from the testes, prostate and other acessory sex glands.

Semi longhair A longhair that does not have an extremely long coat. For example, the Maine Coon is considered a semi-longhair, but the Persian is not.

Seminal plasma The fluid portion of semen which is produced by the prostate gland.

Seminal vesicles Accessory sex glands in the male.

Seminiferous tubules The location in the testes in which sperm are produced.

Seminoma A testicular tumor that usually displays benign biologic behavior.

Semipalmate Webbed only at base (toes).

Semipermeable membrane A membrane that allows water and small molecules to pass through it but prevents passage of large molecules such as colloids. The peritoneal membrane lining the abdominal cavity is an example of a semipermeable membrane.

Semitendinosus The Semitendinosus is a muscle in the human thigh.

Senile iris atrophy Atrophy of the constrictor muscle: poor pupillary light reflexes but normal vision. Pupil margin looks a bit moth-eaten and irregular.

Senior A horse at least five years old. A rider at least 50 years old.

Senna The woody shrub, Cassia senna, contains chemicals which act as strong cathartics. The leaves and the seed pods are used medicinally.

Sensible fluid losses Sensible fluid losses are those that can be easily detected and measured. Sensible losses can occur through the urinary and gastrointestinal tracts. The loss of fluid through the GI tract is negligible in healthy dogs and cats but can be substantial through vomiting or diarrhea. In the adult, healthy dog or cat, sensible loss is through urine and is about 12-20 ml/lb/day. Loss of water through the urinary and GI tracts is usually accompanied by loss of electrolytes (in both health and disease) (an isotonic loss).

Sensitivity Tests Tests used to determine the most effective method of treatment of disease by testing the resistance of the microorganism to classes of antibiotics.

Sensitizing soup Chemical mediators released by cells following tissue damage and inflammation that individually or collectively results in pain sensitivity.

Sensory discriminative dimension of pain This dimension of pain gives the individual information about the location, onset, intensity, type and duration of pain.

Separation anxiety A behavioral condition in which the pet becomes anxious when separated from the owner. Dogs with separation anxiety tend to 'shadow' their owners, greet them exuberantly when they return after being gone, and sometimes vocalize, chew destructively, and urinate or defecate when separated from their owners.

Separator 1.Formerly a centrifuge device used to remove the fat from milk on the farm, but now used primarily at processing plants.

2. A device used to separate manure into solids and effluent and accomplished by trickling manure over a sloped screen or mechanically forcing through a screen.

Sepsis The presence of toxins in the blood or other tissues; the toxins are produced by bacteria or other microorganisms.

Septic A condition caused by an infection e.g., with bacteria or fungi, or toxins they produce.

Septic arthritis A bacterial infection in a joint causing inflammation.

Septicaemia Serious infection in which the bloodstream is invaded by large numbers of causal bacteria which multiply there.

Septicemia A disease affecting many organ systems due to toxins in the blood which are released by bacteria or other microorganisms. Signs include fever, pinpoint bruises on mucous membranes, and lesions in the joints, heart valves, eyes, or other organs.

Septum A septum is a muscular partition seperating the two sides of the human heart.

Sequencing Genes To determine the DNA nucleotide sequence (the genetic code) of a gene.

Serial analysis of the gene expression SAGE is a high throughput differential gene expression methodology that permits the identification of candidate tumor antigen within a subset of differentially expressed genes that are over expressed in cancer cells.

Seroconversion A change in immune status from having no measurable antibodies against an infectious agent to development of measurable antibodies in the blood.

Serology Laboratory testing for antibody-antigen reactions and antibody levels.

Seroprevalence The frequency of occurance of exposure to an infectious agent based on measuring antibodies to the agent in the blood.

Serotype A subdivision of a species of microorganism, e.g., a bacteria, based upon its particular antigens.

Serotype The type of microorganism as determined by the kind and combination of constituent antigens associated with the cell.

Serous Thin and watery.

Serpentine Series of half circles and straight lines crossing from one side of the centerline to the other, requiring a change of direction each time the horse passes over it.

Serrate With teeth like saw (cutting edge of bill).

Serratia A genus of bacteria of the family enterobacteriaceae that is saprophytic on decaying plant and animal materials.

Sertoli cell Cells in the testicle which support the testosterone-producing cells. These cells can produce the female hormone, estrogen.

Sertoli cell tumor A testicular tumor that may produce estrogens and cause signs of feminization in the male dog.

Sertoli cell tumor A type of testicular cancer that may result in a male showing signs of feminization.

Serum alanine aminotransferase SALT (ALT) Also known as alanine aminotransferase (ALT). An enzyme found in hepatocytes (liver cells) released with cellular injury including cellular hypoxia.

Serum alkaline phosphatase SAP (AP) Also known as alkaline phosphatase (AP). An enzyme found in many tissues but most often elevated in serum in response to cholestasis, bone remodeling or glucocorticoid excess.

Serum The clear part of blood that remains after blood is allowed to clot. Very similar to plasma except that plasma is the fluid part of blood when blood is separated into cells and fluid before the blood clots.

Service A term commonly used in animal breeding, denoting the mating of male to female. Also called serving or covering.

Service sire The sire to which a female currently is bred. Service sire information should be reported on DHI barnsheets.

Service/conception Number of AI or natural services needed to achieve pregnancy (conception). Goal is 2-2.5 Svc/con.

Set To keep eggs warm so they will hatch; also called "brood."

Set, Settle To group a bunch of cattle into a quiet, compact herd. In cutting or team penning, a group of competitors that use the same group of cattle.

Setting A group of hatching eggs in an incubator or under a hen; the incubation of eggs by a hen (called "sitting" by some).

Settled A term commonly used to indicate that an animal has become pregnant.

Settling basin Any area that reduces flow velocity and allows particulates to settle from a liquid suspension. With manure suspensions, usually built to allow solids removal on a regular basis.

Settling Pond A manure pit where the flow rate of liquid manure is slowed to allow suspended materials to collect at the bottomed, where they can later be removed.

Set-Up Putting a horse in the proper stance for the judge to evaluate him in a halter or conformation class.

Sex feather A hackle, saddle, or tail feather that is rounded in a hen but usually pointed in a rooster (except in breeds that are hen feathered).

Sexed Newly hatched chicks that have been sorted into pullets and cockerels.

Sex-link A genetic trait that creates a difference (usually in color) between males and females. Most often this is used to refer to traits that make chicks of different genders visibly distinct for ease of sexing. The term may apply to the gene or characteristic, or is often applied to hybrid crosses that display this characteristic such as the Golden Sex-link.

Shade Structures in corrals designed to provide shelter from sun.

Shafts A pair of poles that fit on either side of a horse in a single harness.

Shank Lead rope or "stud" chain. Also the arm extending from the mouthpiece of a curb bit to where the reins attach. Pressure on these reins exerts leverage.

Sharp teeth Molars that have sharp points that injure tongue or cheek.

Sharps Equipment that is used in skin piercing procedures, such as needles or lancets.

Shearing Cutting off the fleece of the sheep. This is done once or twice a year.

Sheath The skin folds that encase a horse's penis.

Shedding Shedding (of organisms): A term used to describe the release of organisms (bacteria, protozoa, viruses) into the environment from an infected animal. The organisms may be in the stool, urine, respiratory secretions, or vaginal discharges. The 'shedding' animal may or may not be showing symptoms of disease.

Shedding blade Metal blade with short teeth to scrape out loose hair.

Sheep 1. A ewe will normally have 1, sometimes twin, lamb during 12 months. The lambs are usually born during the winter or early spring. The mature sheep are sheared of their wool in the spring. The wool production from each animal is from 7 9 pounds annually.

2. The lambs that are being sold will be held for 6 9 months. Their weight at selling time will be about 90 100 pounds.

3. Feeder lambs are purchased at about eight weeks weighing about 20 pounds. They will be in the feedlot for 6 7 months, weighing 90 100 pounds when sold.

Sheet cotton Cotton pressed into thin sheets, used under leg wraps.

Sheet Cover (blanket) for horse made of light canvas or cotton. Useful for putting on after bathing.

Shelf life The time after processing during which a product remains suitable for human consumption, especially the time a food remains palatable.

Shepherd A person who cares for sheep.

Shiatsu A Japanese technique which uses finger and thumb pressure on precise body points to encourage the proper flow of chi.

Shiitake A fungus that grows on the trunks of dead trees. Shiitake mushrooms are often found in Chinese cuisine. The mushroom may have some beneficial effects against cancer.

Shingles See herpes zoster.

Shipping fever A complex seen in cattle, especially feedlot cattle, where the stress of shipping weakens their immune system and they develop viral and then oportunistic bacterial infections.

Shoat Weaned pig 25 -40 pounds, also weaner.

Shoer Horse shoer, farrier.

Shorn A sheep that has had its fleece removed by shearing.

Short bones In human anatomy, short bones are part of the skeleton designed for strength and compactness. They are comprised of a spongy substance surrounded by a thin crust of compact bone.

Shorthair A cat with a relatively short coat. The coat may be very close-lying and sleek, or it may be thick and plush.

Shoulder-In Horse is slightly bent around the inside leg of the rider, and his inside legs pass and cross in front of the outside legs.

Show An exhibition of cats, during which the cats are evaluated by licensed judges and awarded prizes for their conformance to breed standards.

Show animals Any animal used for competition of judging animals against each other. Often related to 4-H or FFA stock show competitions for farmers children. Winner receives prize money and, often, retains the animal. May also be competitions entered by taxpayer or other members of family.

Show cat A cat that is exhibited in show.

Show quality A cat that meets its breed standard closely enough to be competitive in show.

Show year or **show season** The year long period during which show cats accumulate points for regional, national, and international awards. In North America, the show year traditionally runs from May to April.

Showmanship An in-hand class that is judged on the exhibitor's ability to show his horse.

Shrinkage A term used to indicate the amount of loss in body weight, as in dairy steers, when exposed to various conditions and/or slaughter. Also, the decrease in volume of dairy products during storage, and the loss of milk or milk solids in processing.

Shy breeder A male or female of any domesticated livestock that has a low reproductive efficiency.

Shying A horse spooking or becoming startled by a movement or object. It may or may not include a sudden jump sideways, or bolting.

Sib (sibling) In genetics, a brother or sister.

Siberian Ginseng Siberian ginseng is derived from the root of a shrub, Eleutherococcus senticosus, found in the Siberian regions of Russia and China. It stimulates the immune system and increases the body's resistance to disease, stress, and fatigue.

Sibs (Full Sibs) Brothers and sisters from the same sire and dam.

Sickle hocked Describes an animal having a crooked hock, which causes the lower part of the leg to be bent forward out of a normal perpendicular straight line.

Sickles The long, curved tail feathers of some roosters.

SID Giving medication once a day. Example 60 mg SID would be giving 60 mg all at once, one time a day. (Veterinary term only)

Side Effect Undesirable reaction resulting from immunization.

Side pass Full pass moving the horse sideways, with no forward movement, crossing one leg over another. Often used in trail classes.

Side step The maneuver in which a horse moves sideways a step at a time.

Sidebone Inflammation followed by an ossification of the lateral cartilages of the foot.

Signal Transduction The process by which extracellular signals are detected and converted into intracellular signals, that, in turn, generate specific cellular responses.

Signalment This is the physical description of the animal including species, breed, sex, neuter status, age and color and/or markings.

Silage (ensilage) Green forage, such as grass or clover, or fodder, such as field corn or sorghum, that is chopped into a silo, where it is packed or compressed to exclude air and undergoes an acid fermentation (lactic and acetic acids) that retards spoilage.

Silage A feed prepared by chopping green forage (e.g. grass, legumes, field corn) and placing the material in a structure or container designed to exclude air. The material then undergoes fermentation, retarding spoilage. Silage has a water content of between 60 and 80%.

Silage additives Substances added during the ensiling process to enhance the correct and rapid fermentation of the feed.

Silage Bags Large plastic tubes in which forages are fermented. Plastic is removed and discarded as the ensiled feed is fed.

Silicone A polymer of alternating oxygen and silicon atoms combined with other organic groups. Catheters made of silicone are relatively inert and have less stimulation of clot formation compared to other materials.

Silo A vertical cylindrical structure, pit, trench, or other relatively airtight chamber in which chopped green crops, such as corn, grass, legumes, or small grain and other livestock feeds are fermented and stored. See silage.

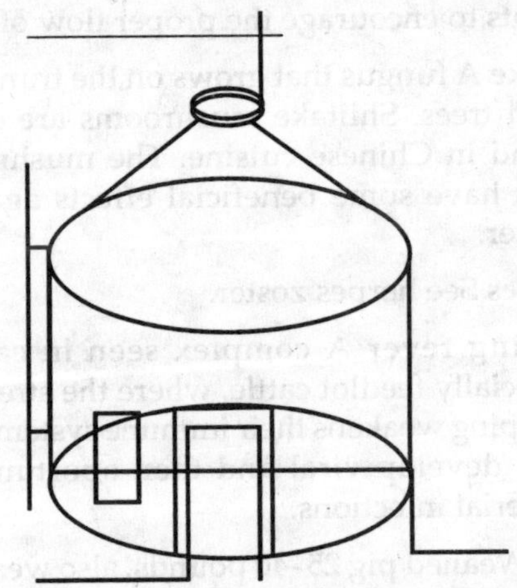

Fig. Silo

Simple Lead Change Change from one lead to another with a walk, trot, or halt in between.

Simultaneous ventilation compression CPR For every compression, you give the patient a simultaneous ventilation. The ventilatory rate is very high and matches the chest compression rate.

Single tree Single whiffletree.

Sinus A sinus is an air-filled space in the diploe of a skull bone.

Sire Father or male parent in a pedigree.

Sire family The offspring of one cock mated to two or more hens, so that all are full or half siblings.

Sire selection Process of identifying bulls to be used as service sires with the goal of increasing the genetic potential of the herd.

Skeleton The skeleton is the hard internal or external framework of bones, cartilage or shell which provides protection for an animals organs, provides fixing points for the muscles and a general frame for the body.

Sketch (photo) A method of permanent identification to be cross-referenced with visible identification. Accurate sketches or photographs of Holsteins, Ayrshires and Guernseys provide unique identification.

Skim milk Milk from which sufficient cream has been removed to reduce its milk fat content to less than 0.5 percent (usually less than 0.1 percent). Skim milk contains as much protein, lactose, minerals, and water-soluble vitamins and only half as many calories as whole milk. Skim milk is practically cholesterol-free.

Skin cytology Examination, with a microscope, of a skin scraping or material from swabbing the skin. The material may be stained and checked for the presence of yeast, bacteria, tumor cells, etc.

Skin In the human body, skin, or Dermoid Tissue, is composed of two layers, the cuticle, epidermis or epithelium and the corium or dermis.

Skin scraping Scraping some material from the surface of the skin and looking at it under a microscope, e.g., to check for skin mites.

Skin tent When the skin of an animal is gently pinched and pulled outward. A dehydrated animal's skin will not rapidly return to its normal position or shape.

Skin turgor Skin elasticity. Skin turgor is used to assess hydration.

Skirt The square or round leather flaps under the saddle seat of the western saddle.

Slack Loose rope or reins, or to loosen. In rodeo, the morning or afternoon performance.

Sleeping sickness Encephalomyelitis.

Slip To abort.

Slit lamp biomicroscopy Provides magnification and depth for examination of the eyelids, puncta, conjunctiva, sclera, cornea, anterior chamber, iris, lens, and anterior vitreous.

Slotted Floor A concrete floor design in which slats are positioned in the floor so that cow traffic may work manure through the slats and into a pit beneath the floor of the barn.

Smegma Accumulation of fatty secretions, dead skin cells, and dirt found in the male's sheath.

Smooth muscle The type of muscle found in the internal organs such as stomach and intestines (not the heart).

Smooth mouth An animal that has lost all of its permanent incisors, usually 7 or more years of age.

Smut Black feathers that are uncharacteristic for the breed, such as black body feathers in a Rhode Island Red.

Snaffle, Snaffle bit Bit with a solid or jointed mouthpiece that has no shanks and works on principles of direct pressure only.

Snatch To jerk the reins sharply.

SNF Solids not fat of milk; proteins, lactose, minerals, and other water-soluble constituents. This is the same as NFS and NMS.

Snip Small white streak above or on nose.

Snots Rhinopneumenitis in foals when thick mucous runs from nose.

Snow nose Loss of pigmentation on the nose, usually in winter.

SOAP SOAP's are progress notes recorded in a medical record.

S = subjective information

O = objective information

A = assessment of information

P = plans for diagnoses, treatment or client information

Sock White above fetlock.

Soilage Freshly cut green forage often fed to animals in drylot. Also called green chop.

Sole The bottom layer of the hoof.

Solid phase epitope recovery SPHERE, a combinatorial; peptide library screening technology that enables the identification of the minimal epitope recognized by T-cells.

Soluble carbohydrate Also, soluble fiber. Easily digested carbohydrates like starch.

Soluble intake protein SIP Portion of the protein intake that is completely soluble in rumen fluid and rapidly utilized by bacteria. Soluble protein forms part (or all) of the degradable intake protein (DIP) value of a feed.

Solvent extracted Fat or oil removed from materials (such as soybean seeds) by organic solvents.

Somatic cell count (SCC) The number of white blood cells per milliliter of milk or measurement of the number of somatic cells present in a sample of milk. A high concentration of more than 500,000 somatic cells per milliliter of milk indicates abnormal condition in the udder. This serves as an indicator of mastitis infection when elevated above 200,000.

Somatic Cell Score A logarithmic representation of the SCC, often referred to as linear scores because they are linearly related to milk production loss.

Somatic cells The cell content of milk is composed of approximately 95 percent leukocytes (white blood cells) from the blood and 5 percent epithelial cells from the secretory tissue of the udder. Leukocytes are present in response to infection or injury, and epithelial cells are present as a result of infection or injury. Collectively, these cells are called somatic cells.

Somatic Relating to the wall of the body as distinguished from the viscera.

Somatosensory Sensory signals from tissues. Somatic usually refers to input from body tissue other than viscera.

Somatotropin A protein hormone produced by the pituitary gland, which stimulates growth of muscle, bone and mammary development in young animals and increases milk production in lactating animals by making available nutrients for milk synthesis and secretion.

Somnolence Sleepiness, a condition of semiconsciousness approaching coma.

Somogyi effect A condition in which the blood glucose level increases if too much insulin is given. It occurs when insulin causes the blood glucose level to go so low it stimulates the production of other hormones in the body such as epinephrine, which promote the breakdown of glycogen (the chemical compound which the body uses to store glucose) and increases the blood glucose level above normal. It is also called rebound hyperglycemia or insulin-induced hyperglycemia.

Sored Having physical evidence of inhumane training practices.

Soremouth A highly contagious (also to humans), viral infection that causes scabs around mouth, nostrils, eyes and may effect udders of lactating ewes.

Sorrel A reddish or copper-red body with mane and tail the same color as the body.

Sound Having no defect, visible or unseen, that affects serviceability; the state of being able to perform without hindrance.

Soundness 1. If there are no weak spots in the wool

2. When an animal is free from disease and lacks structural defects that affect its usefulness.

Source oriented record A record keeping system in which all data of a similar type are clustered together, e.g. all laboratory reports and together.

Sow A female hog which is part of the breeding herd which has produced offspring.

Spasmodic colic Acute intermittent colic as digestive tract spasms (usually involves small intestine).

Spatulate Spoon-shaped (bill).

Spavin An unsoundness of the hock which can involve soft tissues (bog spavin) or bone (bone spavin or jack spavin).

Spay To surgically remove the reproductive organs of the female cat. A "spay" is a spayed female cat.

Spayed To have surgically removed the ovaries of a female.

Spayed mare A neutered female horse.

Specialty A "specialty ring" is a ring where the breeds are separated into categories such as "longhair" and "shorthair" for the purposes of judging and awarding prizes. A "specialty judge" is a judge that is licensed only to judge in a specialty ring, not in an allbreed ring.

Species A distinction for a specific type of animals. For example, geese are a species and ducks are a species. There may be many breeds of each species. Typically species cannot interbreed successfully, for example a duck and a goose can not produce offspring together. If species can cross the offspring are typically sterile like a mule (horse x donkey).

Specific pathogen free pigs SPF pigs The pigs are taken surgically at birth and reared in a pig free environment so they have no contact with other pigs and no opportunity to catch a disease.

Specific treatment Treatment that will eliminate or modify the primary cause of a disease process. For example, surgical removal of a tumor.

Spent No longer laying well.

Sperm Spermatozoa. The male structure that fertilizes an egg.

Spermatogenesis Formation of sperm in the testes.

Spermatozoa Sperm. The male structure that fertilizes an egg.

Speuter An agglomeration of spay and neuter. Another word for alter.

Sphenoid bone The sphenoid bone is situated at the base of the human skull, in front of the temporal bones and the basilar part of the occipital bone.

Sphincter A ring-like band of muscle that constricts a passage or closes an opening, e.g., the anal sphincter constricts to close the anus and relaxes when the animal is passing stool. The urethral sphincter closes the urinary bladder.

Spillover What spillover means is that rabies viral variant isolated from a rabid animal will be the variant from the terrestrial wildlife reservoir in that area. That is why if you have a rabid raccoon in Montana it will be spill over from a skunk because that is the only wildlife reservoir that maintains the virus in that area.

Spinal myelopathy Disease of the myelin, or covering (sheath) of the spinal nerves (the spinal cord).

Spinal tracts — ascending and descending Bundles of nerves the go through the spinal cord from the body delivering sensory information to the brain, ascending, or from the brain delivering motor information to the body, descending

Spinales The spinales are human muscles which extend the vertebral column.

Spinoreticular A tract in the spinal cord leading to behavioral responses that help the individual determine whether a painful input is tolerable or not. Also conveys visceral pain.

Spinothalamic A tract in the spinal cord which conveys impulses associated with pain and temperature sensation, and tactile sensation. Somatic pain pathway.

Spirochete A type of bacteria which is long, slender, and assumes a spiral shape. Leptospira species and the bacteria that causes Lyme disease (Borrelia burgdorferi) are spirochetes.

Spitting off When the female is no longer receptive to the male indicating she has ovulated.

Splay legged A condition in newborn pigs that involves a muscle weakness so they are unable to stand and bear their weight.

Spleen Part of the immune system of an animal. A large, tongue-shaped organ in the abdomen containing many lymphocytes. The spleen filters blood and removes damaged cells. It can also manufacture new blood cells if the animal's bone marrow is damaged.

Splenii The splenii are two muscles in the human body, the splenius capitis and the spelnius cervicis. They are used to move the head backwards, to one side and to rotate it.

Splint Term commonly applied to inflammation of the attachment of the splint bone to the cannon; older cases of splints are identified as bony enlargements at various points along the splint bone.

Splint boots Protective covering worn around the cannons of the front legs to prevent injury.

Spooky An easily startled horse.

Sporotrichosis Cutaneous nodules; draining, ulcerative tracts caused by Sporothrix schenckii. Lesions may be focal or disseminated.

Sport horse A purebred or crossbred horse suitable for dressage, jumping, eventing, or endurance.

Spray The behavior, commonly seen in the tom cat, of urinating everywhere (typically on the walls, floor, etc) to establish territory.

Spread Type of fence that requires jumping the width from front to rear.

Springer A term commonly associated with female cattle showing signs of advanced pregnancy. Often used to refer to heifers close to term with their first calf.

Springer or Fresh Cow/heifer that has recently calved.

Spurs The sharp pointed protrusions on a rooster's shanks.

Squalamine An example of a powerful anti-angiogenic molecule originally isolated from the liver of dogfish sharks.

Squamate Scaly-bodied reptile including lizards and snakes.

SSRI Selective serotonin reuptake inhibitors: Medications which slow down the ability of nerve cells to absorb serotonin, a neurotransmitter (chemical that serves as a messenger between nerves). Example: Prozac.

St. Johns Wort The flowers of this woody perennial have been used externally to help with wound healing. The flowers contain a substance which is germicidal, anti-inflammatory, and antidepressant.

Stablemate See herdmate.

Stades procedureA surgical procedure for correcting upper eyelid entropion.

Stag A cockerel on the brink of sexual maturity, when his comb and spurs begin to develop.

Stage 1 This is the stage of cervical dilation and lasts 6-8 hrs in the bitch and queen.

Stage 2 This is the stage of fetal expulsion in the labor of a bitch or queen and lasts 3-6 hrs.

Stage 3 This is the stage of placental expulsion in the labor of a bitch or queen and lasts 5-15 min.

Stage of lactation Period of milk production during a lactation determined by the length of time since parturition.

Stake out Tie an animal on a long rope or chain to a stake driven in the ground.

Stakeholder A person or group of persons, or an industry, association, organization, etc. with an economic or professional interest/ responsibility in an area or (involuntarily) affected by the developments in the same area. In the field of antimicrobial usage in food animals the farmers, veterinarians, animal feed organizations, pharmaceutical companies, consumers, public health officials, academic and other related groups are recognized as stakeholders.

Stakes class Money-earning class.

Stale A period when an animal does not work or lactate at the normal standards, as opposed to bloom. Also refers to milk products that have deteriorated in storage.

Stall A cow housing cubicle.

Stallion A male horse four years of age and over (not gelded).

Stallion syndicate A financial investment group owning shares in a stallion.

Stanchion A device with two rails that was closed around a cows neck after she entered a stall and to keep her restrained in the stall.

Stanchion barn Stall barn where cows are chained within their stalls.

Standard The term standard is used in several related ways. A Standard is a detailed "official" description of a breed and its recognized varities. In the United States, the American Poultry Association (APA) and the American Bantam Association (ABA) produce the recognized standards for domestic chickens, turkeys and waterfowl. These standards are published in books known as"Standards of Perfection". These books are often called standards. Standard or Standard Bred birds are breeds and varieties that conform to a standard written for them by a recognized authority. Recognized breeds and the standards for them differ from country to country. Only birds conforming to the APA or ABA 'Standard of Perfection" can be placed in an APA or ABA sanctioned poultry show. Note there are some common hybrids such as the Gold Sex-link and the Rock Cornish that may be called standard, but should not be confused with the standard breeds and varieties for exhibition as they are hybrids, not a breed.

Standard drip sets An adminstration set for intravenous fluid administration. The set has a spike to penetrate the container of fluids, a drip chamber and a long flexible tube that connects to the patient's catheter. The end of the drip set vary by manufacturer, requiring anywhere from 10-20 drops to comprise a milliliter.

Standard Sized See Large Fowl

Standard The description of an ideal specimen for its breed; also, a chicken that conforms to the description of its breed in the American Standard of Perfection, sometimes erroneously used when referring to large as opposed to bantam breeds.

Standardbred An American breed of horse developed for harness racing.

Standardization The process of adjusting the milkfat and solids-non-fat content of milk to meet a required standard.

Standby pool An arrangement between cooperatives in markets that have periods of milk shortages and cooperatives in areas of surplus milk production. Cooperatives in the deficit market make monthly payments to certain cooperatives in the surplus regions to assure that they have sources of milk available at reasonable prices when local milk does not supply their Class I needs.

Standing When a stallion is at a breeding farm to breed mares brought to him.

Standing bandage A bandage held up by wraps down to the hoof.

Staphylococcus, staph A type of bacteria. Normally found on the skin and upper respiratory tract, but can occasionally cause localized suppurating infection.

Staple A group of wool fibers.

Starter A feed ration for newly hatched chicks, also called "crumbles".

Started pullets Young female chickens that are nearly old enough to lay.

Starve-out Failure of chicks to eat.

Stasis In the gastrointestinal tract, a condition in which the food does not move through normally, but remains in one section, e.g., food does not pass from the stomach into the intestine.

State Veterinary Service The Government organisation which makes sure that Government policies on animal health and welfare are carried out. SVS staff deal with outbreaks of notifiable diseases and carry out tests for these and certain other diseases. They visit farms and markets to check that animal welfare is protected, that medicines are correctly used and stored, and to advise on disease prevention and control. It became a Government Agency on 1st April 2005.

Statistical significance The probability that an event or difference occurred as the result of the intervention (vaccine) rather than by chance alone. This probability is determined by using statistical tests to evaluate collected data. Guidelines for defining significance are chosen before data collections begins.

Statistically significant It usually refers in research to tests for differences resulting from treatments. The reliability of such differences is expressed as degree of probability or the percentage of time an observation would be expected to fall outside a certain range of variation from normal observation.

Status epilepticus A condition in which the animal exhibits one severe (Grand Mal) seizure right after another, with no time to recover in-between.

Status Status epilepticus is defined as more than 30 minutes of 1. Continuous seizure activity or

2. Two or more sequential seizures without full recovery between seizures. More than 3 major seizures within a 24 hour period should be considered a serious condition that may evolve into status and should be treated. The 30 minute duration in the above definition was chosen because detrimental effects begin to occur after this time. These effects include systemic effects such as abnormal breathing, blood pressure and heart rate, and blood glucose, in addition to body temperature. Also, prolonged abnormal electrical activity within the brain can cause persistent brain damage. These changes tend to be reversible during the 30 to 60 minute period of continuous seizure activity but after 60 minutes, death of nerve cells occurs.

Steer Male cattle that have been neutered or castrated when young. Young bull calves are castrated to make their meat taste better and be more tender when they are old enough for market.

Stem cells Young cells that have the capacity to become other cell types

Stem Cells, Hematopoietic and Mesenchymal Stem cells are of embryonic origin and possess the properties of both self-renewal and differentiation into a wide variety of tissue types. There are many different types of stem cells among which include Hematopoietic and Mesenchymal. Hematopoietic Stem Cells (HSCs) have the properties to give rise to all known cell types in the blood-forming and immune (hematolymphoid) systems. The bone marrow also contains other non-hematopoietic cells termed mesenchymal stem cells (MSCs), that are capable of both self renewal and differentiation into bone, cartilage, muscle, tendon, and fat. MSCs are similar to HSCs in that they are very rare, existing at an estimated frequency of about 1 in 100,000 bone marrow cells.

Stenosis A narrowing or contraction of an opening. aortic stenosis obstruction of the blood flowing from the left ventricle to the aorta. mitral stenosis narrowing of the mitral valve that separates the left atrium and the left ventricle. pulmonary artery stenosis narrowing of the outflow from the lungs. subaortic

Step A beat.

Step-Up Parlor Cows step onto raised platforms for milking. The milking units are attached from the side.

Sterile Clean, free of any living organisms. Also means unable to reproduce.

Sterilizable syringe Either all plastic or all glass syringe with steel needle. This type of syringe is designed for re-use after proper cleaning and sterilization in a steam sterilizer or autoclave.

Sterilize Destroy all microorganisms; usually not possible with chemical disinfectants, and requires physical disinfection.

Sternal Laying down on the chest and belly.

Sternocostalis The sternocostalis is a muscle in the human body.

Sternohyoid The sternohyoid is a muscle in the human body which dpresses the hyoid bone.

Sternomastoid The sternomastoid is a muscle in the human neck.

Sternum In anatomy, the sternum is a long flat bone which forms the median portion of the anterior wall of the thorax. The top of the sternum supports the clavicles.

Steward A show official who assists the judge in or out of the show pen.

Stillborn Born lifeless; dead at birth.

Stirrup The leather covered (in the western saddle) or metal (in the English saddle) part of the saddle used to support the riders feet.

Stock horse A Western-style horse of the Quarter Horse type.

Stocking rate (per acre) The number of animals that can be pastured on one acre, or the number of acres required to pasture one animal.

Stocking White leg marking above the cannon.

Stomach tube Tube passed usually through the nose into the stomach.

Stomatitis Inflammation of the mouth including the gums and tongue.

Stones A mass, usually formed from mineral salts, occurring within the hollow organs: kidney, gallbladder, urinary bladder.

Storage diseases Diseases in which cells of the body accumulate (store) a substance that causes the cells to malfunction. For example cells may store too much fat or sugar.

Stover Fodder; mature cured stalks of grain from which seeds have been removed, such as stalks of corn without ears.

Straight bit A simple bar bit with no breaks, joints, or projections.

Straight run Newly hatched chicks that have not been sexed; also called "unsexed" or "as hatched."

Straight stall Stall with two walls and manger where horse is tied.

Straightbred Purebred.

Strain A specific version of an organism. Many diseases, including HIV/AIDS and hepatitis, have multiple strains.

Strangles Bacterial respiratory disease caused by Streptococcus equii causing swollen abscessed glands.

Stranguria Straining to urinate.

Strategic worming Worming during the times of year that infection is most likely to occur.

Stratified As applied to the sheep industry, this means that different types and breeds of sheep are kept on different sorts of land – hill, uplands, and lowlands - and used for different purposes. For instance, upland farms commonly cross-breed older ewes from hill farms (such as the Swaledale) with a longwool breed (like the Blueface Leicester) to produce a hybrid ewe. These hybrids are sold to lowland farms for further breeding to produce prime lamb.

As applied to a survey, it means that the number of individuals included in the survey is in proportion to different sections in the population being studied. For example, a survey for a disease in dogs might look at blood samples from 1,000 animals. If we knew that, say, 85 % of dogs lived in towns and 15 % lived in rural areas, a stratified survey would look at 850 urban dogs and 150 rural ones.

Stratum corneum The outer layer of skin.

Strawberry roan A mixture of red and white hairs all over a horse's body, with red, black, or flaxen mane and tail. Also called red roan.

Streak canal Small canal located in the end of each teat, through which the milk passes immediately prior to expulsion. Also called the teat meatus.

Streptococcus A genus of bacteria of the family lactobaccillaceae occurring regularly in the mouth and intestines of humans and other animals. Some species are Pathogenic.

Stress An unusual or abnormal influence causing a change in an animal's function, structure, or behavior.

Stress induced hyperglycemia A condition in cats in which the blood glucose level becomes abnormally high when the animal is stressed, e.g., in the veterinarian's office.

Stria Streaks in the cornea caused by the cornea stretching from increased pressure.

Stricture The narrowing of an organ of passage such as a blood vessel or intestine.

Stride The distance traveled in a particular gait, measured from the spot where one hoof hits the ground to where it next lands. Ten to twelve feet is the normal length of stride at a canter, for example.

Strike When horse reaches up, out, and down with front foot.

Striking A bad habit of reaching out with a front foot so as to hit the handler, equipment, or another horse. A problem calling for professional help.

String A group of animals within a larger group, or herd.

String out To move without engaging the hindquarters, so hind end looks "strung out" from the forehand.

Strip To remove residual milk from the mammary gland (udder).

Strip Cup A small cup or device to collect forestrippings and which makes abnormal milk easier to observe.

Stripe White streak down face.

Stroma Thickest layer of the cornea.

Strongyle "Blood worm".

Structural carbohydrates Complex carbohydrates (fiber)including cellulose, hemicellulose, lignin and pectin that form the plant cell wall. Measured in the laboratory as neutral detergent fibre (NDF).

Structural correctness Free from any conformational abnormalities.

Struvite A chemical compound, magnesium ammonium phosphate, which is made by the body and can form crystals and stones in the urinary bladder.

Stub Down on the shank or toe of a clean-legged chicken.

Stud A unit of selected animals kept for breeding purposes (e.g., bulls).

Stud cat A whole male cat that is part of a breeding program.

Stud fee The charge for breeding to a stallion.

Stud, Stud farm Farm where mares are bred.

Stylish Attractive, possessing a pleasing conformation or way of movement.

Subalbinotic Animals with blue irises.

Subclavius The Subclavius is a muscle in the human body between the clavicle and the first rib. It steadies the clavicle during movements of the shoulder.

Subclinical A disease condition without clinical manifestations.

Subclinical infection The presence of infection without symptoms. Also known as inapparent or asymptomatic infection.

Subcorneal Just under the stratum corneum.

Subcorneal pustular dermatosis SPDA rare condition characterized by the formation of pustules which are subcorneal in location.

Subcutaneous (sq) injections Are accomplished by inserting the needle just under the skin and not into the muscle. This is important because SQ injectables are designed for a slower rate of absorption or are highly irritating to muscle tissue

Subjective information Information told to the physician by a patient. Not relavent to veterinary patients.

Subluxation A partial dislocation of a joint in which the bones become out of alignment, but the joint itself is still intact.

SubQ Subcutaneous, under the skin shot (sometimes written as SQ or sq).

Substance Strength and density of bone, muscle, and tendons or an indication of large body size.

Substrate Relative to the husbandry of reptiles, amphibians, and small mammals, the substrate is the material that lines the bottom of a cage.

Subunit vaccineA vaccine that use parts of a pathogen rather than the whole organism.

Subway An area beneath the milking pit that houses milk meters, pipelines, vacuum lines and transfer tanks to reduce noise and improve the milker's ability to move around in the pit.

Succession The orderly replacement of one plant or animal by another.

Succulence A condition of plants characterized by juiciness, freshness, and tenderness, making them appetizing to animals.

Suck wind The action of a mare taking air into her genital tract.

Suckling A foal that is still with its mother; it has not been weaned; usually it is under four months of age.

Sudden Acquired Retinal Degeneration Syndrome SARDSAcute (2 days-2 weeks) degeneration of the photoreceptors followed by the other retinal layers affecting both eyes simultaneously.

Sudden Infant Death Syndrome (SIDS) The sudden and unexpected death of a healthy infant under 1 year of age. A diagnosis of SIDS is made when an autopsy cannot determine another cause of death. The cause of SIDS is unknown. Also known as "crib" death.

Suffering An unpleasant emotional state, but the external expression of suffering through behavior is distress.

Suffix The cattery name at the end of the cat's name, if any, indicating the cattery in which the cat resides. Usually preceded by "of." In the name "CH Sheenah's Ashley of Ashmanor, DM" the suffix is "Ashmanor" ("DM" is a title) which indicates that this cat lives at the Ashmanor cattery.

Suitability Appropriateness for a particular purpose and/or a type or size of rider.

Sulfonamides A class of antibiotics which contain sulfur. They are bacteriostatic (they stop the growth (reproduction) of bacteria, but do NOT kill them).

Sulky Two-wheeled cart.

Sull To move slowly, to resist moving forward.

Sullen Sulky, resentful, or withdrawn.

Superfecundation Having a litter with more than one father (or breeding).

Superficial cells Epithelial cells exfoliated from the vagina during estrus. They are also called cornified or anucleated cells and are the largest of the epithelial cells present during estrus. The nuclei of these cells appear faded or absent. These cells stain lightly, may appear multi-layered, and with folded borders. If 80-90% of the cells in the smear are superficial cells that can be used as an indication to start breeding.

Superficial intermediate cells Epithelial cells exfoliated from the vagina during late proestrus to early estrus. They are larger than parabasal cells and have small nuclei and irregular/folded borders.

Superhutches Calf housing structures, often open on one side, designed for a small number of calves when first grouped immediately after weaning.

Supinator The Supinator is a muscle surrounding the upper one-third of the radius in the human arm. It is used to rotate the radius, thereby turning the palm of the hand forwards.

Supplement Feed or feed mixtures rich in one or more of protein, energy, vitamins, minerals or antibiotics. Combined with other feeds to produce a more complete feed.

Support Price The equivalent price of milk as set by prices of NDM, cheese, and butter offered by the Commodity Credit Corporation of USDA. These prices effectively set a minimum price for milk and intermitantly provide milk producers an indirect government subsidy.

Supportive treatment Supportive treatment corrects or modifies abnormalities that occur secondary to a disease process. For example fluid and electrolyte therapy for a patient with hypoadrenocorticism.

Supraventricular tachycardia A condition in which the heart beats very rapidly because of signals coming from the atria (chambers of the heart that receive the blood) or near the junction of the atria with the ventricles (the chambers of the heart that pump the blood to the body or lungs).

Surcingle The strap that encircles the heart girth. A belt or girth of leather or nylon webbing that is passed around the horse at the girth line and firmly fastened down.

Surplus milk The quantity of grade A fluid milk in excess of that needed for Class I purposes.

Surprise tests These are tests for verification performed on cows whose projected 2X (twice daily milking), 305D (305-day lactation), ME (mature equivalency) records exceed certain levels of milk and/or fat as established by breed associations.

Surrogate marker An indirect measure of disease progression.

Surveillance Systems The ongoing systematic collection and analysis of data. The data may lead to actions taken to prevent and control an infectious disease.

Susceptible Unprotected against disease.

Suture A suture is an anatomical term for an articulation found only in the skull, where the margins of the bones articulate with one another, but are separated by a thin layer of fibrous tissue (sutural ligament) and is continuous externally with the periosteum on the outside of the skull and internally with the fibrous layer of the dura mater.

Sutured Caslick operation having been performed.

SVECCS Society for Veterinary Emergency Medicine and Critical Care.

Swamp fever Equine infectious anemia.

Swan A large elegant species of waterfowl with breeds native around the world. Some breeds are raised for their ornamental qualities, adding a stately grace to ponds and waterways.

Sweat A mild liniment put under a waterproof wrapping to "draw" swelling and infection.

Sweat scraper Metal blade to scrape sweat and water off horse's coat.

Sweating out The process of placing a group of sheep in an enclosed area and letting the body heat generated cause the wool grease to heat. This helps to reduce second-cuts.

Sweet butter Unsalted butter.

sweet feed A commercial feed sweetened with molasses to improve palatability.

Sweetened condensed milk The food obtained by partially removing water from a mixture of milk and a safe and suitable nutritive sweetener.

Swells Exterior projection of the fork of a Western saddle.

Swine 1. A sow will average two litters a year. The litters will varyfrom 4 12 piglets each. The average size of a litter over the productive live of the sow is about eight.

2. A sow is usually kept for 3 4 years or 6 8 litters before being sold.

3. Feeder pigs are held by farmer for 6 8 weeks. They are then sold at a weight of 40 60 pounds.

4. Usually, butcher hogs are sold when they reach 220 280 lbs which occurs about 5 6 months after birth.

Swing Parlor Parlor characterized by having the milking units positioned in the middle of the parlor for use by cows on both sides.

Switch The brush of hair on the end of a bovine's tail.

Symbiosis Parasitic state in which the parasite and animal survive in a beneficial relationship – e.g. bacteria within the rumen.

Symblepharon Adherence of the conjunctiva to the cornea.

Sympathomimetic Producing effects similar to the 'flight or fight' response, which means the body is alerted to a danger of some sort and prepares to basically run or fight. Sympathomimetic effects include increased heart rate, sweating, and increased blood pressure.

Symptomatic treatment symptomatic treatment eliminates or suppresses clinical signs without affecting or knowing the underlying cause of the sign. For example antiemetics to suppress vomiting.

Synapse The location at which a nerve impulse is transmitted from one neuron to another.

Synchronization A management practice used to cause the goats to cycle at the same time.

Syncope The temporary loss of consciousness; fainting.

Syndactyl Two front toes partially joined, as in kingfishers.

Syndecans and Glypicans Integral membrane proteins in the family of heparan sulfate proteoglycans.

Syndrome A condition in which two or more different signs of disease regularly occur together in individual animals or in a population, suggesting that they are both part of the same disease.

Synergetic model (Synonymous to synergistic) coordinated or correlated action of two or more structures, agents, or physiological processes so that the combined action is greater than the sum of each acting separately.

Synergist An agent that enhances the action of another.

Synergistic Two or more drugs which enhance the effectiveness of each other.

Synovial fluid Fluid made by the synovial cells that lubricates joints

Synovial joint In anatomy, a synovial joint is one where the bones are covered with articular cartilage but are not attached to each other. These joints allow extensive movement.

Synovial Pertaining to a joint made up of bone ends covered with cartilage, ligaments, a cavity filled with synovial fluid (joint fluid) and an outside fibrous capsule, e.g., hip joint, elbow joint.

Systemic Body-wide process (e.g. systemic infection).

Systemic Disease A disease where more than one portion of the body is affected; often the whole body or one or more systems.

Systemic lupus erythematosis, SLE An autoimmune disease in which the immune system sees its own body as foreign matter. Characterized by polyarthritis, hemolytic anemia, skin disease, among many other symptoms.

Systemic lupus erythematosus SLEA multisystemic autoimmune disorder.

Systemic Throughout the body.

Systole Part of the normal beating of the heart where blood is pushed from the ventricles of the heart. This is known as the contraction phase of the heartbeat.

T

T cell Also called 'T lymphocytes.' The type of lymphocyte which is responsible for cell-mediated immunity. T cells may directly kill a cell or produce chemicals called lymphokines that activate macrophages which will kill the cell. Compare with 'B cell.'

T cytotoxic cells TC cellsTheir function is to - use perforins and cytotoxins to destroy target cells that are carrying foreign proteins on their surface.

T helper 1 cells A subset of CD4 cells that make the cytokines IFN-g and TNF on recognition of antigen. Their major function is the activation of macrophages and are sometimes called inflammatory CD4 T cells.

T helper 2 cells A subset of CD4 T cells that are characterized by the cells they produce. They are mainly involved in stimulating B cells to produce antibody, and are often called helper CD4 cells.

T lymphocyte proliferation assay A test used to measure the memory of T cells to antigens.

T Touch The Tellington Touch is a method of training developed by Linda Tellington-Jones. It is a technique which uses a combination of specific touches, lifts, and movement exercises. It is believed to enable an animal to learn new behavior more easily, promote optimal health and correct inappropriate behavior by eliminating fear and reactive responses.

T'ai chi A martial art involving meditation and slow, flowing self-guided movements that follow set forms. This is intended to bring about physical self-awareness and affect the flow of chi.

Tachycardia An abnormally rapid heart rate.

Tachypnea Rapid breathing.

Tack Equipment used on a horse (brushes, blankets, saddle, halter, bridle, etc..).

Tacrolimus A compound with similar actions as cyclosporine (inhibition of IL-2 through inhibition of calcineurin). Available as a topical ointment (0.1%).

Tagging Trimming or shearing the wool away from the tail or dock area.

Tail Bands Used for marking treated cows. Rubber bands are sometimes used to dock cow's tails.

Tail enders Cow producing low levels of milk at the end of their lactation.

Tail rope Rope attached to horse's tail by a half hitch, then tied forward to neck or harness.

Tail rubbing A habit that may originate from anal or skin itch or a dirty sheath or udder. Even when the cause is removed, the habit often persists.

Tail wrap Material to wrap tail during breeding or examination and foaling.

Tail-Set How the base of the tail is set on the rump.

Take To accept a male in coitus. Also a lay term meaning to become pregnant.

Talus In human anatomy, the talus is the principle connecting link between the foot and the bones of the leg and has an important part in the formation of the ankle.

TAN SAL Tannic acid solution used as a topical drying agent.

Tanbark trail A term often associated with those who exhibit animals in competition at fairs and livestock shows.

Tandem Parlor Parlor design where cows line up head to tail in individually opening stalls.

Tankerload In milk collection and distribution, large quantities of milk in a large stainless steel tank borne on a transport truck—the method of transporting milk.

Tapadero A leather hood fixed to the front of the stirrup. A covering over the stirrups in a western saddle to prevent the riders foot from slipping through and to give a decorative effect.

Tapetum A highly reflective layer located in the dorsal half of the choroid in most domestic species (pig and llama being exceptions).

Tapetum Lucidum The highly reflective portion of the interior of the canine eyeball that aids in night vision.

Tapetum The tapetum is the irregular sector in certain animal's eyes which shines owing to an absence of black pigment. Tapetum is found in the eyes of cats.

Tapeworms long, ribbon-like segmented flatworms that can inhabit the gastro-intestinal tract of animals.

Targeted surveillance This involves carrying out specific projects or surveys to collect information about a particular disease. The aim is usually to estimate how much of the disease there is in a given population of animals, or to provide sound evidence that the disease does not occur.

Tarsal plate A plate of cartilage that gives rigidity to the eye.

Tarsal See "tarsus"

Tarsi Plural of tarsus.

Tarsometatarsus The bone underlying the tarsus.

Tarsorrhaphy Suturing together of the eyelid margins partially or totally to make the palpebral fissue smaller or to protect the cornea.

Tarsus In human anatomy, the tarsus comprises 7 short bones which make up the skeleton of the posterior half of the foot.

Tartar A build-up of bacteria, saliva, and food on the teeth which becomes mineralized, forming a hard coating and eventually causing gum disease and tooth loss. See also 'Plaque.'

Tattoo A method of permanent identification to be crossreferenced with visible identification. Permanent ink used with tattoo numbers creates a lifetime record of identification in the ears of dairy cattle.

Tawny Used, along with white, to describe Ibizan Hounds, this color is the color of lions (sandy yellow). Also referred to as Lion Tawny. Color definitions may vary by breed. Always check the breed standard for the definitive color description.

Taxol A drug derived of Taxanes, chemically known as Paclitaxel. Derived from a natural/semi-synthetic extract of the bark of the western yew (Taxus brevifolia or Taxus baccata). Emerging as the most powerful anti-cancer drug in the treatment of breast, ovarian, Kaposi's sarcoma and AIDS-related lung cancers. Acts by disrupting the microtubule equilibrium thereby inhibiting cell replication.

T-cell This population has been trafficked through the thymus and is important in cellular immunity.

TDN Total Digestible Nutrients. Indicates the usable amounts of various nutrients found in feed.

Tea Tree Oil Volatile oil from the leaves of Melaleuca trees was used treat cuts, abrasions, burns, insect bites and minor skin problems. The oil is extracted from the leaves by steam distillation.

Tease The action of a mare in heat; the action of a stallion when he sees mares; to bring a teaser stallion near mares to determine if they are in heat.

Teaser A bitch used to get a male dog sexually aroused in order to collect semen.

Teaser bitch A bitch which is used to excite a male dog in order to collect a semen sample for semen analysis or artificial insemination.

Teaser ram A ram incapable of inseminating the ewe (eg vasectomized).

Teasing In heat.

Teat The projecting organ through which milk is drawn from the udder of female mammals in suckling young.

Teat Dip Pre and Post-milking Substance that kills bacteria and helps to seal the teat end to prevent entry of bacteria into the udder between milkings. May contain emollients to improve teat end condition for use in cold, winter conditions.

Teat meatus Small canal located in the end of each teat; also called a streak canal.

Teat orifice The opening at the bottom of the teat where milk exits. This opening serves as a potential route for bacteria to enter the teat.

Teat Sealant A product that forms a mechanical barrier on the teat end to protect the teat. Generally used at dry-off after antibiotic infusion.

Telogen The resting phase of the hair cycle before it is shed.

Telophase Telophase is the 4th stage of mitosis cell reproduction. The nuclear membrane and the nucleolus reappear and the cytoplasm undergoes constriction around the equator of the achromatic spindle. The constriction deepens and the original cell is gradually divided.

Temperament The general consistency with which a horse behaves.

Temperature Normal adult temperature varies among horses, but will usually range in degrees from 99.5°F to 100.5°F.

Temple In anatomy, the temple is the flat part either side of the head between the forehead and the ear.

Temporal association Two or more events that occur around the same time but are unrelated, chance occurrences.

Temporal bones The temporal bones are situated at the sides and base of the human skull. They assist in the protection of the cerebrum and the transmission of sound waves to the ear.

Temporalis The temporalis is the human facial muscle which raises the mandible, closing the mouth.

Temporomandibular joint The joint between the lower jaw and the skull.

Tendon A tendon is a connective tissue that joins muscles to bone in vertebrates.

Tensor A tensor is a type of muscle which tightens or stretches a part of the body.

Terete Round in cross section.

Term The gestation period.

Terminal Sires Sires that are used in a crossbreeding program where all offspring are marketed. This system allows for maximum heterosis and breed complementarity. Usually an F1 female with strong maternal traits is bred to a terminal sire that imparts carcass quality and growth ability to the offspring to be marketed. But, a supply of F1 females is necessary.

Terrestrial rabies Rabies in terrestrial mammals, mammals that walk on the ground like a skunk or raccoon.

Terrier Front Straight front as found on fox terriers.

Terrier Group A group of dogs used originally for hunting vermin.

Tertials Flight feathers attached to upper arm (humerus).

Tertiary hyperparathyroidism Tertiary hyperparathyroidism is a relatively uncommon event occurring in some chronic renal failure patients, which may result in a moderate increase in calcium.

Tertiary waste treatment Usually, the final treatment of waste water to reduce pollution potential or health hazard allowing discharge into bodies of water. Not economically practical with animal manure waste waters.

Test To evaluate the producing ability of a lactating animal; to determine the percentages of various components of milk, such as milk fat; to examine the blood of an animal for specific pathogens.

Test interval The interval, in days, between successive DHI tests. As a routine procedure, a test interval shall not consist of less than 15, or more than 45 days. For Official DHI/ DHIR records, the test interval shall not exceed 75 days.

Test jump To allow a teaser to mount a mare before the actual breeding stallion is risked.

Tester One who weighs, samples, and tests milk. Also called a test supervisor.

Testes Structures that produce sperm.

Testicle Testicle is another name for testis.

Testicles The male gonads, which produce spermatoza. AKC regulations specify that a male that does not have two normal testicles normally located in the scrotum may not compete at any show and will be disqualified, except that a castrated male may be entered in obedience trials, tracking tests, field trials (except Beagles), as a stud dog in a Stud Dog class, and Veterans class at an independent specialty.

Testicular degeneration The deterioration of the testicular tissue with resultant decrease in function.

Testicular hypoplasia Testicles that are smaller than normal.

Testis The testis is the male organ in which sperm are produced. Most mammals have two testis enclosed in the scrotum.

Testosterone A potent androgenic hormone produced chiefly by the testes; responsible for the development of male secondary sex characteristics.

Tetanus Bacterial disease caused by Ciostridium tetani.

Tetany A condition in an animal in which there are localized, spasmodic muscular contractions.

Tether To tie an animal with a rope or chain to allow grazing but prevent straying.

Texas gate Gate of barbed wire.

Thalamus The thalamus is the interior region of the brain where certain important sensory nerves, especially the optic nerve, originate.

Thalidomide A sedative and hypnotic drug C 13 H 10 N 2 O 4 that has been the cause of malformation of infants born to mothers using it during pregnancy. Thalidomide acts as an antiangiogenic agent and therefore can be inhibitory for bone formation.

Theca In anatomy, a theca is a case or sheath which encloses some organ or part.

Thenar The thenar is the ball of muscle at the base of the thumb.

Therapeutic touch A method of healing which does not involve actual physical contact. The practictioner aligns and balances the patient's natural energy fields by moving his/her hands above the patient's body. The healer consciously attempts to focus energy to the reciever to balance and unblock energy flows.

Therapeutic use Application of antimicrobials in curative does in an adequate period of time to combat an established infection.

Therapy Medical treatment.

Thiamin Also known as vitamin B_1. A component of the B complex group of vitamins. It is found in various foodstuffs and present in the free state in blood plasma and cerebrospinal fluid.

Thigh The hindquarter from hip to stifle.

Third eyelid Nictitating membrane, pink membrane in inner corner of eye that can extend across eyeball.

Third generation A description of medications developed from an earlier form of the medication. First generation medications were developed from the original form of the drug; second generation medications are adaptations of first generation drugs; third generation drugs are adaptations of second generation, etc.

Thoracic pump theory CPR performed in patients over 7 kg positioned in dorsal recumbency likely uses the thoracic pump theory which says that when the chest is compressed, the heart underneath the chest wall is not directly compressed but rather the chest compression is causing an increase in intrathoracic pressure. The increase in intrathoracic pressure collapses veins, prevents retrograde blood flow back towards the abdomen and compresses arteries which pushes blood forward towards the heart and brain. The heart is just acting as a passive conduit and doesn't change shape very much at all.

Thoracic vertebrae In anatomy, the thoracic vertebrae are the 12 vertebrae following from the cervical vertebrae. They provide articulation for the ribs.

Thorax The thorax in vertebrates is the part of the body containing the heart and lungs and protected by the rib cage.

Thorough Pin Swelling in the web of the hock that may be an unsoundness or a blemish.

Thoroughbred The breed of horse registered with the Jockey Club. Not meant to be used as a synonym for purebred. All individuals can trace ancestry back to one of five Arabian stallions.

Three in one formula A formula for partial parenteral nutrition that can be tailored to the individual patients by compounding the formula. Most, if not all, commercial solutions provide amino acids and dextrose but don't typically provide lipids.

Threshold See Seizure Threshold.

Throatiness An excess of loose skin under the throat.

Throat-latch The part of the bridle passing under the horse's head holding the bridle on over the horse's poll.

Thrombocytopenia A lower than normal number of platelets in the blood. Platelets, which are actually fragments of specific types of cells, are necessary for blood to clot. Signs of thrombocytopenia include bruising and bleeding from the nose, into the gastrointestinal tract, etc.

Thrombocytopenic purpura A disease characterized by the formation of platelet clots in the microcirculation (very small vessels). Exact cause is unclear but thought to be due to infections, inherited conditions or immunologic abnormalities. Results in bleeding with a low platelet count, anemia, neurologic symptoms kidney disease and fever.

Thromboemboli A blood clot which forms in a blood vessel, then breaks loose into circulation and may lodge and obstruct other blood vessels.

Thrombophlebitis Inflammation of a vein associated with thrombus formation. The thrombus may break loose as a thromboembolis and then plug other blood vessels.

Thrombosis The formation of blood clots in blood vessels.

Thrombus Clot in, or blocking, a blood vessel.

Throughput The number of cows that can be milked in a parlor in a given period of time.

Thrush A foul-smelling disease of the hoof which causes decomposition of the frog and other hoof structures. It is often associated with unsanitary conditions, but a more likely predisposing cause is lack of exercise and neglected foot care.

Thumb Marks Black spots on the region of the pastern.

Thymus The thymus is a ductless glandular body situated near the base of the neck in vertebrates. Its function is uncertain, and in man it disappears or diminishes soon after childhood.

Thyroid gland See "Thyroid"

Thyroid The largest of the hormone secreting (endocrine) glands located in the neck; it regulates metabolism. 1. Hyperthyroid excessive production of thyroid hormones, often seen in older dogs, causing excessive thirst, weight loss, increased appetite and restlessness.

2. Hypothyroid decreased production of thyroxine, causing poor coat, weight gain, mental dullness, fatigue, cold intolerance, and infertility.

Thyroprotein See Iodinated casein

Thyrotropin releasing hormone Hormone produced by the hypothalamus that stimulates the pituitary gland to produce thyrotropin (thyroid stimulating hormone-TSH), which in turn stimulates the thyroid gland to produce thyroid hormone. Also called TSH releasing factor or TSH releasing hormone.

Tibia The tibia is the medial and stronger of the two bones of the leg. It is prismoid in form, and posesses a shaft and two ends. Its purpose is to support the weight of the body.

Tibiotarsus In birds, the tibiotarsus is the equivalent of the tibia, but it is fused at the lower end with some of the bones of the tarsus.

TID Giving medication three times per day. Example 30 mg TID would be giving a total of 90 mg a day.

Tie Stall Parlor Facility is frequently used for both housing and milking. Cows are tied and milked with the cow and operator on the same level.

Tiedown A strap that connects to the noseband and the cinch or breastcollar; a control device to limit the height of the horse's head. Western version of the standing martingale. A strap from the girth to the noseband or bosal to keep the horse from tossing his head.

Time recording device/monitor A mechanical/electronic device that automatically monitors the interval between milkings. The time is expressed in hours plus minutes, and the device must display the starting and ending time of the previous milking.

Times milked Cows are normally milked twice per day with records being labeled 2x; however, cows may be milked more frequently (3x, 4x, etc.).

Timothy Grass hay, Phleum pratense.

Tissue A group of specialized cells that together perform a particular function, e.g., muscle tissue, nerve tissue, bone.

Titer A measurement of the amount of antibodies in the blood. The test to measure antibodies is usually performed by making a number of dilutions of the blood and then measuring at what dilution there is sufficient antibody to react in the test. For example, a titer of 1:8 (one to eight) means the blood can be diluted to one part blood and seven parts saline and still produce a positive reaction in the test. The higher the titer (1:16 is higher than 1:8), the more antibody is present. (NOTE: The word 'titer' may also be used when discussing the amount of antigen present, e.g., a high titer vaccine has a large number of virus particles.)

Titer(s) The immune system's response to a particular disease. The higher the titer number, the stronger the immune response. Titers are used to determine if an animal has been exposed to a specific virus or bacteria. If the titer numbers are near zero, the animal has not been exposed to that organism recently

Title An award earned by a cat that may be added to the cat's name according to the rules of a cat registering association. Depending on the particular title, it may be earned either by defeating other cats in one or more shows, earning some number of year-end points, or producing some number of offspring that earn titles themselves. Typically, a title is added to the beginning of the name of the cat, before the cattery name prefix, but some titles are added to the end of the cat's name. For example, in the name "CH Sheenah's Ashley of Ashmanor, DM" there are two titles. The title "CH" (Champion) is at the beginning of the name. The title "DM" (Distinguished Merit) is at the end of the name.

TMR Total mixed ration. See complete ration.

TMS See total milk solids.

TNF-alpha, beta Abbreviation for tumor necrosis factor. A cytokine produced by macrophages and T cells that has multiple functions in the immune response. It is the defining member of the TNF family of cytokines. These cytokines function as cell-associated or secreted proteins that interact with receptors of the tumor necrosis factor receptor via components known as TRAF's (tumor necrosis factor receptor associated factors).

TNTC Too numercus to count. Used primarily to describe the number of red or white cells observed per high power field when performing a urinalysis.

Tobiano A Paint and Pinto coat pattern of spots that are regular and distinct.

Toe out To walk with the feet pointed outward. Also called splay-footed.

Tolerance Tolerance is the failure to respond to an antigen; when that antigen is borne by self-tissues, tolerance is called self-tolerance.

Tolerance levels 1/1000th the level where birth defects were induced by a drug and 1/100th the level where other side effects were induced.

Tom A whole male cat.

Tomium Cutting edge of both maxilla and mandible.

Tongue The tongue is a muscular organ in the mouth of a tetrapod.

Tonic Clonic See Generalized Seizure.

Tonic The phase of a generalized seizure where the dog falls, loses consciousness and extends its legs rigidly. In a mild generalized seizure, the dog may not lose consciousness and could have little or no extension of the legs.

Tonometry Measuring pressure in the eyeball.

Tonopen tonometer An applanation tonometer used to caloculate IOP from the force required to flatten (applanate) the cornea.

Tonsils The tonsils are a pair of small organs on either side of the root of the tongue composed of lymphatic tissue and instrumental in protecting the throat from infection.

Tooth A tooth is a hard structure in the mouth of vertebrates.

Top side The sire's side of the pedigree.

Topical To be used on the skin.

Topline The proportion and curvature of the outline of a horse's neck, back, and croup; a line from poll to tail-head.

Torsion Twisting of a body part. For example, a retained testicle may twist, cutting off its blood supply.

Total body water Total body water accounts for ~ 60 to 70% of an animal's body weight. Total body water is distributed across interconnected compartments. 2/3 of total body water is located within cells and 1/3 in extracellular locations including plasma and interstitial locations

Total digestible nutrients (TDN) A standard evaluation of the nutritional merit of a particular feed for farm animals which includes all the digestible organic nutrients—protein, fiber, nitrogen-free extract, and lipids.

Total milk solids (TMS) Primarily milk fat, proteins, lactose, and minerals.

Total Mixed Ration (TMR) Complete ration consisting of concentrate, roughage, and supplements necessary to meet the daily nutrient and energy nutritional requirements of the cow or heifer.

Total parenteral nutrition TPN Providing 100% of a patient's caloric needs by the intravenous route through a central catheter.

Total protein TP All the proteins in the blood stream including albumin, immunoglobulins and other globulins. TP can be measured with a refractometer or by chemical methods.

Totipalmate All 4 toes connected by web.

Totipotent stem cells Totipotent cells can become all types of cells.

Tovero A Paint coat pattern that has markings of both the overo and the tobiano.

Toxemia Capacity of parasite to produce toxins (endotoxins or exotoxins). Be cautious about differentiating this from a toxic substance, such as lead poisoning from old batteries, or toxic plants.

Toxic Harmful.

Toxic epidermal necrolysis TEN Cutaneous lesions with 2 forms in humans: Staphylococcal scalded skin syndrome (SSSS) which is seen generally in children and is caused by the elaboration of an exfoliating toxin from S. aureus. TEN (Lyell's disease) is the adult form which is identical clinically, but thought to be caused by a different factor.

Toxic shock syndrome An acute, sometimes fatal, intoxication by an infectious agent during which organ activity is blocked causing severe shock and hypotension.

Toxicity Referring to medical treatments, the degree to which they produce unwanted, adverse effects.

Toxicology The study of poisons (toxicants).

Toxin Any poisonous substance of biological origin.

Toxins The poisons produced by certain microorganisms. They are products of cell metabolism. The symptoms of bacterial diseases, such as diphtheria, tetanus, botulism, and staphylococcal food poisoning, are caused by toxins.

Toxoid Inactivated toxin from a particular bacteria that is injected and generates antibodys to the toxin.

TPR A common medical abbreviation for temperature, pulse, and respiration.

Trace Heavy strap that attaches the harness to the vehicle or load being pulled.

Trace minerals (TM) Minerals that are required in very small amounts.

Trachea The trachea (windpipe) carries air from the larynx to the bronchi.

Tracheobronchitis Inflammation of the trachea and bronchi.

Tracing Finding out where an animal has come from or where it has gone, particularly when investigating outbreaks of disease. We need to find the farms which have sent any animals to the affected farm so we can check whether they were the source of the disease. Animals which have left the affected farm may be carrying the disease, so we need to find them so they can be checked.

Track A path. Also to follow.

Tractable A quality in a horse's disposition that makes him cooperative and trainable.

Tractor Heavy duty vehicle, low geared, used to carry, push, and/or pull implements for tillage, planting, and harvesting crops.

Trade barriers Rules and regulations that hamper the trade of commodities. Tariffs, fees for imported goods and import limits or quotas are barriers to trade.

Trailer Vehicle towed to move horses; long extension on heel of horseshoe.

Trainer Person who specializes in training horses.

Trait Any measurable or observable characteristic of an animal.

Tranquilizer A drug that calms an animal without affecting consciousness.

Transabdominal ultrasonography Passing sound waves through the belly to see internal organs and structures.

Transcription The process of constructing a messenger RNA molecule using a DNA molecule as a template. The messenger RNA (mRNA) is the unstable intermediate in the formation of a protein. (If the DNA is the cookbook, the mRNA is the recipe copied from the cookbook to make the protein (the cake)).

Transdermal Absorption of a drug across the intact skin.

Transfaunation When rumen juices and flora from a healthy animal are placed in an animal where normal rumen function has been compromised.

Transforming Growth Factor-Beta Receptors A receptor on cell membranes that binds TGF-beta, a growth factor involved in a number of biological events important in normal and abnormal growth of cells and tissues.

Transgenic Having chromosomes into which one or more "foreign" genes (genes from a different organism and/or genes that have been modified) have been incorporated either artificially or naturally.

Transgenic models Genetic manipulation of an animal's genes, usually mice

Transient Temporary.

Transition Cow A cow that is from 2 months before 1 month after expected calving date.

Transition Housing Barns designed especially for transition cows, often including a maternity area.

Transition Upward or downward change between gaits, speed, direction, or maneuvers.

Transitional cell carcinoma TCC A tumor originating from the transitional epithelium lining the urinary tract. The most common location for development of transitional cell carcinoma tumors is in the trigone of the urinary bladder.

Transmissibility/contagiousness Capacity of parasite to spread between animals – e.g. Salmonella dublin is regard as highly contagious between heifers and calves via feces.

Transmissible Spongiform Encephalopathies A group of diseases which includes BSE in cattle, scrapie in sheep and variant Creutzfeld-Jakob Disease (vCJD) in people.

Transplacental Transplacental means crossing the placenta. The placenta is the in-utero connection between the mother and the fetus. Transplacental means something (a drug, antibodies, an infectious agent, etc.) crosses from the mother to the fetus before birth. This can be good in the case of antibodies that protect the newborn from disease early in life or bad if it is an infectious agent that transfers from mother to baby.

Transport host An animal or insect which carries an immature parasite from one mammalian host to another.

Transposons (Jumping Genes) Mobile elements of DNA that can insert into new locations in the chromosomal DNA and that can affect the function of genes at or near the insertion site.

Transrectal ultrasonography Placing the ultrasound probe into the rectum in order to more clearly recognize internal organs and structures

Transtracheal wash When fluid from the lungs is collected and then evaluated.

Transverse Cross sectional view of a structure.

Transverse Myelitis The sudden onset of spinal cord disease. Symptoms include general back pain followed by weakness in the feet and legs that moves upward. There is no cure and many patients are left with permanent disabilities or paralysis. Transverse Myelitis is a demyelinating disorder that may be associated with Multiple Sclerosis (MS). Also see demyelinating disorders.

Trapezium The trapezium is a small bone in the human hand below the little finger.

Trapezium bone The trapezium bone is one of the bones in the human wrist.

Trapezius The trapezius is a human muscle. It is a flat, triangular muscle, covering the back of the neck and shoulder.

Trapezoid bone The trapezoid bone is one of the bones in the human wrist.

Trappy Course with sharp turns.

Travasol An amino acid solution used in TPN and PPN.

Travel The path of the flight of each limb during movement.

Travers Haunches-in The horse is slightly bent around the inside leg of the rider. Its outside legs pass and cross in front of the inside legs. The horse is looking in the direction in which it is moving. Performed along the wall or on the centerline, at an angle of about thirty degrees to the direction in which the horse is moving.

Tree The basic framework of the saddle over which the leather is laid and attached.

Trematode A parasitic fluke.

Triceps The Triceps are muscles situated on the back of the upper arms in the human body.

Trichiasis Condition in which hairs originating from normal locations turn inward and cause irritation.

Trichogram This is a hair "plucks". The trichogram is useful to evaluate the integrity of hair shafts and also serves as a test for demodicosis and dermatophytosis.

Tricuspid valve defect A defect in the heart valve that separates the right atrium and the right ventricle.

Tricyclic antidepressant A class of antidepressants which work by decreasing the amount of certain chemical transmitters taken up by specific nerve cells. The tricyclic antidepressants include clomipramine, amitriptyline, and nortryptyline and are often used to treat behavioral problems in small animals.

Triple Bar Ascending staircase jump consisting of three bars that add spread and increase in height.

Triquetral bone The triquetral bone is one of the bones in the human wrist.

Tris EDTA solution A combination of EDTA, tromethane [hydroxy-methyl] aminomethane) and sodium dodecyl sulfate used intreatment of Pseudomonas otitis.

Trocar An instrument used in an emergency to relieve the gas from a distended rumen.

Trochanter The trochanter is a protuberance in

the upper part of the femur to which the muscles attach.

Trochoides In anatomy, a trochoides is a pivot joint.

Trombiculidiasis Chiggers.

Trot A two-beat diagonal gait.

Trough Level Either the results from,or the testing of the AED blood serum values just before the next medication dosage is given. It is at this time that the AED is at its lowest level in the blood.

TRP-2 Abbreviation for tyrosine related protein-2, a melanogenesis- related protein shown to be immunogenic in animal model and humans.

Trypsin Trypsin is an enzyme present in pancreatic juice. It converts proteins into peptones.

Tubule Microscopic ducts. The tubules in the kidneys help to concentrate the urine.

Tucked-up Hunchbacked and empty bellied.

Tumor a. A swelling; a morbid enlargement. b. A neoplasm; i.e., a mass of new tissue, physiologically useless, growing independently of its surroundings.

Tup A male sheep.

Tupping Putting the rams and ewes together for mating. Joining is the same thing.

Turgor Normal state of distention and resiliency of the skin.

Turkey A large game bird native to the Americas. Wild turkeys are found throughout North and South America and there are a number of domesticated breeds. Males are called toms, females called hens and chicks are known as poults.

Turmeric An ingredient of Indian curries which is thought to have medicinal properties. It is derived from the root of the plant Curcuma longa which has spongy, orange bulbs and yellow, trumpet-shaped flowers. Turmeric is used in Ayurvedic medicine as a digestive aid.

Turn on the Forehand Maneuver in which the horse's hindquarters rotate around his forehand.

Turn on the Haunches (hindquarters) Maneuver in which the horse's forehand rotates around his hind end.

Turnout Overall appearance of a horse (and rider).

Twitch A means of restraint. A nose twitch is often a wooden handle with a loop of chain, applied to the horse's upper lip.

Two hand To ride with one rein in each hand.

Two point To rise from the saddle, so you contact the horse with only your thighs, not your seat.

Two tooth or yearling A sheep of either sex from about 1 year to 1 ½ years old and showing two permanent incisor teeth. Sheep usually get 2 adult front teeth every 12 months for the first 4 years of life; after this they are then known as full-mouthed sheep

Two-track A lateral movement, where the horse's forefeet and hind feet move on separate tracks. Also called the half-pass.

Tying up A form of metabolic muscle stiffness caused from irregularity in feed and work schedules.

Tympanum The tympanum (middle ear) is a cavity in the temporal bone filled with air, closed externally by the tympanic membrane and containing a chain of small bones which convey sound vibrations to the inner ear.

Type A particular style of horse with certain characteristics that contribute to its value and efficiency for a particular use.

Type classification A program sponsored by breed associations whereby a registered animal's conformation may be compared with the "ideal" or "true" type animal of that breed by an official inspector (classifier).

Type I diabetes A form of diabetes in which so little insulin is produced that supplemental insulin must be given for the animal to live. Also called insulin dependent diabetes mellitus (IDDM).

Type II diabetes A type of diabetes mellitus in which although the blood glucose levels are higher than normal, they are not immediately life-threatening, and the animal can survive without supplemental insulin. Also called non-insulin dependent diabetes mellitus (NIDDM).

U

Udder The encased group of mammary glands provided with teats or nipples as in a cow, ewe, mare or sow. Also referred to as a bag.

Ulcer Loss of continuity of the epidermis. Often slow to heal.

Ulna The ulnar is one of the two long bones which form the human lower arm. It connects with the humerus at the elbow.

Ultrasonography Passing sound waves through a structure or organ in order to see its internal structure and consistency.

Ultrasound US An imaging technique in which sound waves are passed through body tissues in order to view the size, shape, location and internal structure of an organ or tissue.

Umbilical cord Naval cord. Attaches foal to mother, at the navel, through which nutrients and waste pass between the mare's placenta and the foal.

Umbilical Hernia A usually self-correcting hernia of the intestines in which protrusion occurs through the abdominal wall in the region of the navel.

Umbilicus The area where the umbilical cord was attached during gestation. This is commonly known as the "belly button."

Unavailable protein/heat damaged protein Portion of the protein irreversibly bound to the fibre fraction in feedstuffs. It is usually a small fraction of the total protein, but can be greatly increased by heat.

Unciform The unciform is a small bone in the human hand below the first finger.

Undegradable intake protein UIP Portion of ingested protein that escapes rumen degradation and is digested directly in the other stomachs or small intestine; generally a more expensive source of protein. Commonly referred to as 'bypass' protein.

Under shot or bull dog mouth The lower jaw is longer than the upper jaw, and the teeth extend forward past the dental pad on upper jaw.

Underage Dam Dam under eight months of age at the time of mating.

Underage Sire Sire under seven months of age at the time of mating.

Undercoat Dense, soft, short coat concealed by a longer top coat.

Underline The length and shape of the line from the elbow to the sheath or udder.

Undershot The front teeth (incisors) of the lower jaw overlapping or projecting beyond the front teeth of the upper jaw when the mouth is closed.

Undifferentiated A cell that has not yet developed into the type of cell it will eventually be. An un-differentiated cell may be able to develop into different cell types (that is, it may be a stem cell), or its fate may already be determined (lineage restricted).

Unilateral Involving one side.

Unilateral Cryptorchid See Cryptorchid

Unit livestock method Applicable to livestock raised or purchased before maturity. Livestock must be grouped into class and age. A value is set for each year of the animal's life to maturity. The total of these amounts should equal the cost of raising the animal to maturity.

United Kennel Club (UKC) An official registry in the United States for purebred dogs.

Unsaturated fat Any fat that is not completely hydrogenated. Unsaturated fats are liquid at room temperature. Examples: corn oil, vegetable oil.

Unsound A dog incapable of performing the functions for which it was bred.

Unsoundness A defect that may or may not be seen but that does affect serviceability.

Unthrifty Unhealthy appearing and/or failing to grow at a normal rate.

Ununited anconeal process, UAP The anconeal process never unites with the ulna, can detach and form a loose body in the joint, called a joint mouse.

up until it touches the horse's throat.

Upper Arm The humerus or bone of the foreleg, between the shoulder blade and the forearm and associated tissues.

Upright silo Storage unit for high moisture feed, generally silage, either upright.

Urate A chemical compound which contains uric acid and is made by the body, and can form crystals and stones in the urinary bladder. Uric acid is a waste product from the breakdown of certain proteins.

Urea Wasteproduct of protein metabolism that is removed from the body by the kidneys.

Urease An enzyme that breaks down urea. Urea is a wasteproduct of protein metabolism that is removed from the body by the kidneys.

Ureter A small tubular structure leading from the kidney to the bladder. There are 2 ureters, one from each kidney.

Urethra The tubular structure through which urine flows after it leaves the bladder. During ejaculation sperm are transported to the outside through the urethra.

Urethroliths A general term referring to mineral deposits that form an obstruction in the urethra of male dogs.

Urethroscopy An examination of the urethra using an endoscope.

Urinary bladder The sac-like structure that holds urine until the animal passes the urine.

Urinary Calculi Metabolic disease of male lambs characterized by the formation of stones within the urinary tract. It is caused primarily by an imbalance of dietary calcium and phosphorus.

Urinary incontinence A phrase used to describe the inability to control urination.

Urinary obstruction A blockage in the urinary system, most often occurring in the urethra, the tube that leads from the urinary bladder to the outside of the body.

Urinary retention A condition in which the urinary bladder does not rid itself of all urine it contains during the process of urination.

Urination To pass urine.

Urine Liquid wastes.

Urine specific gravity USG The weight of urine compared to an equal volume of pure water. USG can be used as a measure or kidney function.

Uro vagina Presence of urine in the vagina.

Uroliths or urolithiasis Describing a variety of stones that are found in the urinary system. These include kidney and bladder stones.

Uropygial gland Papilla on top of uropygium that secretes oils for preening.

Uropygium The fleshy posterior end supporting the tail.

Urticaria An allergic reaction of the skin characterised by reddened irregular, elevated patches and severe itching. Also called hives.

USP United States Pharmacopeia - a drug regulating agency.

Uterine inertia Ineffective or absence of uterine contractions during delivery.

Uterine prolapse A side effect that may occur after a difficult birth where the the uterus comes out the birth canal.

Uterine torsion Twisting of an organ, in this case, twisting of the uterus.

Uterine tubes Tubes that connect the ovarian bursa to the uterus. Eggs are transported through these tubes to the uterus.

Uteroverdin A green pigment present in the placenta attached to the endometrium of a bitch. As placental separation occurs during whelping the pigment is discharged.

Uterus The uterus (womb) is the organ in which young are conceived, develope and are protected until birth.

Uticaria The eruption of red marks on the skin that are usually accompanied by itching. This condition can be caused by an allergy (e.g. to food or drugs), stress, infection or physical agents (e.g. heat or cold). Also known as hives.

Utility Utility breeds are the traditional "barnyard" birds, bred for a combination of egg laying abilities and meat production capabilities. These are all-purpose breeds.

Utility Dog (UD) A title awarded to a dog that has been recorded a Utility Dog by the AKC as a result of having won certain minimum scores in Utility classes at a specified number of AKC licensed or member obedience trials. This title may be combined with the TD or TDX title and shown as UDT or UDTX, respectively.

Uvea The vascular layer of the eye comprised of the iris, ciliary body, and choroid. The function is nutritio.n

Uveodermatologic syndrome, Vogt-Koyanagi-Harada-like syndrome depigmentation of the skin and hair, and of the nose, lips, eyelids, footpads and anus. (In humans this disease is believed to be immune-mediated.)

V

V.E.E Venezuelan equine encephalomyelitis.

V Vaccine Product made from disease-causing organisms and used to produce immunity.

Vaccination The act of giving a vaccine. See also 'immunization,' since the two words have different meanings and are often confused.

Vaccine A preparation of a weakened or killed pathogen, such as a bacterium or virus, or of a portion of the pathogen's structure that upon administration stimulates antibody production or cellular immunity against the pathogen but is incapable of causing severe infection.

Vaccine Adverse Event Reporting System (VAERS) A database managed by the Centers for Disease Control and Prevention and the Food and Drug Administration. VAERS provides a mechanism for the collection and analysis of adverse events associated with vaccines currently licensed in the United States. Reports to VAERS can be made by the vaccine manufacturer, recipient, their parent/guardian or health care provider.

Vaccine failure A term often used to describe a condition in which an animal who was vaccinated against a disease still gets the disease. In truth, there is usually nothing wrong with the vaccine, but for some reason, the animal's immune system did not adequately react to it.

Vaccine Safety Datalink Project (VSD) In order to increase knowledge about vaccine adverse events, the Centers for Disease Control and Prevention have formed partnerships with four large health Management Organizations (HMOs) to continually evaluate vaccine safety. The project contains data on more than 6 million people. Medical records are monitored for potential adverse events following immunization. The VSD project allows for planned vaccine safety studies as well as timely investigations of hypothesis.

Vaccine Suspension of attenuated or killed microbes or toxins administered to induce active immunity.

Vaccinia virus Virus causing cowpox, used by Edward Jenner in the successful vaccination against smallpox, which is caused by the related variola virus.

Vagina The part of the female reproductive tract connected to the vulva on one end and the cervix on the other.

Vaginal cytology Taking samples of the epithelial cells lining the vagina in order to help determine the state of the bitches cycle.

The appearance of the cells changes in response to estrogen.

Vaginal prolapse Prolapse of the vagina through the lips of the vulva. Vaginal prolapse most often occurs during proestrus or early estrus, during the time of estrogen stimulation.

Vaginal speculum Instrument to enable dilation of vagina so it and cervix may be examined visually.

Vaginitis Inflammation of the vagina.

Valerian The root of Valeriana officinalis has been used as a mild tranquilizer and sleep aid.

Van Horse truck with large box holding several horses.

Van or **van pattern** A color pattern which restricts color to the head and the tail, leaving the body and most of the extremities white. Most standards for this pattern allow for no more than two small spots of color on the body. The name comes from the Turkish Van breed, which always exhibit this pattern.

Variable Accreditation Program VAPA set of standards set by the American Animal Hospital Association (AAHA) which serve as a yardstick for measuring quality of patient care and a vehicle for setting specific goals for the hospital staff.

Variant Creutzfeld-Jacob disease A form of CJD which is believed to result from people eating meat from cattle with BSE.

Variation The amount of difference observed or measured for a trait in a group of animals.

Varicella Chickenpox

Variety within a breed, there may be specific variations known as varieties - For example, a Golden Laced Wyandotte and a Silver Laced Wyandotte would both be recognizable as part o the Wyandotte breed, but each variety has a different color pattern. Typically the term variety is used in reference to a "recognized" variety (see standard). A bird can recognizable as a member of a breed, but not be in a recognized variety.

Varminty A keen, very bright or piercing expression.

Vascular Of, characterized by, or containing vessels that carry or circulate fluids, such as blood, lymph, or sap, through the body of an animal or plant.

Vasculitis Inflammation of the endothelial lining of a blood vessel.

Vasoconstriction A decrease in the diameter of blood vessels.

Vasodilator Agent which dilates, or increases the diameter of blood vessels.

Vasopressin An extremely potent vasoconstrictor. It may replace the use of epinephrine in treatment of refractory ventricular fibrillation.

Vasopressor A drug that stimulates the contraction of the muscle in the walls of capillaries and arteries causing vasoconstriction and an increase in blood pressure.

Vat pasteurization The heating of milk, while stirring in a vessel, to a temperature of at least 62.8°C (145°F) for 30 minutes.

VCAPP Veterinary and Comparative Anatomy, Pharmacology and Physiology.

VCS Veterinary Clinical Sciences.

Veal A calf (usually male) that is raised on milk and is intended to be used for meat at a young age. Veal meat is served at many restaurants and is very popular in cultural cuisine.

Veal calf A calf used for meat when 4 to 8 weeks old.

Vector A sequence of genetic material used to introduce specific genes into the genome of an organism. A carrier molecule.

Veil The portion of the dog's forelock hanging straight down over the eyes or partially covering them.

Vein A blood vessel that carries blood back to the heart. The pressure in veins is lower than in arteries. Veins contain less oxygen and nutrients than arteries and contain waste products that they carry to the lungs or other organs for disposal.

Vena cava Either of two large veins carrying blood to the right atrium of the heart. The cranial vena cava brings blood from the head region, front legs, and upper chest to the heart; the caudal (or posterior) vena cava carries blood from the areas of the abdomen and hind legs to the heart.

Venereal Sexually transmitted. Transmissible venereal tumors occur on the genital organs; penis or vagina, and are transmitted from dog to dog by sexual contact.

Venous Referring to the system of veins.

Vent The outside opening of the cloaca, which is a common passageway for feces, urine, and reproduction.

Ventilator A device that is used to control breathing.

Ventricle A chamber of the heart that pumps blood to the lungs and the rest of the body. A sheep or goat's heart has two ventricles, left and right.

Ventricular arrhythmia A heart condition in which the heart beats irregularly and/or at an abnormal rate because of signals coming from the ventricles (chambers of the heart that pump the blood).

Verification test A special test conducted on Official DHI/DHIR herds to verify production records of cows and herds or for investigation of rule violations. A supervised preliminary milking prior to the verification test is required to determine a 24-hour milking interval. (Tests may be ordered by breed organizations, state DHI boards of directors, state DHI managers and/or the Extension dairy specialist for NCDHIP.)

Verified identification program (VIP) A program sponsored by the National DHIA, Inc., in which a DHIA supervisor verifies the required identification information for an animal. NDHIA issues an identification certificate, permanently identifying the animal and its parentage.

Verminous pneumonia Pneumonia caused by worms.

Vertebra The vertebrae are the bones of the vertebral column. Vertebrae are irregular bones comprised of two distinct parts, an anterio termed the body, and a posterior part termed the vertebral arch.

Vertebrae The segments of the backbone. Each vertebrae is separated from adjacent vertebrae by a spongy structure called a disk.

Vertebral column The vertebral column is the central axis of all vertebrate animals. It is comprised of a number of independant irregular bones (vertebrae), which are firmly connected to one another, but are capable of a limited amount of independant movement.

Vertebrate Animal with a vertebral column (spine); includes such animals as fish, birds, turtles, reptiles, amphibians, and mammals.

Vertical Straight or upright fence.

Vertical transmission Ways an infection is spread from a parent to its offspring.

Vesicle Small elevated area on the skin filled with a clear fluid.

Vestibular Pertaining to balance. The inner ear and the cerebellum of the brain are responsible for maintaining balance.

Vestibular system Portions of the inner ear, nerves, and brain which help the body maintain balance.

Vestibulum The area of the female genital tract between the vulva and the vestibular sphincter that opens into the vagina cavity and has on it's floor the opening of the urethra.

Veterinary Investigation Diagnosis Analysis A database which records the results from samples sent to the laboratories of the VLA and SAC.

Veterinary Laboratories Agency An Executive Agency of Defra. It provides specialist veterinary services and advice to the UK Government, and advisory services to farmers and vets. These include post-mortem examinations, laboratory tests and on-farm investigations of disease problems.

Veterinary Officer A veterinary surgeon who works for the State Veterinary Service.

VFA (volatile fatty acids) Commonly used in reference to acetic, propionic, and butyric acids produced in the rumen of cattle, goats, and sheep, in the cecum of sheep, the cecum and colon of swine, the colon of the horse, and the cecum of the rabbit.

Vice Abnormal behavior in the stable environment that results from confinement or improper management and can affect a horse's usefulness, dependability, and health. Examples are cribbing and weaving.

Vicryl rapide An absorbable suture which breaks down in about 2 weeks.

Villi Microscopic projections which cover the intestine, greatly increasing the surface area and therefore, increasing the ability to absorb nutrients. Singular: Villus.

VIN Veterinary Information Network (on-line veterinary community).

Vinblastin A chemotherapeutic drug derived from Vinca rosea that arrests cell division in mitosis and exhibits antimetabolic activity. Used in the treatment of Hodgkin's disease, choriocarcinoma, acute and chronic leukemia and other neoplastic diseases.

Virgin Never been bred.

Virucide A substance that kills viruses.

Virulence factor A specific factor possessed by an organism rendering the organism pathogenic, or established in the host E.g. enzymes, toxins and so on.

Virulence The ability that a microorganism has to cause an infection or disease. Microorganisms which have the ability to cause more severe disease are said to be highly virulent.

Virus Any of various simple submicroscopic parasites of plants, animals, and bacteria that often cause disease and that consist essentially of a core of RNA or DNA surrounded by a protein coat. Unable to replicate without a host cell, viruses are typically not considered living organisms.

Virus-like particle An assembly of capsid proteins into a shell like structure without nucleic acid and thus non- infectious. These empty shells can display conformational epitopes that are not present on individual purified capsid proteins.

VIS Veterinary Information Systems.

Viscera A general term for the abdominal organs which are also called viscera.

Viscerocutaneous Pertaining to the internal organs and skin.

Viscosity Thickness of a fluid, e.g., molasses is more viscous than water.

Visera The internal organs of the body.

Visible identification A readily visible, numbering system attached to the animal that is used to identify the animal easily on test day.

Vital signs The signs of life which are pulse, respiration, and temperature.

Vitamin An organic substance found in foods and essential in small quantities for growth, health and survival. The body needs vitamins as well as other food constituents such as proteins, fats, carbohydrates, minerals and water. Vitamins serve as coenzymes or cofactors in enzymatic reactions. They are required only in trace quantities because they are not consumed in the reactions.

Vitamin A A fat-soluble, organic alcohol formed in animal tissues from carotenoids found in plants. Also called retinol. It is formed from carotenoids, principally carotene, in the intestinal epithelium, except by cats, and stored in the liver. It is essential for proper growth and maintenance of surface epithelium, for the accurate sculpting and proper growth of bones, and for the maintenance of light-sensitive pigments in the eye.

Vitamin B A group of water-soluble substances. Excess amounts of B vitamins are eliminated from the body in the urine. B vitamins include biotin, choline, folic acid, niacin, pantothenic acid, pyridoxine, riboflavin, thiamin, and vitamin B_{12}.

Vitamin B_1 See thiamin

Vitamin B_{12} Generic term describing all corrinoids with biological activity of cyanocobalamin. Required by all cells for nuclear maturation and cell division but required particularly for erythropoiesis. The vitamin is produced by ruminants who require only cobalt in sufficient quantities in their diet.

Vitamin B_2 See riboflavin

Vitamin B_6 A group of methylpyridine derivatives that include pyridoxine, pyridoxamine, pyridoxal.

Vitamin C See ascorbic acid

Vitamin D A group of closely related steroids that have antirachitic properties. They commence as provitamins in both plants and animals and are converted by exposure to ultraviolet light. In animals the provitamin 7-dehydrocalciferol is irradiated to form vitamin D_3.

Vitamin E An alpha-tocopherol, one of the three tocopherols found in wheat germ. It is an important nutrient with a number of physiologic and pharmacologic effects. As a potent antioxidant, it reduces fat oxidation, and it increases the production of HDL cholesterol. At higher doses, it also reduces cyclooxygenase and lipooxygenase activities thus decreasing the production of prostaglandins and leukotrienes. As such, it is a potent anti-inflammatory drug. It will, however, reduce platelet function and prolong the bleeding time slightly in healthy individuals. Levels greater than 100 IU/day can create hepatolipidosis in cats.

Vitamin K Group of fat-soluble compounds which are required for the formation of prothrombin and therefore play an important role in blood clotting. They are present in most green feeds and are not likely to be absent from natural diets.

Vitamins Small organic compounds, necessary for proper metabolism, that are found in feed in minute amounts. Deficiencies result in distinct diseases or syndromes.

Vitiligo Depigmentation.

Vitreocentesis Obtaining a sample of fluid from the vitreous for cytology or culture.

Vitreous Clear, jellylike substance filling the vitreous chamber, the most posterior cavity in the eye, comprising two-thirds of the volume of the eye. Maintains the shape of the globe.

Vivonex By Norwich Eaton. A hypoallergenic elemental diet.

VMP Veterinary Microbiology and Pathology.

Vogt Koyanagi-Harada syndrome Uveodermatologic syndrome or "uveitis with poliosis and vitiligo". Syndrome of uveitis, alopecia, depigmentation and whitening of the hairs.

Volatile fatty acids VFABy products of digestion in the rumen that make an acidic environment and keep pathogenic bacterial populations down.

Volatilization The loss of gaseous materials, such as ammonia nitrogen, from animal manures to the atmosphere.

Volte Circle with a 6-meter diameter (20 feet).

Volvulus Twisting of the stomach or intestine, which often has the effect of cutting off the blood supply to it.

Vomer The vomer is a thin flat bone which forms the hinder and lower part of the septum of the human nose.

Vomeronasal organ Sensory organ also called 'Jacobson's organ,' which detects pheromones.

Von Willebrand's disease Von Willebrand's disease deficiency of coagulation factor VIII causing prolonged bleeding time. This can be an autosomal dominant trait, but Bernese Mountain Dogs have Type I, which is an autosomal recessive trait.

Von Willebrand's factor A blood factor that promotes platelet adhesion.

VPRD Office Of Veterinary Public Relations and Development.

VTH Veterinary Teaching Hospital.

Vulva The opening into the female genital tract from the outside of the animal.

W

W.E.E Western equine encephalomyelitis.

WADDL Washington Animal Disease Diagnostic Laboratory.

Waist The waist is the part of the body between the ribs and the hips.

Walk Gaiting pattern in which three legs are in support of the body at all times, each foot lifting from the ground one at a time in regular sequence.

Walking dandruff Common name for Cheyletiella infestation.

Walk-Through Parlor Upon completion of milking, cows walk through the front of the stall to exit.

Walleye An eye with a whitish iris; a blue eye, fisheye, pearl eye.

War bridle Restraining rope placed under nose, over gums, and up over poll.

Warm-blooded Having a relatively high body temperature that is regulated internally and is independent of the environmental temperature. Mammals and birds are warm-blooded.

Warrigal A wolflike yellowish-brown wild dog of Australia.

Wart Benign growth caused by a virus.

Wash pen A corral or pen with a solid floor and permenent sprinklers or other washing devices for cleaning cows collectively prior to milking. Usually associated with a holding area.

Wash racks Area set aside for bathing of animals.

Wasting Loss of muscle mass due to decreased food intake or increased metabolic rate.

Wasty a. Too much fat on a carcass; b. An animal that has a paunchy middle.

Water soluble vitamins Includes B complex vitamins and vitamin C. Not normally supplemented for ruminants after two months of age because rumen microbes are able to manufacture enough to meet the animal's requirements.

Watershed A region or area that has drainage ultimately into a particular watercourse or body of water.

Wattles Pieces of red flesh that hang under the chickens' beaks.

Wax Colostrum coming from or coagulated on mare's teats just prior to foaling.

Waxing Showing evidence of wax.

WBC White blood cell. There are several types of WBCs including, neutrophils, lymphocytes, eosinophils and monocytes.

Wean To take the young animal away from their mother so they are not able to get milk. This is done so the animal will learn to eat on its own.

Weaner An animal that has been weaned from its mother or has stopped suckling its mother (usually 5 to 7 months old).

Weaning A weaned foal.

Weanling A foal that has been separated from its mother; usually 4–12 months of age.

Weaving Rhythmic swaying of weight from one front foot to the other when confined. Can be socially contagious.

Web of Life The concept that all organisms are interrelated. If one part of the "web" is broken, the entire web is affected.

Webbed Connected by a membrane.

Webbed Toes Toes connected by a skin membrane; important for water-retrieving dogs, providing help in swimming.

Weedy An insufficient amount of bone; light boned.

Weighing Procedure used by supervisors and dairy producers to determine the amount of milk given by a cow on test day.

Weight averaged molecular weight The sum of the number of molecules at each number-averaged molecular weight divided by the total number of molecules in solution. The weight-averaged molecular weight gives an indication of how long a solution will exert an oncotic effect. Generally, the larger the weight-averaged molecular weight, the longer it lasts.

Weimaraner A large breed of hunting dog that originated in Germany, having a smooth grayish coat.

Well Let Down Having short hocks; refers to short metatarsals.

Welsh Corgi Either of two breeds of dog that originated in Wales, having a long body, short legs, and a foxlike head.

West Highland White Terrier A small white terrier with upright ears and tail, developed in Scotland from Cairn, Scottish, and Skye terriers.

Western Banding A grooming technique using tiny rubber bands to make thirty or forty little pony tails out of the mane.

Western Referring to riding with Western tack and attire.

Western white-face A term used to describe the typical ewe utilized on large commercial range sheep operations in the United States. Historically they are comprised predominately of the Rambouillet breed, ,with Columbia or Targhee genetics in their makeup.

Wet cow average Average milk production by lactating cows. Goal is 70 to 80 lbs/day, 21,000-24,000 per year.

Wet ewe A ewe that is nursing a lamb.

Wet Neck Loose or superfluous skin; with dewlap.

Wether Castrated male sheep.

Wethers Uterus.

Wheal A circumscribed raised lesion of edemma of the dermas. A large number of wheals is urticaria.

Wheaten Pale yellow or fawn color. The color of wheat. Color definitions may vary by breed. Always check the breed standard for the definitive color description.

Wheel Back A marked arch of the thoracic and lumbar vertebrae.

Whelp Date The date of birth of a litter.

Whelping The act of birthing puppies.

Whey The water and solids of milk that remain after the curd is removed. It contains about 93.5 percent water and 6.5 percent lactose, protein, minerals, enzymes, water-soluble vitamins and traces of fat.

Whiffletree (whippletree) A device, usually wooden with metal rings or hooks, to which traces are attached; may also be double to hold two single whiffletrees.

Whip Tail Carried out stiffly straight and pointed.

Whip training Training horse to respond to touch of whip.

Whipworm Common name for a roundworm often parasitic in the human intestines.

Whiskers Vibrissae or sensory organs (hairs) on the sides of the muzzle.

White The color of dog that lacks pigmentation.

White blood cells Cells in the blood whose major role is to defend the body against invading organisms such as bacteria, viruses, and fungi. There are different types of leukocytes: lymphocytes are part of the immune system; monocytes, eosinophils, and neutrophils eat or engulf organisms; basophils contain histamine and are involved in inflammatory reactions.

White line White border between sole and wall of horse's.

White matter Outer part of the spinal cord, looks white because of the myelinated (a white fatty substance that wraps axons) spinal tracts running through this area

White muscle disease A disease caused by a deficiency of selenium, Vitamin E or both that causes degeneration of skeletal and cardiac muscles of lambs.

White Muscle Disease A disease caused by a deficiency of selenium, Vitamin E or both that causes degeneration of skeletal and cardiac muscles of goats.

Whitelies Body color white with red or dark markings. Color definitions may vary by breed. Always check the breed standard for the definitive color description.

WHO World Health Organization.

Whole milk Milk as collected from the cow.

Whole Not neutered or spayed.

Whooping cough An acute infectious disease caused by Bordetella Pertusis with recurrent spasms of coughing ending in a sonorous and convulsive respiration. SYN pertussis

Wind sucker Cribber, a horse that holds an object with its teeth and sucks in air.

Wind up Sensitization of the central nervous system in response to sustained pain. With sustained pain, new receptors (NMDA receptors)are formed in the central nervous system. These receptors use a very fast neurotransmitter and cause a marked increase in the amount of pain transmitted to the brain. They also prevent opioids from working to their full effectiveness.

Window of susceptibility A time period in the life of a young animal in which the maternal antibodies are too low to provide protection against a certain disease, but too high to allow a vaccine to work and produce immunity.

Wing shoulder A condition in which the shoulder joint is away from the rib structure and skeleton (much of the skin is tucked in behind it).

Wink Opening and closing of the mare's vulva exposing the clitoris.

Winter Baby Syndrome Crias born in the winter months that are deficient in vitamin D.

With calf Terminology designating a cow that is pregnant.

Withdrawal Period (or time) The time when a drug must not be administered prior to marketing to insure that no drug residues remain in the meat or milk.

Withdrawal periods The amount of time it takes for a drug to be broken down in the body until it is at a level safe for human consumption.

Withdrawal Time Time required after the last drug treatment to lower drug residues to acceptable levels. These times are established using healthy animals according to label directions. An amount of time required following use of a medication in an animal before milk or meat can be entered into the human food supply. Ensures residues are maintained at levels approved by the USDA.

Withers The part of the horse's spine where the neck joins the back.

Withholding period The time after a drug is administered, before the animal can be marketed (or the milk used for human consumption).

Withholding time Time milk must be withheld from sale following treatment to avoid appearance of residues in milk.

Wohlfahrtia A genus of flies parasitic in animal tissue, belonging to the family Sacrophagidae, order Diptera.

Wolf teeth Small vestigial first pre-molar.

Wood chewing A common vice that damages facilities and can cause abnormal wear of teeth and possible complications from wood splinters.

Wood's light An ultraviolet light filtered through nickel oxide. Of the common dermatophytes, only M. canis fluoresces, 25 to 50% of the time.

Wool blind A term applied when the wool around the eyes has excessive growth and interferes with the sight of the sheep.

Wool The "hair" of sheep that is cut off and made into cloth for clothes. Wool is very wavy and is made up of many tiny scales.

Woolsorter's disease A pulmonary form of anthrax that develops in those who handle wool contaminated with Bacillus anthracis.

Work of digestion See heat increment.

Working Gait In dressage, a gait that is regular and unconstrained, energetic but calm, with even, elastic steps.

Worms Internal parasites.

Wright's stain A combination of eosin and methylene blue used in studying blood cells and revealing malarial parasites.

Wry tail Tailhead set either to the right or left of center.

X

Xanthopsis Yellow pigmentation seen in certain cancers and degenerating tissue.

Xeno A combining form meaning 'strange or referring to foreign matter'.

Xenoimmunisation To deliberately induce an immune response using foreign antigen, from a different species.

X-ray The x-ray is the high energy beam that produces a "picture" of a body part which is called the radiograph. Radiographs are commonly, but incorrectly, referred to as x-rays.

Y

Yaws An infectious nonvenereal disease caused by a spirochete, Treponema pertenue. Mainly found in humid, equatorial regions. Symptoms include febrile disturbances, rheumatism, eruption of tubercles with a caseous crust on hands, feet, face and external genitals. SYN bouba; frambesia; tropica; parangi; pian.

Yearling A male or female farm animal (especially cattle and horses) during the first year of life.

Yogurt Fermented milk, lowfat milk, or skim milk, sometimes protein-fortified. Lactobacillus bulgaricus and Streptococcus thermophilous are the fermenting bacteria. Fruit, flavors, and sugar may be added.

Yeast A single cell fungi which improves feed digestion by stimulating microbial activity and stabilizing digestive tract pH. Products packaged as "yeast" consist of cells only; "yeast culture" includes live yeast cells plus growth media.

Yellow body Corpus tuteum.

Yellow fever An acute infectious disease characterized by jaundice, epigastric tenderness, vomiting, hemorrhages, and a febrile course consisting of two paroxysms. There are two forms of yellow fever urban, in which the transmission cycle is mosquito; and sylvan, in which the reservoir is wild primates. Also, in sylvan yellow fever, the mosquito will remain infected for life. Except for a few cases in Trinidad in 1954, urban yellow fever has not been reported in North or South America since 1942. Outbreaks do occur in Africa adjacent to rain forests. Yellow fever has not been reported in Asia or eastern coast of Africa. Sylvan yellow fever is enzootic in South America and parts of Africa.

Yersin's serum An antitoxic serum for the plague.

Yersinia pestis Etiologic agent of plague.

Yin and Yang Concepts used in traditional Chinese medicine to understand the dynamic nature of all the interrelationships in life. Yin and Yang are two stages of a cyclical motion which represent the dual opposite and interdependent aspects of everything in the universe. Everything is paired with its opposite and is represented as Yin (night, darkness, rest, moon, dimmness, cold, weakness) or Yang (day, light, activity, sun, brightness, heat, strength). Disease occurs when there is imbalance in the rhythmic cycling between Yin and Yang.

Yolk The yolk is part of an embryo which serves as nutrition for the rest of the embryo.

Yorkshire Terrier A breed of toy terrier developed in Yorkshire and having a long, silky, bluish-gray coat.

Young's rule A method for calculating the dose of medicine a child should receive. Divide the age by the age plus 12. The result represents the fraction of the adult dose suitable for the child. Named after Thomas Young.

Youth An exhibitor eighteen years of age and under. Additional age divisions are often created to separate children further.

Z

Zona pellucida The envelope surrounding the egg or ovum.

Zoonoses These are diseases which can affect people as well as animals. Some such as Salmonella are spread by food being contaminated. These are called food-borne zoonoses. Others can be caught by contact with infected animals (like ringworm) or being bitten by them (like rabies). Some diseases (like West Nile Fever) are carried by insects. These are called vector borne zoonoses.

Zoonoses Action Plan A voluntary scheme developed by the pig industry to reduce the amount of salmonella in pigs. Samples are taken from pigs when they are slaughtered. Tests for antibodies to salmonella are used to identify the herds with the worst problem. The farmer is then given advice on how to deal with it.

Zoonotic A disease which can be transmitted between animals and people.

Zoonotic bacteria Bacteria that are present in animal reservoirs, that can be transferred to, and cause infections in humans.

Zoonotic disease Infectious diseases naturally transmitted from vertebrate animals to humans. Some of these diseases can be harbored in a vertebrate animal but there might be a vector involved in transmission, so that is still a zoonotic disease because it is harbored in a vertebrate animal. Additionally the disease may be food or water borne, so you don't need to have direct contact with an animal to acquire a zoonotic disease.

Zoonotic Infection Refers to infectious microorganisms that have the potential to cause disease in humans. Public Health is the study of zoonotic infections.

Zoosmosis Process of passage of living protoplasm into the tissues from blood vessels.

Zygodactyl Two toes in front and two behind, as in woodpeckers.

Zygomatic Arch A bony ridge extending posteriorly (and laterally) from beneath the eye orbit.

Zygomatic bone In a human, the zygomatic bone is the bone in the skull responsible for the prominence of the upper and anterior part of the cheek. It forms the lateral part of the lower margin of the orbital opening.

Zygote The product of fertilization, ie. a cell formed from the union of an oocyte and a spermatozoan.

Zyme An enzyme or ferment; An agent that produces an infectious disease.

Zymoid Resembling an enzyme.